FOLK NAME & TRADE DISEASES

Folk Name & Trade Diseases

E. R. Plunkett, M.D.

Illustrated by Lynn Sabol

Barrett Book Company
Stamford, Connecticut
1978

Library of Congress Card Catalog Number: 78-72537

ISBN: 0-932684-00-9

Copyright © 1978 by E. R. Plunkett. All rights reserved, including the right of reproduction in whole or in part, in any form or by any means, electronic or mechanical, including photocopying, recording, or by any information storage and retrieval system, without permission in writing from the Publisher.

Manufactured in the United States of America

BARRETT BOOK CO.
388 Summer Street
Stamford Connecticut 06901

PREFACE

From food gathering and hunting in prehistoric periods to the sophisticated and specialized occupations of today, vocational endeavors have dominated man's activities. It is logical to presume that the association between hazardous occupational acts and physical incapacities arising therefrom must have been apparent quite early. Names applied to such disabilities would correctly and simply tend to identify both the vocational pursuit and the physical impairment as a folk or common name entity as distinct from disease terminology imposed by medical or scientific disciplines for the less well understood afflictions. As social activities and occupations evolved through the centuries, so would the related occupational disabilities and their folk appellations or designations, dictated by common terminology rather than a scientific vocabulary.

A review of the development of names for occupational diseases over several hundred years brings into focus the exquisite distinction of terminology for these illnesses as compared with frequently used medical eponyms. To the uninitiated, the Crigler-Najjar Syndrome (congenital hyperbilirubinemia associated with brain damage) is meaningless; but who would question that "glass workers' cataract" was anything but what the phrase says—the occurrence of lenticular cataracts among glass workers. Perhaps no other branch of medicine enjoys the closeness to folk and common names for illness as does occupational medicine for diseases of the workplace. Many of these names, such as "black lung", were immediately adopted and widely used from their inception, and continue to be used today in our modern vocabulary.

Although a good number of trade disease names are archaic, unused or obsolete, they continue to convey a message of work conditions of bygone years, and for this reason alone should not be forgotten. They represent part of the history of the technical evolution of trades and occupations with brevity, variety, clarity and sparkle. And the coining of such phrases continues today as in the past, meeting modern needs as the older phrases suited the technology of the past. "Jeep disease" is as meaningful to modern soldiers with a sore behind as "knights' disease" was to the mediaeval horsemen. Time changed only the hardware!

This collection ranges from old to new, obsolete to fresh, quaint to common, and somber to ridiculous. For those engaged in the occupational disciplines the names will be meaningful and the source citation may be useful. Every reader, whatever his vocation or avocation, will probably be able to find some reference to a condition which he has suffered from, has observed in someone else, or may yet fall prey to. Historically, each entry represents a new concept pertinent to the community of the period. Even those names which appear repetitious seem to represent transitions in phraseology of the times.

A reasonably thorough search of the English medical literature promising a fair yield of these names was made in an attempt to locate the first reference in which the designation appeared, and the emphasis has been on the disease appellation. Attention was directed primarily to those names involving the trade or activity combined with the affected part of the body or organ; e.g. "Pall-bearer's palsy". In some instances the adopted name did not appear in the first description of the disease, but was coined by a subsequent author or even by an editor who felt the condition deserved special mention. Rarely, the special name showed up for the first time in the annual index of a journal. Occasionally, such terms are also found in popular publications. Many widely used terms such as "air pain", "bean weevil allergy", "fiberglass dermatitis", "Kwok's quease" were deemed not close enough to the intent of the publication; i.e., the "activity-body" concept, although a few have been included. The citations given are for the earliest reference found for that particular phrase. It may be very likely that earlier references were missed, or that disease names have been overlooked. A note from any reader about a missing name and its original source would be appreciated. Most of the foreign citations are secondary references and have not been verified. The reader should keep in mind that the definitions reflect simplification for this publication and do not necessarily represent current scientific opinions.

After searching through so many dusty volumes, the addition of one new phrase seems justified, and so the disease "index readers' syndrome" has been included.

For convenience, a rather complete listing of major body parts has also been included as an appendix.

ACKNOWLEDGEMENTS

Most of the research for this volume was completed at the Yale Medical Library and I am indebted to the library staff for their sympathetic help and assistance during the year 1977. It is doubtful that the work could have been completed without the dedication, help and suggestions of George Simonson and Peggy Delaney who also spent many hours in the tedious chore of screening journal indices. Mrs. Susan Baye cheerfully devoted her attention and demonstrated remarkable skill in producing an impeccable manuscript.

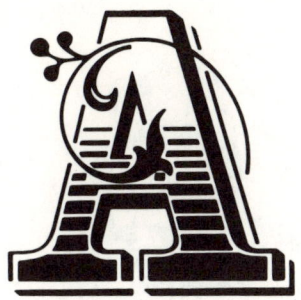

ACADEMY HEADACHE

intense frontal headache, sleeplessness and nervous prostration from studying collections of pictures in art galleries

Brit. Med. J. 1:936, 1880

ACCIDENT PRONENESS

increased susceptibility to accidents because of psychologic reasons

Farmer, E. The Causes of Accidents. London, 1932

ACID BITES

irritation and/or ulceration of the skin among workers handling chromic acid or chromate salts

Ann. Surg. 63:155, 1916

ACNE ARTIFICIALIS

acneiform eruption of the skin caused by contact with crude petroleum in Carpathian mines

Brit. Med. J. 2:86, 1887

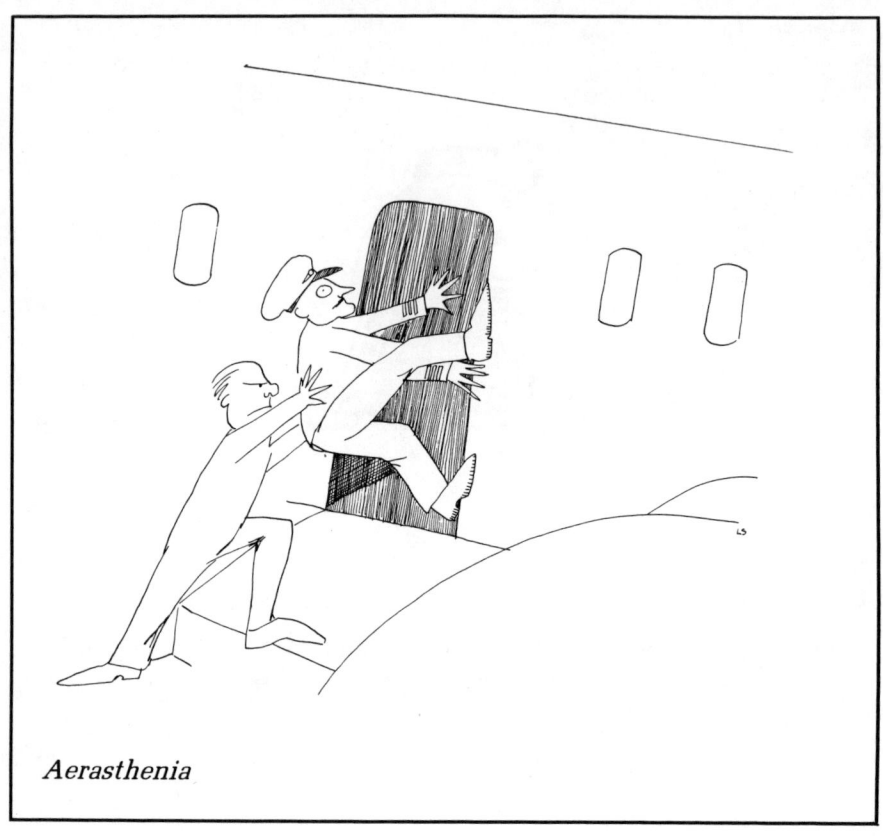

Aerasthenia

AERASTHENIA

a general inability to adapt to flying an airplane

Brit. Med. J. 1:389, 1916

AERODONTALGIA

dental pain among persons who fly, brought about by lowered temperature and barometric pressure at high altitudes

Bull. of U.S. Army Med. Dept. 73:62, 1944

AERODROMOPHOBIA

morbid fear of traveling by air

Dorland's Medical Dictionary. 25th ed. Phila.: W. B. Saunders, 1974

AERONEUROSIS

FLYING SICKNESS (motion sickness)

Dorland's Medical Dictionary. 25th ed. Phila.: W. B. Saunders, 1974

gastric distress, nervous irritability, insomnia and emotional instability among pilots

JAMA 106:1347, 1936

AEROPHOBIA

fear of flying

Dorland's Medical Dictionary. 25th ed. Phila.: W. B. Saunders, 1974

AEROSINUSITIS

affection of the paranasal sinuses produced by changes in barometric pressure

Arch. Otol. 35:107, 1942

AESTHETE'S FOOT

an implication that gout afflicts people of higher intelligence and education

Morris Dictionary of Word & Phrase Origins. N.Y.: Harper & Row, 1977

AIR CONDITIONER PNEUMONITIS

allergic inflammatory response of the lungs to the spores of Thermophilic *actinomycetes* contaminating the air conditioning system

Exxon Med. Bull. 33:32, 1973

AIR CONTROLLERS' SYNDROME

peptic ulcer occurring among air traffic controllers as a result of job stress

Illinois Med. J. 142:111, 1972

AIR HAMMER DISEASE

blanching of the fingers with the loss of sensation, pain and occasional joint changes caused by the use of an air hammer

JAMA 129:672, 1945

AIRMAN'S PTOSIS

drooping of an upper eyelid alleged to flying in an open cockpit airplane without wearing a helmet or goggles

Lancet 2:873, 1954

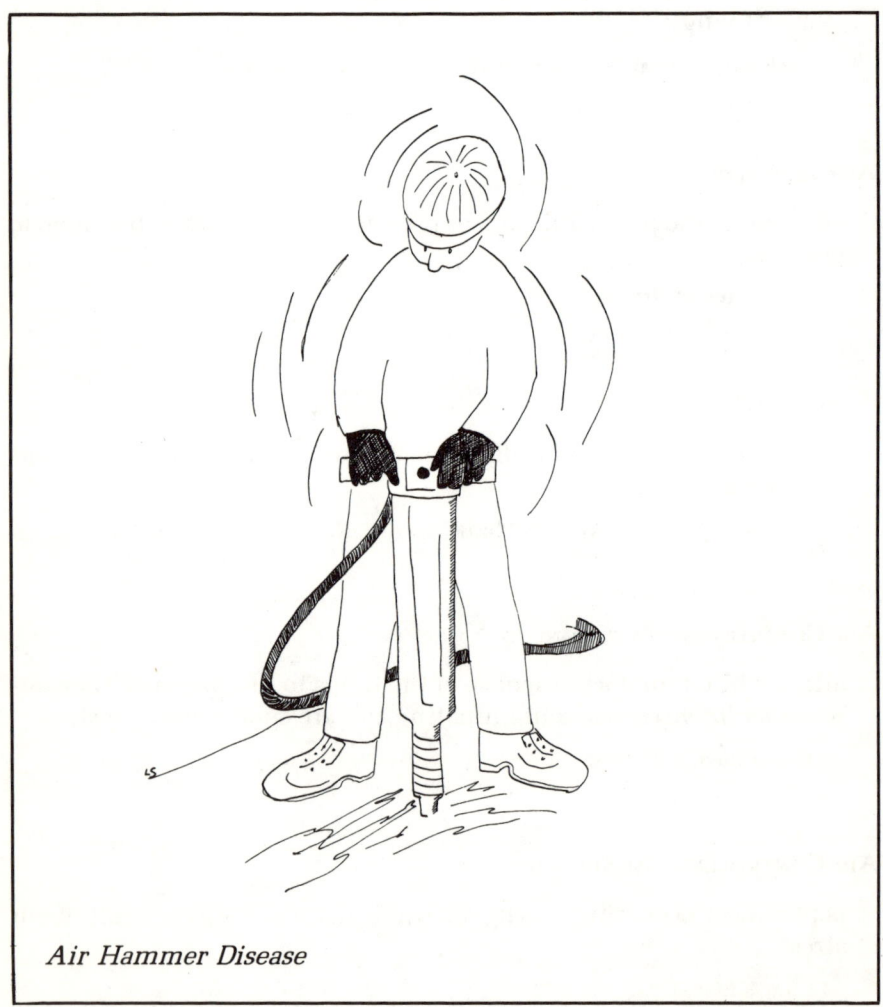

Air Hammer Disease

Airmens' Breakdown

irritability, fatigue, weakness and anxiety among aviators

Lancet 1:714, 1928

Airplane Sickness

motion sickness from air travel

International Classification of Diseases. 8th rev. USDHEW. Pub. Hlth. Serv. Pub. No. 1963, 1968

Alkali Itch

irritation of the skin by caustic used in nickel plating

White, R. P. The Dermatogoses or Occupational Affections of the Skin. London: H. K. Lewis, 1928

Alpine Sickness

ALTITUDE SICKNESS

International Classification of Diseases. 8th rev. USDHEW. Pub. Hlth. Serv. Pub. No. 1963, 1968

Altitude Sickness

dizziness, nausea, shortness of breath, headache, thirst and fatigue from a combination of decreased oxygen and atmospheric pressure

Bert, P. (1878). La Pression Barometrique. Paris: Masson (tr. by Hitchcock, M. A. and F. A.) Columbus, OH: College Book Co., 1943

Aluminum Dust Lung

fibrotic lung disease caused by chronic inhalation of aluminum dust

Kobe J. Med. Sc. 4:91, 1958

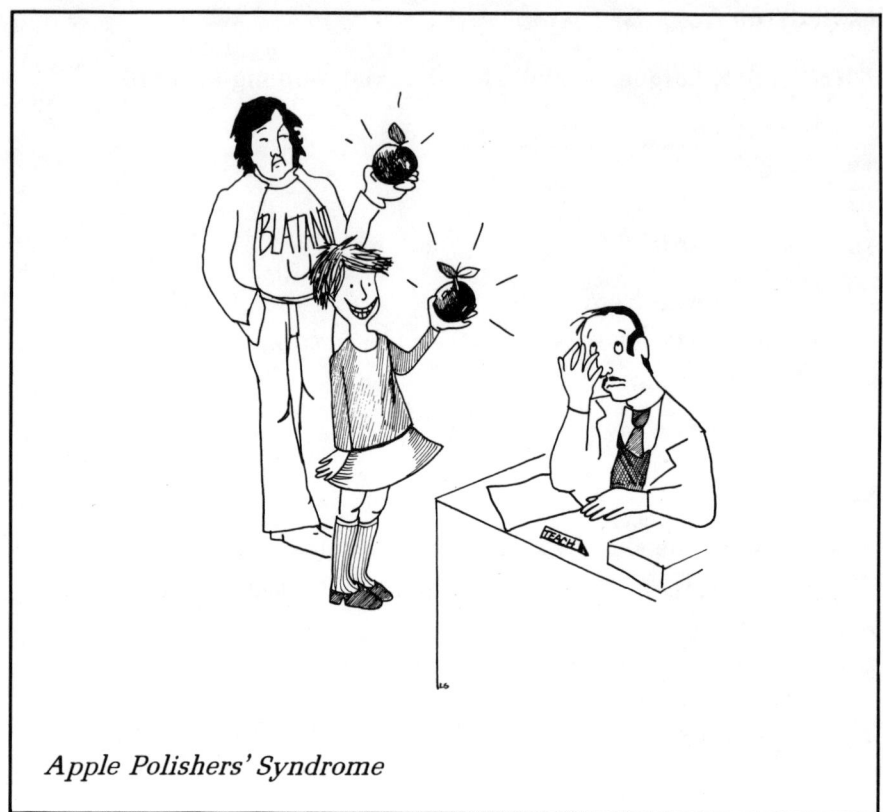

Apple Polishers' Syndrome

Aluminum Lung

ALUMINUM DUST LUNG

Brit. J. Ind. Med. 1:160, 1944

Ampoule Snapper's Thumb

thumb injury from the penetration of glass spicules produced by snapping open medicinal ampoules

Lancet 1:1412, 1976

Anatomic Wart

tuberculosis of the skin seen in pathologists and morgue attendants

Stedman's Medical Dictionary. 23rd ed. Baltimore: William & Wilkins, 1976

Angel Eyes

the observation of hazy halos around lights observed by workers exposed to hypochlorite dust

Indust. Med. 12:885, 1943

Angina Electrica

irregular cardiac rhythm and chest pain which sometimes follows electrical shock

ILO Encyclopedia of Occupational Health and Safety. N.Y.: McGraw Hill, 1972

Aniline Cancer

cancer of the urinary bladder in workers of chemical dye factories and dyeing establishments

Lancet 2:1117, 1934

Apple Packers' Epistaxis

inflammation of the nasal mucous membrane with bleeding, seen among apple packers who used blue-dye apple trays made from recycled newspapers

N. Eng. J. Med. 276:413, 1967

Apple Packers' Nosebleeds

APPLE PACKERS' EPISTAXIS

JAMA 197:165, 1966

Apple Pickers' Disease

bronchitis among apple pickers exposed to the residue of a fungicide, Ziram, following the spraying of apple trees

N. Eng. J. Med. 276:413, 1967

Apple Polishers' Syndrome

favor-currying among students

original source not identified

Apple Sorters' Disease

dermatitis of the hands of apple sorters caused by orthophenylate salts which had been used to prevent mold growth

Occup. Hlth. 12:199, 1952

Apple Thinners' Disease

mild intoxication from parathion, an insecticide, by orchard workers exposed to recently sprayed trees

Brit. Med. J. 2:1132, 1966

Arc Burn

inflammation of the cornea of the eye or the facial skin from ultraviolet light produced by arc welding

original source not identified

Arc Eye

ARC BURN

Arch. Ophth. 23:34 1894

Arc Flash

irritation of the eye caused by a welder's electric arc and characterized by redness, swelling, light sensitivity and a feeling of sand in the eye

JAMA 122:734, 1943

Arctic Anemia

anemia among Arctic expedition crew members during exposure to low temperatures and strenuous exercise

Brit. Med. J. 1:353, 1959

Arctic Temper

extreme irritability developing among arctic explorers exposed to darkness, monotony, isolation and sensory deprivation (compare WHITE-OUT SYNDROME)

Lancet 1:1283, 1910

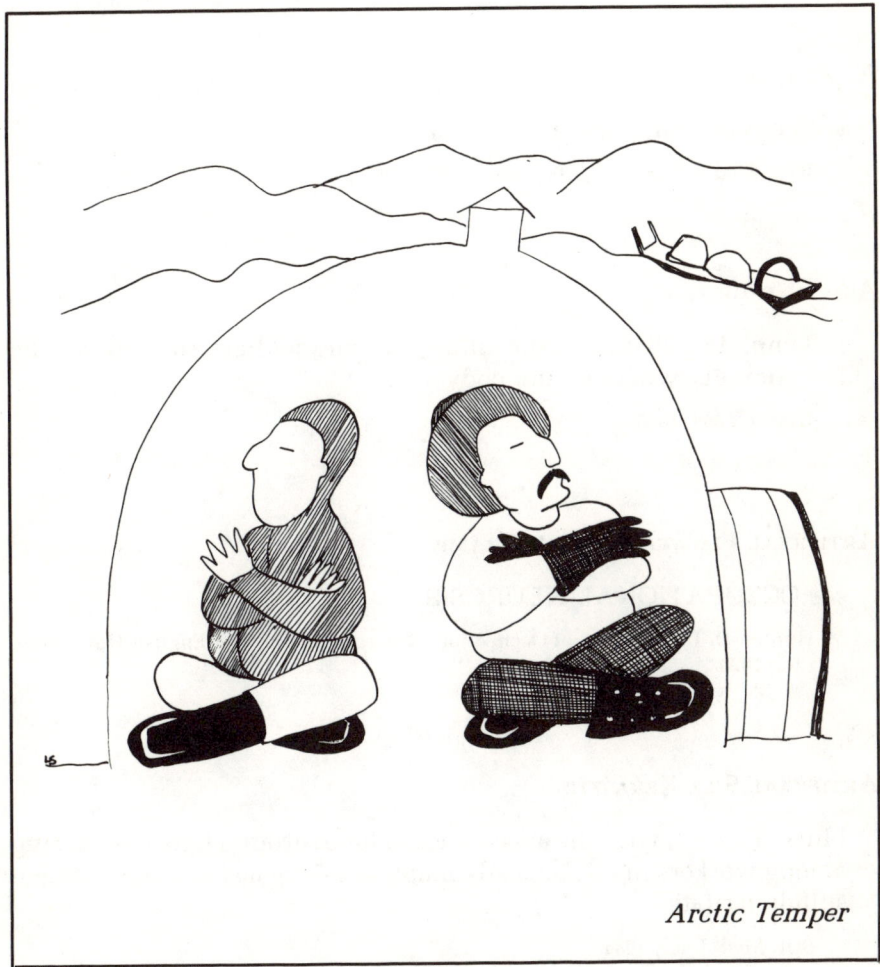

Arctic Temper

TRADE DISEASES

Arc Welder's Lung

deposition of iron in the lung due to the inhalation of iron oxide fumes generated by the welding process

Brit. Med. J. 2:921, 1957

Arc Welder's Siderosis

ARC WELDER'S LUNG

Indust. Med. 13:598, 1944

Army Itch

scabies occurring among soldiers

Bost. Med. & Surg. J. 74:107, 1866

Army Nephritis

inflammatory disease of the kidneys among soldiers, secondary to an infection elsewhere in the body

Lancet 1:495, 1918

Artificial Flower-Maker's Cramp

see OCCUPATIONAL NEUROSIS

Hunter, D. The Diseases of Occupations. 5th ed. London: The English Univ. Press Ltd., 1975

Artificial Silk Keratitis

blurred vision, with the appearance of halos around lights, occurring among workers in artificial silk manufacturing and due to hydrogen sulfide irritation

Brit. Med. J. 2:6, 1936

Asbestos Corns

small, hard nodules on the fingers or hands of asbestos workers caused by asbestos particles which penetrate the skin

Lancet 1:252, 1933

Asbestos Warts

ASBESTOS CORNS

Arch. J. Dermat. Syph. 161:1, 1930

Assembly Headache

headaches due to exhaustion and poor ventilation in crowded theatres, exhibitions, galleries, etc.

Lancet 1:1171, 1884

Athlete's Albuminuria

albumin in the urine following strenuous athletic activity

Stedman's Medical Dictionary. 23rd ed. Baltimore: William & Wilkins, 1976

Athlete's Foot

fungus infection of the foot

Lit. Digest 16:1, 1928

Athlete's Heart

aortic incompetence due to strain in athletic exercise

Dorland's Medical Dictionary. 25th ed. Phila.: W. B. Saunders, 1974

Athlete's Kidney

albumin or blood in the urine following body trauma or marked physical exertion

J. Urol. 83:321, 1960

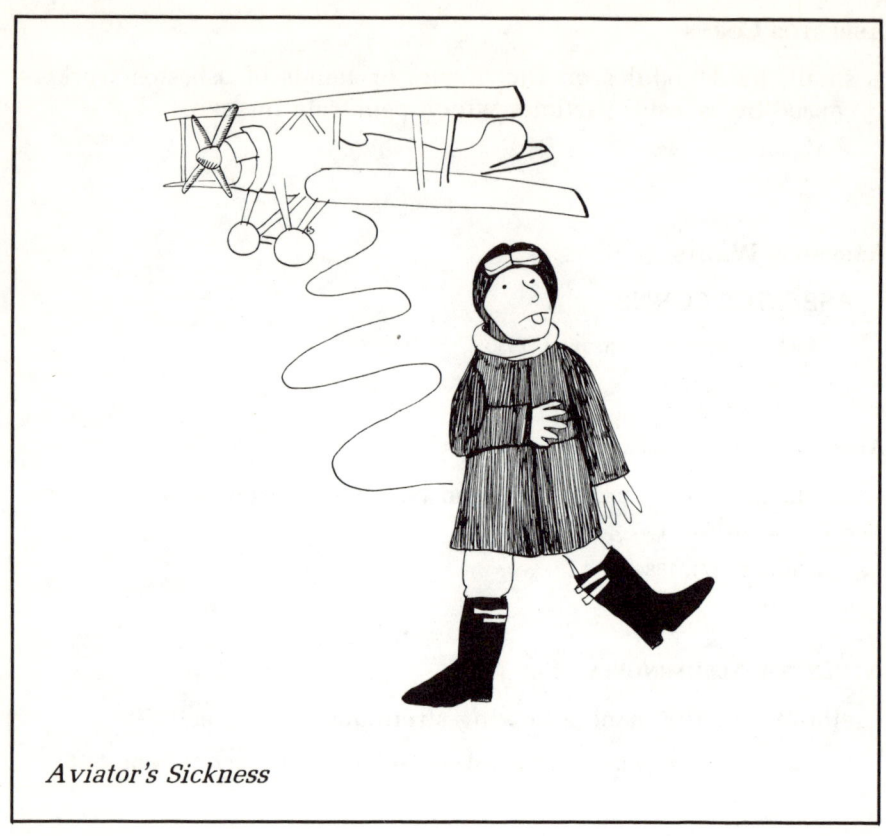

Aviator's Sickness

ATHLETE'S SICKNESS

weakness, blurred vision, nausea and headache following a short period of intense physical exercise

Dorland's Medical Dictionary. 25th ed. Phila.: W. B. Saunders, 1974

ATHLETIC HEART SYNDROME

enlargement of the heart in athletes

Louvain Med. 93:517, 1974

ATHLETIC PSEUDONEPHRITIS

ATHLETE'S KIDNEY

JAMA 161:1613, 1956

Atom Bomb Disease

loss of appetite, vomiting, bloody diarrhea, fatigue and other signs of radiation sickness from exposure to atom bomb radioactivity

Lancet 2:14, 1946

Aviation Deafness

loss of hearing in aviators from noise exposure, barometric pressure changes or faulty ventilation of the middle ear

Arch. Otolaryng, 32:417, 1940

Aviation Otitis

inflammation of the ear resulting from a difference between atmospheric pressure and the air pressure in the middle ear

Dorland's Medical Dictionary. 25th ed. Phila.: W. B. Saunders, 1974

Aviation Sickness

drowsiness, weakness and dizziness among aviators produced by changes in altitude

Presse Med. 24:69, 1916

Aviator's Asthenia

weakness, drowsiness and faintness while flying, ascribed to adrenal gland exhaustion

Brit. Med. J. 2:663, 1918

Aviators' Astragalus

fracture dislocation of the ankle commonly seen in pilots following a crash

J. Bone & Joint Surg. 34B:545, 1952

Aviators' Bends

decompression sickness in pilots subjected to a rapid lowering of atmospheric pressure

Aviat. Space Environ. Med. 46:1186, 1975

Aviator's Blackout

shock-like symptoms associated with high centrifugal forces in airplane dives and recoveries

Lancet 2:267, 1949

Aviators' Cancer

nasopharyngeal carcinoma among bush pilots alleged to be related to frequent barometric pressure changes combined with some other factor

Lancet 2:91, 1968

Aviator's Disease

shortness of breath, fatigue, buzzing in the ears and headaches attributed to rapid changes in altitude and temperature

J. de Physiol. et Path. Gen. 13:387, 1911

Aviator's Ear

AVIATION OTITIS

JAMA 1:419, 1937

Aviator's Heart

enlargement of the left ventricle of the heart proportional to the altitude habitually flown by the pilot

Lancet 2:250, 1918

Aviators' Neurosis

fatigue among aviators related to low oxygen pressure and the stress of flying

J. de Med. de Bord. 90:399, 1918

Aviator's Sickness

ALTITUDE SICKNESS

Sci. Amer. Suppl.3 2:357, 1916

general incapacity of airmen due to changes in barometric pressure, oxygen supply and acceleration forces

JAMA 121:696, 1943

Aviator's Stomach

air sickness

Dorland's Medical Dictionary. 25th ed. Phila.: W. B. Saunders, 1974

Aviators' Vertigo

spatial disorientation in pilots

Aerosp. Med. 31:189, 1960

Ax Grinder's Disease

chronic fibrosis of the lungs due to the inhalation of silica dust

original source not identified

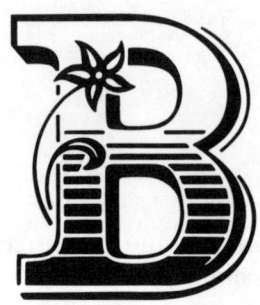

BACKFIRE FRACTURE

CHAUFFEUR'S FRACTURE

Brit. Med. J. 2:1187, 1926

BACKPACKER'S DIARRHEA

gastroenteritis caused by an intestinal parasite *Giardia lamblia* in contaminated drinking water

Rocky Mt. News No. 167, p. 7, 6 Oct. 1977

BACKPACK MERALGIA

altered sensation in the thigh from compression of the lateral femoral cutaneous nerve by a backpack waistband

N. Eng. J. Med. 292:702, 1975

BACKPACK PALSY

motor and sensory changes in the upper extremities from compression of the brachial nerves by a backpack harness

original source not identified

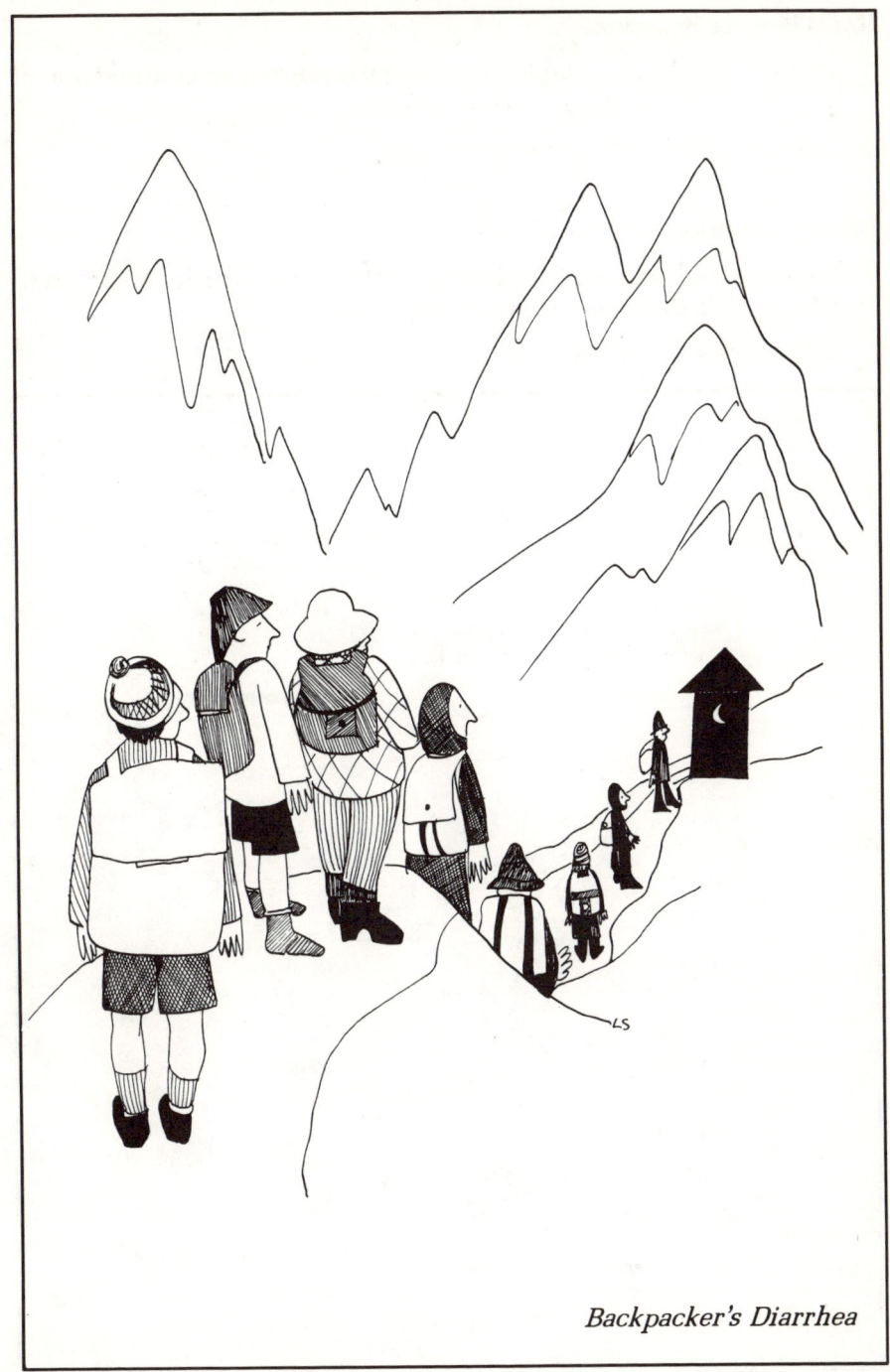

Backpacker's Diarrhea

Back Pocket Sciatica

sciatic nerve pain in the lower extremity caused by compression of the nerve by objects in a back pocket

N. Eng. J. Med. 290:633, 1974

Back-to-School Syndrome

tiredness and weight loss among mothers who rush to and from school with their young four times a day

Brit. Med. J. 2:1106, 1958

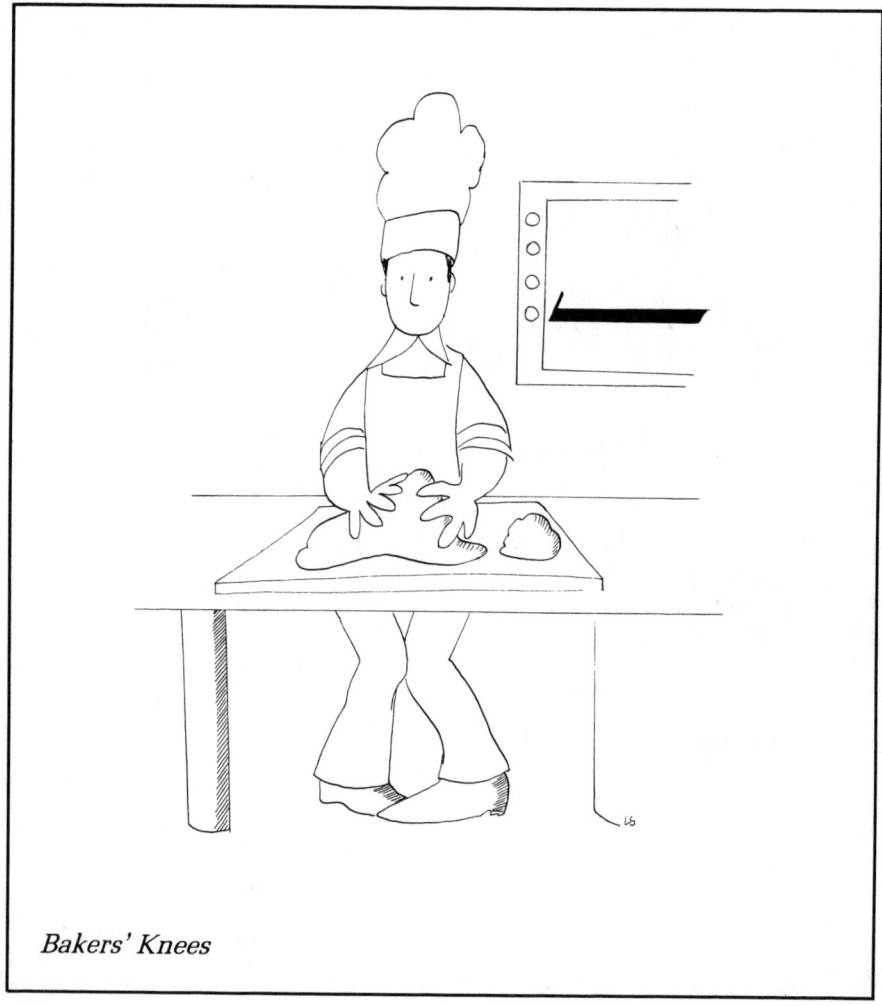

Bakers' Knees

BAGASSOSIS

allergic inflammatory response of the lungs caused by the dust of sugar cane refuse; i.e. bagasse

N. Orleans Med. & Surg. J. 93:580, 1941

BAKERS' ACNE

BAKERS' ECZEMA

Munch. Med. Wchensch. 38:1636, 1903

BAKERS' ASTHMA

asthmatic reaction provoked by the inhalation of flour

Med. Welt. 24:1381, 1969

BAKERS' DERMATITIS

BAKERS' ECZEMA

Lancet 1:80, 1923

BAKERS' ECZEMA

skin irritation from cereal parasites

Act. Derm. Venereol. 27:217, 1947

irritation of the hands and forearms of bakers by the potassium persulfate in the flour

Lancet 2:279, 1923

BAKERS' ITCH

redness, cracking and peeling of the hands and wrists of bakers

Lancet 2:821, 1843

BAKERS' KNEES

knock knees in bakers alleged to be the result of standing in one position for long periods while kneading dough

Morris Dictionary of Word & Phrase Origins. N.Y.: Harper & Row, 1977

BAKERS' PSORIASIS

BAKERS' ECZEMA

Schwartz, L. Occupational Diseases of the Skin. Phila.: Lea & Febiger, 1957

BALLAST FEVER

sickness in merchant seamen caused by the odors arising from ballast consisting of sewage-polluted dredgings (Apparently such material was used to avoid taxation on "marketable" ballast, like rocks.)

Lancet 2:648, 1868

BALLET DANCER'S CRAMP

see OCCUPATIONAL NEUROSIS

Lancet 2:333, 1886

BALLET DANCER'S TOE

partial dislocation and inflammation of the great toe from ballet dancing

Arlidge, J. T. The Hygiene, Diseases and Mortality of Occupations. London: Percival, 1892

BALLOON DISEASE

ALTITUDE SICKNESS

original source not identified

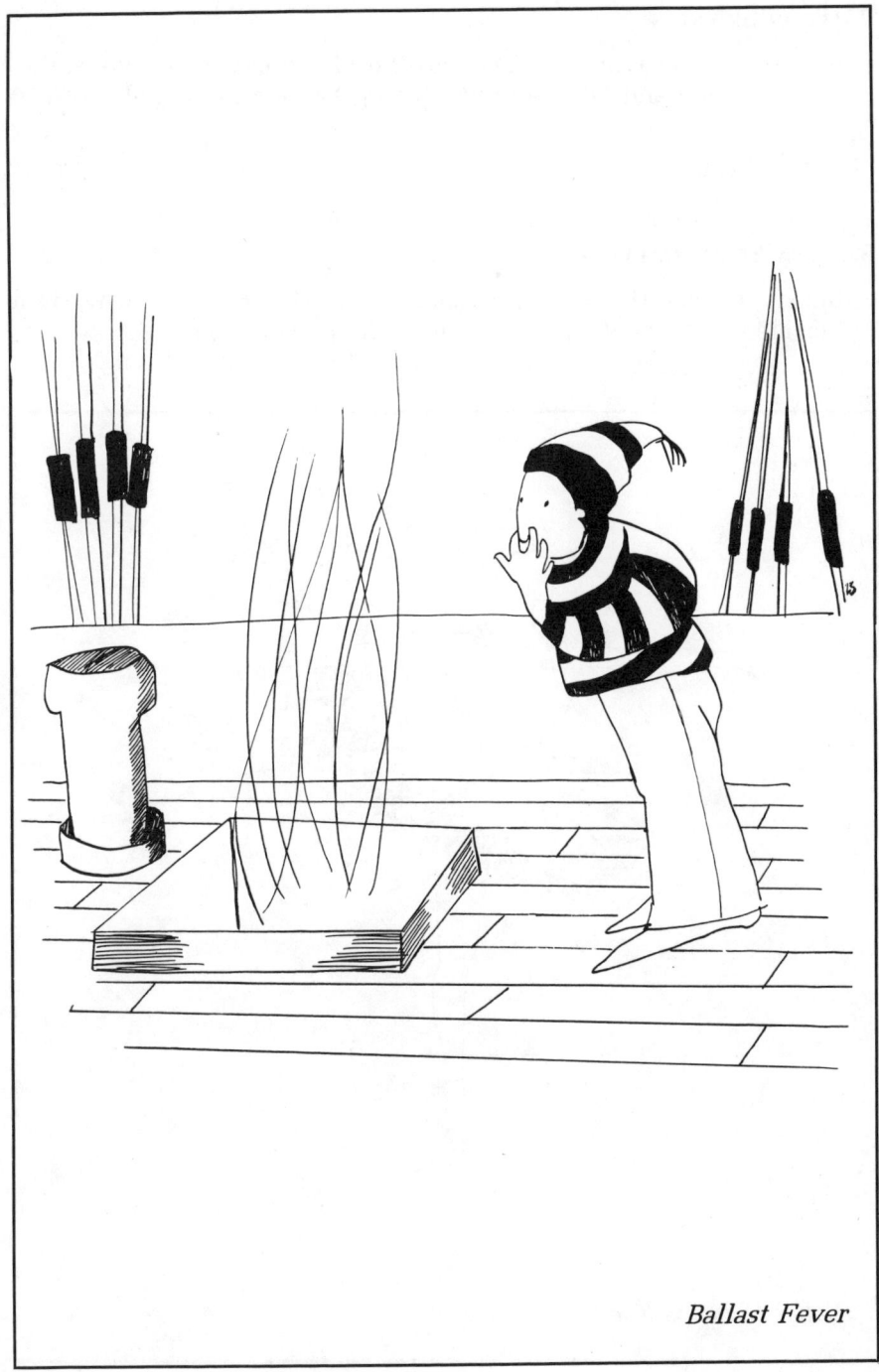

Ballast Fever

TRADE DISEASES

BALLOON SICKNESS

pain in the head and neck, congestion of the face, drowsiness, disturbed vision and fatigue noted during balloon ascents above 4000 meters

Lancet 2:845, 1908

BANANA SEAT HEMATURIA

bloody urine without pain, associated with riding on a narrow, rigid bicycle seat, caused by contusion of the prostate gland

N. Eng. J. Med. 287:311, 1972

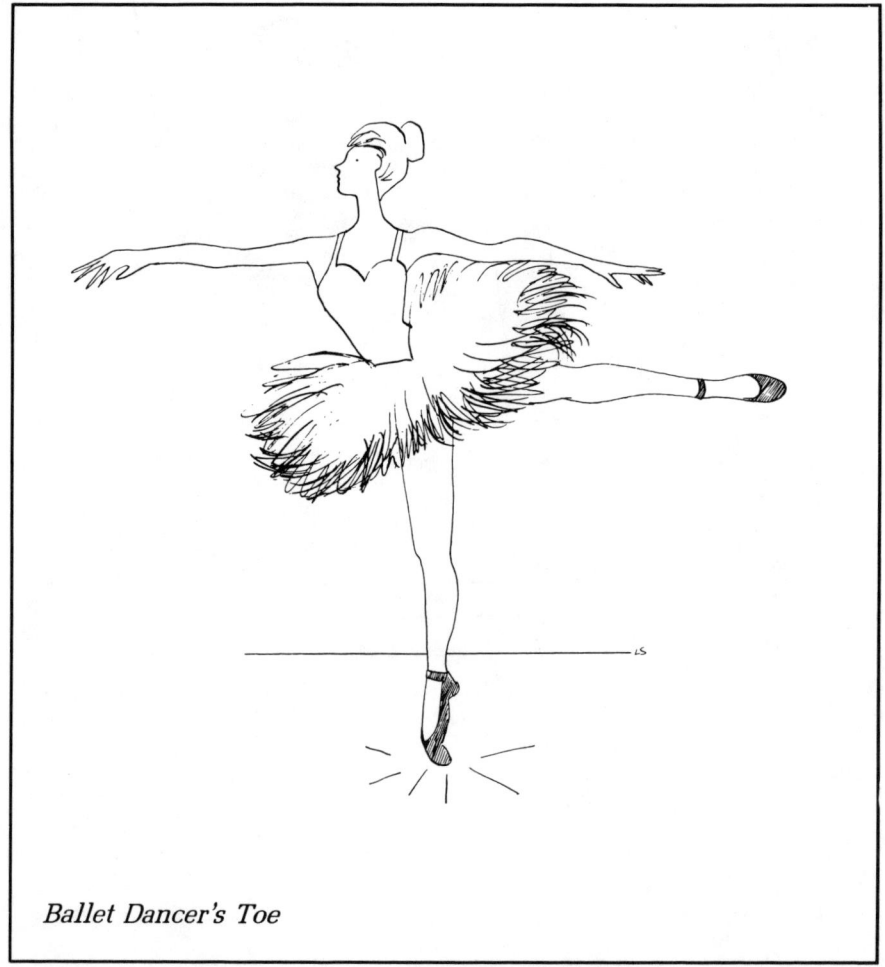

Ballet Dancer's Toe

Banking Clerk's Dyspepsia

sneezing, metallic taste in the mouth, nausea and constipation alleged to the handling of copper and silver coins

Brit. Med. J. 1:435, 1879

Barbed Wire Disease

prisoner-of-war neurosis characterized by irritability, restlessness, depression and memory impairment

Vischer, A. L. Barbed Wire Disease. London: John Bale, 1919

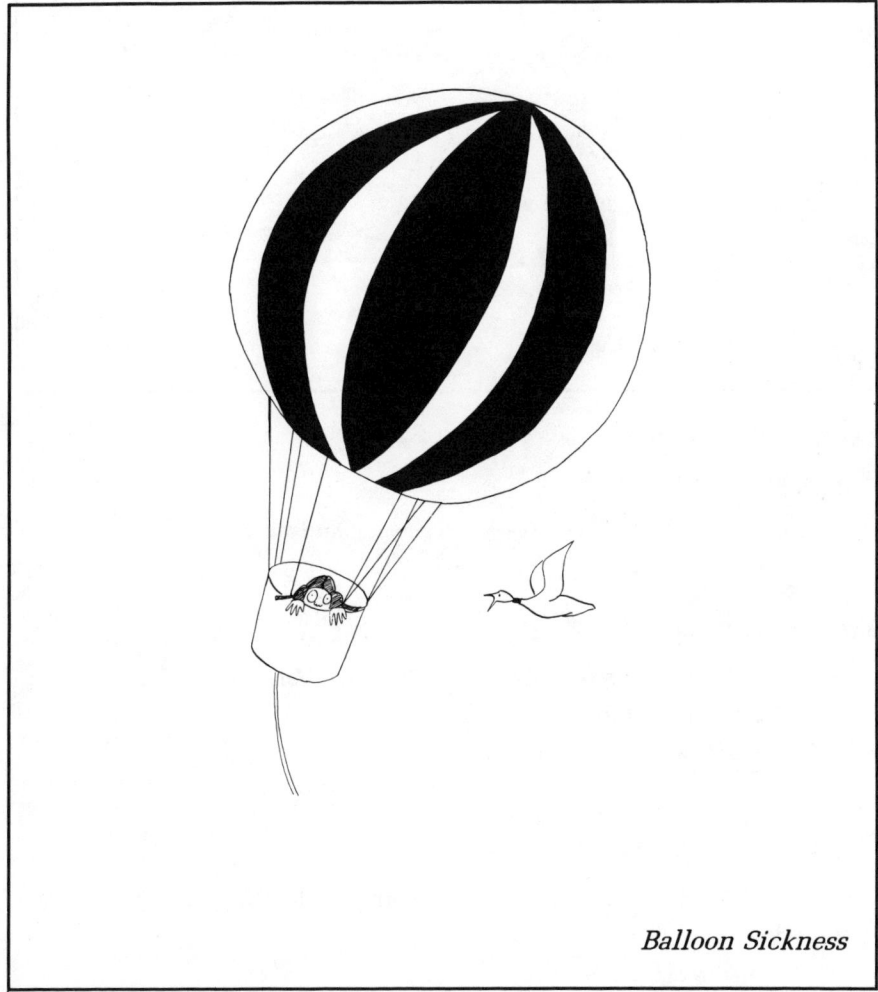

Balloon Sickness

TRADE DISEASES

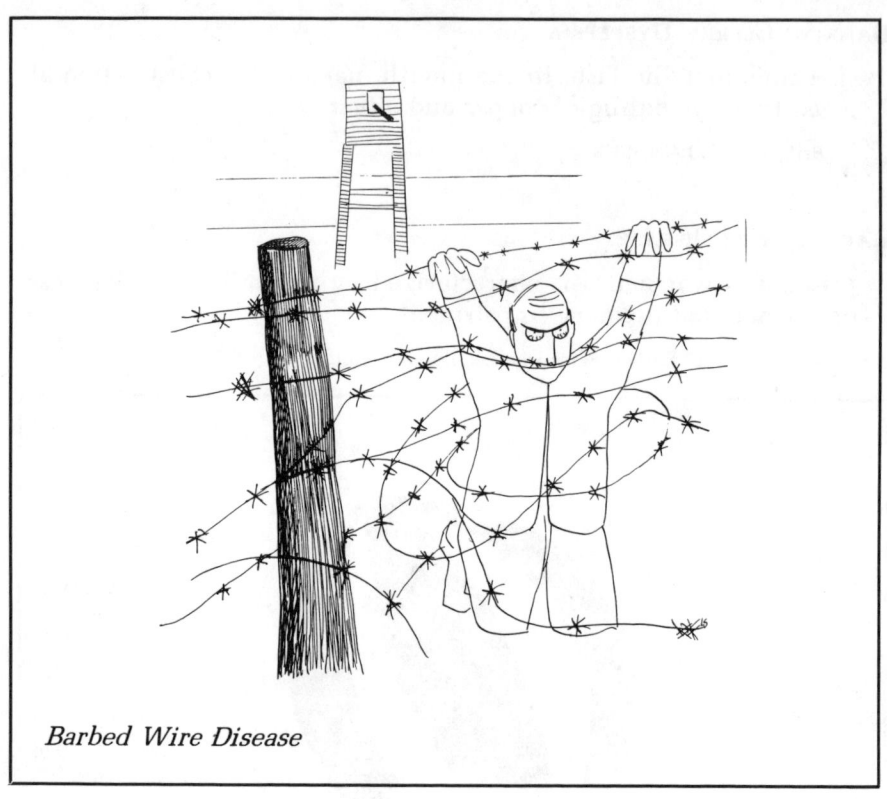

Barbed Wire Disease

BARBED WIRE NEUROSIS

BARBED WIRE DISEASE

Vischer, A. L. Barbed Wire Disease. London: John Bale, 1919

BARBERS' DISEASE

tissue nodules and cysts of the hands of barbers caused by the penetration of hair clippings

Ind. Med. & Surg. 22:111, 1953

BARBER'S INTERDIGITAL HAIR SINUS

skin irritation of the finger webs from penetrating short hair fragments

Arch. Derm. 112:523, 1976

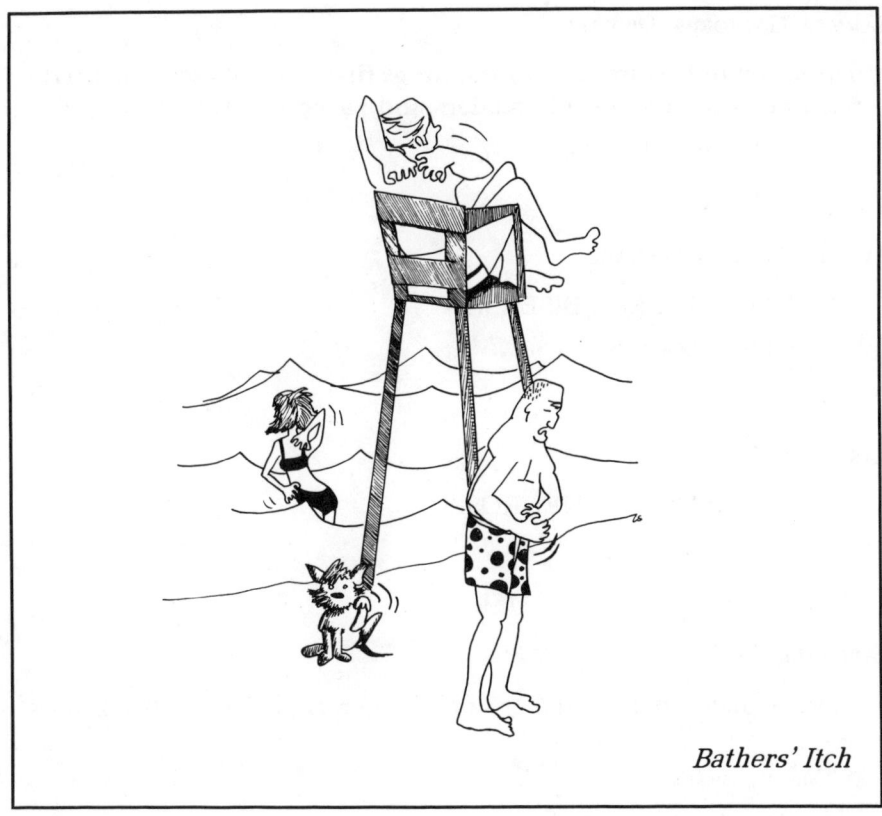

Bathers' Itch

BARBERS' NODULES

localized abscesses of the hands of barbers from the penetration of hair clippings

Arch. Derm. & Syph. 45:614, 1942

BARBERS' PILONIDAL SINUS

BARBERS' DISEASE

JAMA 148:1501, 1952

BAROMETER MAKER'S DISEASE

chronic mercurialism

original source not identified

TRADE DISEASES

BARYTA GRINDERS' DISEASE

deposition of barium dust in the lungs (usually not associated with respiratory symptoms) of grinders and packers of barium sulfate

original source not identified

BARYTA MINERS' DISEASE

BARYTA GRINDERS' DISEASE

Med. Lavoro 24:461, 1933

BASEBALL ARM

see OCCUPATIONAL NEUROSIS

JAMA 57:1698, 1911

BASEBALL FINGER

upward dislocation of the tip of a finger from being struck by a baseball

Lancet 2:958, 1968

disruption of the tendon to the tip of a finger caused by the ball striking the finger

Ann. West. Med. & Surg. 6:154, 1952

BASEBALL PITCHER'S ELBOW

fracture of bone or cartilage from the head of the radius at the elbow due to strenuous baseball pitching

JAMA 95:404, 1930

BASEBALL SHOULDER

calcium deposits in the shoulder from over exertion in throwing a baseball

JAMA 171:1659, 1959

BASKETBALL HEEL

stippled black, tender dermatitis of the heel from trauma to the feet while playing basketball (compare BLACK HEEL)

Arch. Derm. 104:452, 1971

BATHER'S CRAMP

BATHING CRAMP

Brit. Med. J. 2:82, 1883

BATHERS' ITCH

skin irritation among swimmers caused by the snail parasite *Schistosoma cercariae*

Lancet 2:451, 1935

BATHING CRAMP

painful muscular spasm, usually of the lower extremity, occurring while swimming

Brit. Med. J. 2:82, 1883

BATTERY REFINER'S DISEASE

mercury poisoning incurred during the process of extracting mercury from batteries

Neurology 20:401, 1970

BATTLE EXHAUSTION

BATTLE FATIGUE

Brit. Med. J. 2:788, 1950

BATTLE FATIGUE

physical and emotional fatigue among soldiers from the strain of combat

J. Nerv. & Ment. Dis. 101:442, 1945

BATTLE NEUROSIS

BATTLE FATIGUE

original source not identified

BAUXITE FUME PNEUMOCONIOSIS

BAUXITE WORKERS' LUNG

Brit. Med. J. 2:135, 1955

BAUXITE WORKERS' DISEASE

BAUXITE WORKERS' LUNG

Occup. Med. 4:56, 1947

BAUXITE WORKERS' LUNG

fibrosis of the lung with shortness of breath and cough in workers who manufacture corundum

Occup. Med. 4:56, 1947

BEACH EAR

inflammation of the external ear canal occurring among swimmers (compare TANK EAR)

original source not identified

BEAT ANKLE

inflammatory reaction of the ankle bursa of coal miners

Tr. A. Indust. M. Off. 4:122, 1955

BEAT ELBOW

inflammation of the elbow skin and bursa among miners from using the elbow as a brake or lever in sliding over coal faces (compare COAL MINER'S ELBOW)

Lancet 2:867, 1924

BEAT HAND

inflammation of the hand in coal miners from trauma by the pick handle

Lancet 2:867, 1924

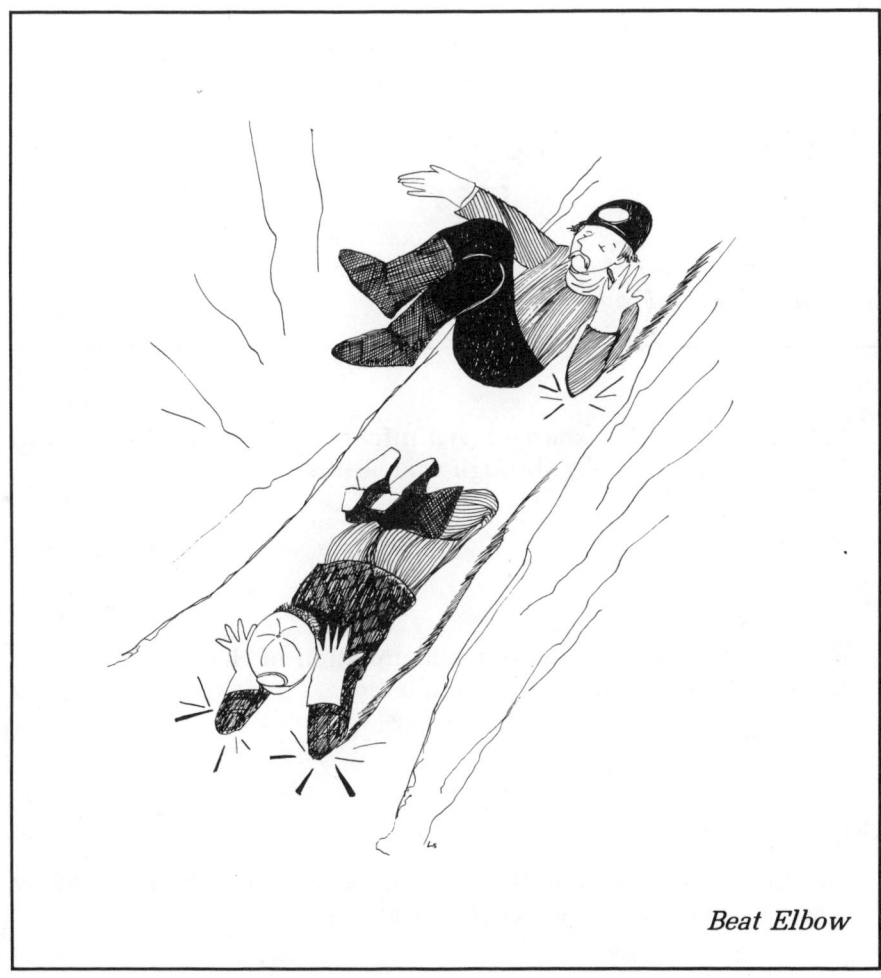

Beat Elbow

TRADE DISEASES

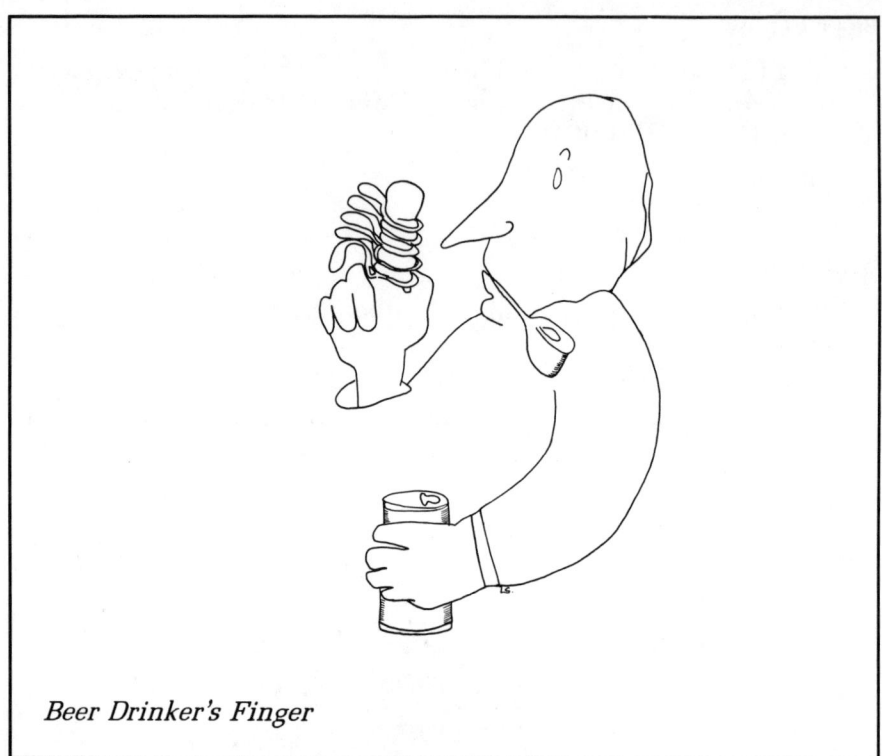

Beer Drinker's Finger

BEAT KNEE

inflammation of the knees of coal miners from repeated trauma in maneuvering the body through coal seams

Brit. Med. J. 1:708, 1912

BEAT SHOULDER

pigmentation of the skin and inflammation of the shoulder bursa from pushing coal tubs at the mine face

Brit. Med. J. 19:222, 1962

BEER DRINKER'S FINGER

swelling, bluish discoloration and maceration of a finger caused by placing pop-top beer can rings on the finger

JAMA 203:1076, 1968

Beet Sugar Worker's Neuritis

functional disturbance of the lower extremity caused by nerve pressure from the squatting position used in transplanting beets

Deutsch. Med. Wchnschr. 18:669, 1934

Bends

pains in the extremities and abdomen among divers suffering DECOMPRESSION SICKNESS

Westm. Gaz. 16 October 1894

Bicycle Heart

palpitation and temporary dilation of the heart from overexertion on a bicycle

Brit. Med. J. 1:908, 1898

Bicyclists' Hump

humped back resulting from the curved posture assumed by bicyclists

JAMA 32:445, 1899

Bikini Dermatitis

dermatitis from contact with an anthraquinone dye used in bathing suits

Arch. Derm. 112:1445, 1976

Billingsgate Hump

FISH PORTER'S BURSITIS

Hunter, D. The Diseases of Occupations. 5th ed. London: The English Univ. Press Ltd., 1975

BIRD BREEDERS' LUNG

allergic inflammatory response of the lungs to avian proteins among those who rear birds

Lancet 1:445, 1966

BIRD FANCIERS' LUNG

BIRD BREEDERS' LUNG

Lancet 1:445, 1966

BIRD FEATHER PICKERS' DISEASE

allergic inflammatory response of the lungs to feather proteins, seen among those who clean and sort goose feathers

Hunter, D. The Diseases of Occupations. 5th ed. London: The English Univ. Press Ltd., 1975

BIRD REARERS' LUNG

BIRD BREEDERS' LUNG

Cas. Lek. Ces. 112:859, 1973

"BIRD'S EYES"

small skin ulcers about the knuckles of tanners caused by contact with chemicals used for dehairing pelts

Paris. Med. 55:270, 1925

BIRD STUFFERS' DISEASE

chronic infective lip ulcers from bird beak bites among professional *gaveurs* who pre-chew grain and fruit and then feed it to quail by mouth

JAMA 93:1396, 1929

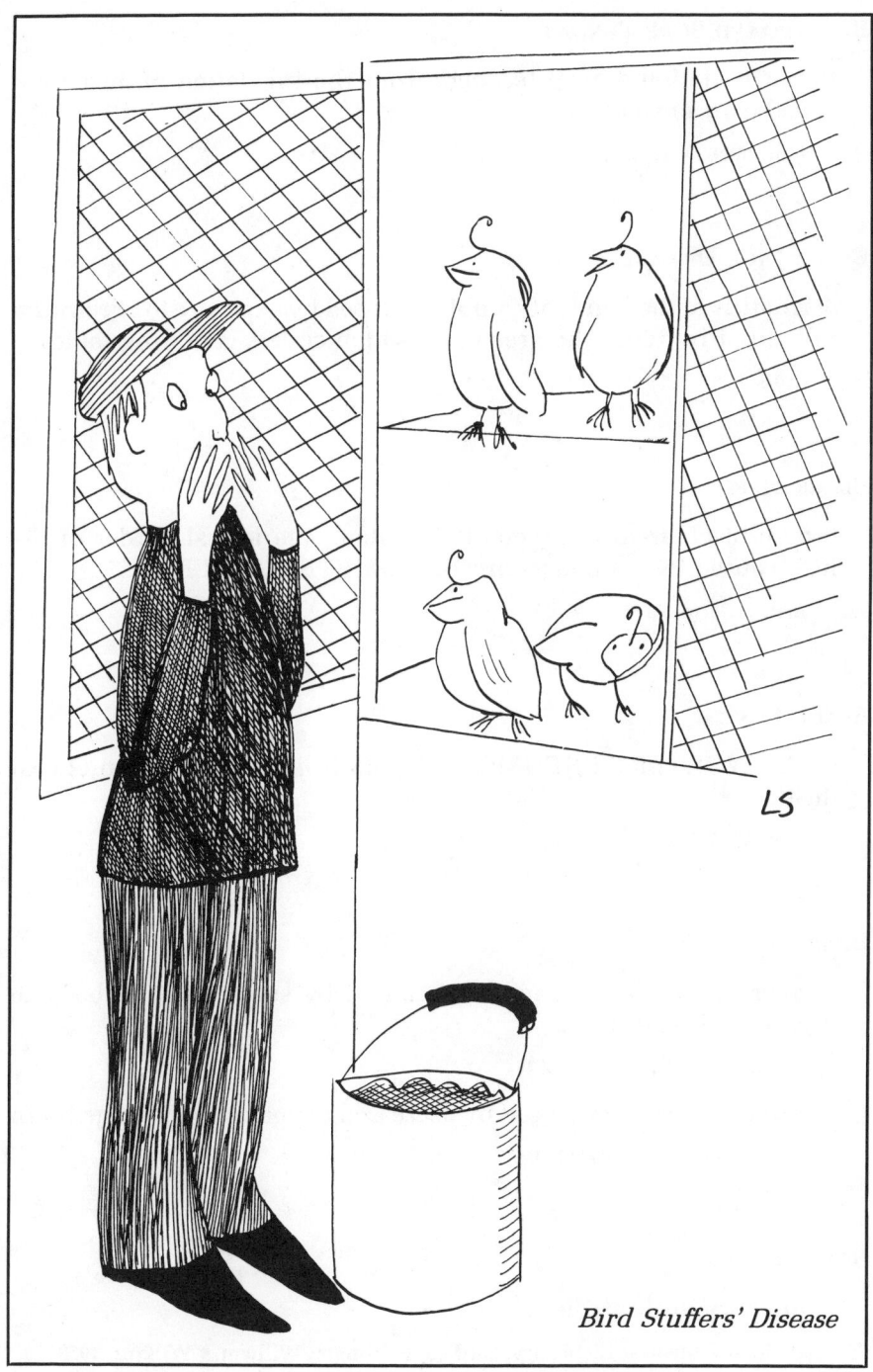

Bird Stuffers' Disease

TRADE DISEASES

BLACKBOARD SORE THROAT

throat irritation among teachers from the inhalation of dust from blackboard dusters

Lancet 1:920, 1889

BLACK JACK DISEASE

dermatitis of the hands of gamblers caused by exposure to chromium salts used in dying the green felt which covers gambling tables

Cutis 18:21, 1976

BLACK HEEL

brown-black areas of pigmentation along the lateral border of the heel caused by trauma (compare BASKETBALL HEEL)

Brit. J. Derm. 79:654, 1967

BLACK LUNG

COAL WORKER'S PNEUMOCONIOSIS from the inhalation of coal dust

Brit. Med. J. 1:425, 1857

BLACKOUT

temporary loss of consciousness caused by subjecting the body to high centrifugal forces

Atlantic Month. 350/1, 1934

loss of consciousness caused by decreased oxygen supply to the brain

J. Appl. Physiol. 3:204, 1950

BLACK PHTHISIS

pulmonary anthracosis

Stedman's Medical Dictionary. 23rd ed. Baltimore: William & Wilkins, 1976

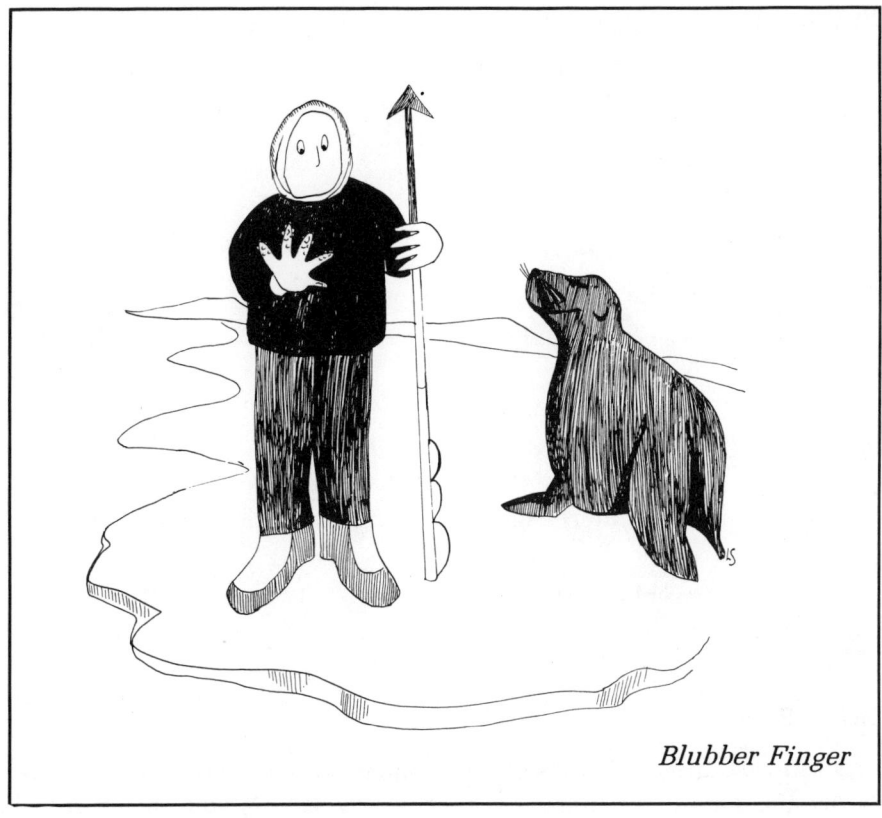
Blubber Finger

BLACKSMITH'S CATARACT

cataract resulting from prolonged exposure of the eye to infrared radiation

<small>Am. J. Ophth. 14:1098, 1931</small>

BLACKSMITH'S DEAFNESS

hearing loss resulting from noise exposure

<small>Lancet 1:645, 1831</small>

BLACKSMITH'S DISEASE

BLACKSMITH'S DEAFNESS

<small>original source not identified</small>

BLACK SPIT

COAL WORKERS' PNEUMOCONIOSIS
> Brit. Med. J. 1:491, 1857

BLAST BLINDNESS

loss of vision due to blast concussion
> original source not identified

BLAST CHEST

concussion and hemorrhage of the lungs from the shock waves of a blast
> Dorland's Medical Dictionary. 25th ed. Phila.: W. B. Saunders, 1974

BLAST EARS

auditory damage, frequently associated with perforation of the ear drums, among military personnel exposed to concussion shock waves
> Brit. Med. J. 1:93, 1944

BLAST INJURY

injury to the chest or abdominal contents resulting from concussion shock waves
> Brit. Med. J. 1:944, 1941

BLAST LUNG

BLAST CHEST
> original source not identified

BLAST SYNDROME

BLAST INJURY

International Classification of Diseases. 8th rev. USDHEW Pub. Hlth. Serv. Pub. No. 1963, 1968

BLUBBER FINGER

skin infection (erysipeloid) of the finger occurring among Scandinavian seal hunters

Acta. Path. et Microbiol. Scand. 26:407, 1949

BLUE GUM

bluish discoloration of the gum at the base of the teeth seen in lead intoxication

Dorland's Medical Dictionary. 25th ed. Phila.: W. B. Saunders, 1974

BLUE HALOS

sensation of blue halos around lights experienced by workers who handle atebrin, an antimalarial drug

Brit. J. Ophth. 31:40, 1947

BLUE LIP

dark blue discoloration of the lips due to lack of oxygen seen in TNT workers

Schwartz, L. Occupational Diseases of the Skin. Phila.: Lea & Febiger, 1957

BLUE MEN

workers whose skin is slate gray due to argyria; i.e., abnormal silver absorption

ILO Enclyclopedia of Occupational Health and Safety. N.Y.: McGraw Hill, 1972

Blue Sweat

blue-green discoloration of the sweat sometimes seen in copper workers

   Dorland's Medical Dictionary. 25th ed. Phila.: W. B. Saunders, 1974

Boilermaker's Deafness

loss of hearing from prolonged noise exposure

   Arlidge, J. T. The Hygiene, Diseases And Mortality of Occupations. London: Percival, 1892

Boilermaker's Ear

BOILERMAKER'S DEAFNESS

   Hunter, D. The Diseases of Occupations. 5th ed. London: The English Univ. Press Ltd., 1975

Boilermaker's Laryngitis

loss of the voice from overuse by constantly shouting in a noisy environment

   JAMA 123:958, 1943

Bolster Finger

swelling of the tissues around the finger nails seen in sugar workers as a result of a fungus infection *(monilia)*

   Brit. Med. J. 2:77, 1936

Bomb Happy

BATTLE FATIGUE

   Brit. Med. J. 2:788, 1950

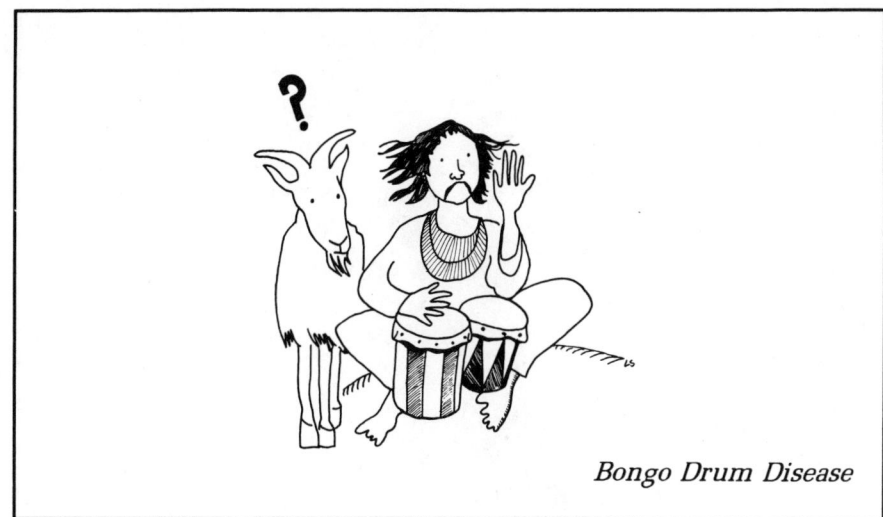

Bongo Drum Disease

BONE BUTTON MAKERS' DISEASE

inflammation of the fingers of button workers from small wounds made by bone fragments

<small>Schwartz, L. Occupational Diseases of the Skin. Phila.: Lea & Febiger, 1957</small>

BONGO DRUM DISEASE

anthrax infection contracted from goat hide bongo drums made in Haiti

<small>Lancet 1:1152, 1974</small>

BOO-HOO FEVER

generalized aching, loss of appetite, fever, and loss of efficiency among overseas troops, associated with their decided wish to be sent home

<small>Brit. Med. J. 2:1706, 1898</small>

BOTTLE FINISHER'S CATARACT

cataract of the eye following prolonged exposure to heat and light at the glass furnace

<small>Brit. Med. J. 1:191, 1903</small>

TRADE DISEASES

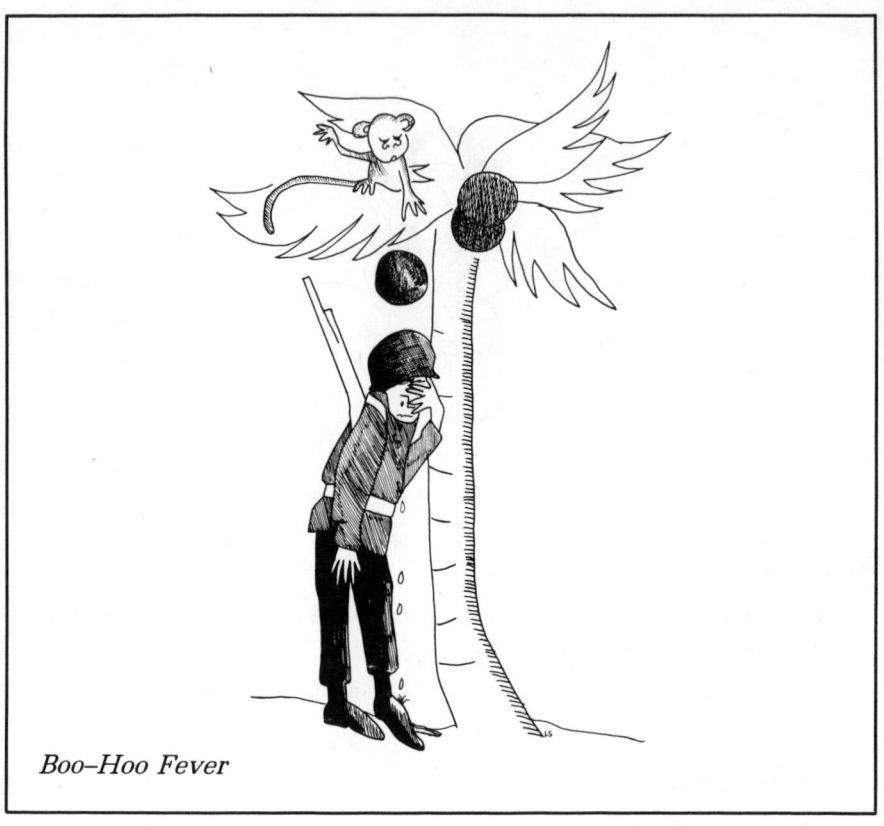

Boo–Hoo Fever

BOTTLE MAKER'S CATARACT

BOTTLE FINISHER'S CATARACT

JAMA 3:381, 1907

BOTTLE WORKER'S CATARACT

BOTTLE FINISHER'S CATARACT

original source not identified

BOWLER'S CRAMP

see OCCUPATIONAL NEUROSIS

Hunter, D. The Diseases of Occupations. 5th ed. London: The English Univ. Press Ltd., 1975

BOWLER'S THUMB

inflammation of the digital nerve of the thumb caused by pressure from the bowling ball

J. of Trauma 6:282, 1966

BOXER'S BRAIN DAMAGE

degenerative disease of the brain from repeated head trauma

Lancet 2:1270, 1974

BOXER'S EAR

deformity of the ear from repeated trauma

Hunter, D. The Diseases of Occupations. 5th ed. London: The English Univ. Press Ltd., 1975

BOXER'S ENCEPHALOPATHY

BOXER'S BRAIN DAMAGE

World Wide Abst. 5(11):18, 1962

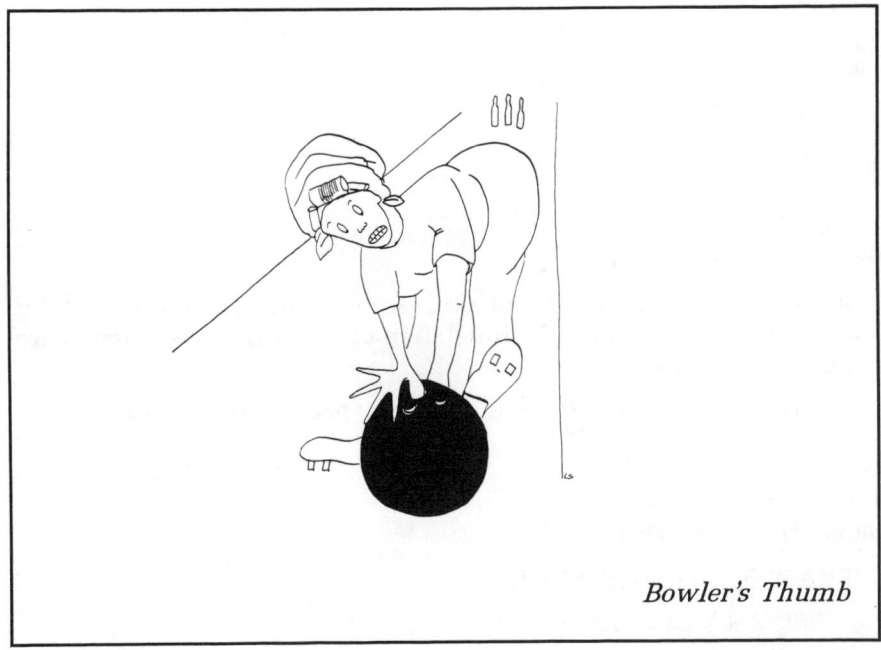

Bowler's Thumb

TRADE DISEASES

BOXER'S FRACTURE

fracture dislocation of the first metacarpal bone of the hand

Dublin J. M. Sci. 73:72, 1882

BOXERS' HEMORRHAGE

bleeding into the brain stem in boxers and fighters following head trauma

Calif. & West. Med. 51:227, 1939

BOXERS' THUMB

partial dislocation of the first metacarpal bone of the hand of boxers

Brit. Med. J. 2:9, 1930

BOXING BRAINS

BOXER'S BRAIN DAMAGE

Lancet 2:1064, 1973

BRASS CHILLS

BRASS FOUNDER'S AGUE

original source not identified

BRASS FOUNDER'S AGUE

headache, chills, fever, cough, profuse sweating, generalized aching and marked thirst from the inhalation of volatilized metal (compare COPPER COLIC)

Thackrah, C. T. The Effects of Arts, Trades and Professions On Health and Longevity. London: Longman, 1832

BRASS FOUNDER'S DISEASE

BRASS FOUNDER'S AGUE

Brit. Med. J. 2:335, 1911

Brass Founder's Fever

BRASS FOUNDER'S AGUE

Ann. Hyg. 34:222, 1845

Brass Molder's Ague

palpitation, chest and abdominal pain, tremors and chills from the inhalation of brass fumes

JAMA 43:465, 1904

Brass Worker's Ague

BRASS FOUNDER'S AGUE

Lancet 1:653, 1934

Brass Worker's Ataxia

muscular weakness and altered sensation of the extremities believed due to copper intoxication

Brit. Med. J. 2:1334, 1888

Brass Worker's Disease

any of the diseases related to brass fume inhalation (B. CHILLS, B. FOUNDER'S AGUE, B. FOUNDER'S FEVER, etc.)

Brit. Med. J. 2:1334, 1888

Brassy Eye

mechanical irritation of the eye among brass workers caused by small brass particles in the eye

original source not identified

BRAZIER'S AGUE

BRASS FOUNDER'S AGUE occurring in a brass worker

JAMA 90:1811, 1928

BRAZIER'S CHILL

BRASS FOUNDER'S AGUE

original source not identified

BRAZIER'S DISEASE

BRASS FOUNDER'S AGUE

Hunter, D. The Diseases of Occupations. 5th ed. London: The English Univ. Press Ltd., 1975

BREAD BAKERS' ITCH

BAKERS' ECZEMA

J. State Med. p. 55, Dec. 1924

BREAK-OFF

sensation of contact severance or physical detachment from the earth when flying at high altitudes

Lansberg, M. P. A Primer of Space Medicine. Amsterdam: Elsevier, 1960

BRICKBURNERS' ANEMIA

hookworm disease contracted by brick workers via unsanitary work conditions (compare TILE BURNERS' ANEMIA)

Lancet 1:1091, 1884

BRICKLAYER'S CRAMP

see OCCUPATIONAL NEUROSIS

Lancet 1:585, 1875

BRICKLAYER'S ELBOW

inflammation of the tissues at the elbow (olecranon bursa) from repeated trauma

>Hunter, D. The Diseases of Occupations. 5th ed. London: The English Univ. Press Ltd., 1975

BRICKLAYERS' ITCH

dermatitis of the hands of brickmasons from contact with hexavalent chrome salts in mortar.

>Hunter, D. The Diseases of Occupations. 5th ed. London: The English Univ. Press Ltd., 1975

BRICKLAYER'S SHOULDER

shoulder bursitis from overuse and trauma of the shoulder

>Hunter, D. The Diseases of Occupations. 5th ed. London: The English Univ. Press Ltd., 1975

BRICKMAKER'S ANEMIA

hookworm disease due to unsanitary work conditions in the brickyards

>Brit. Med. J. 2:640, 1883

BRICKMASON'S ECZEMA

eczematoid skin irritation caused by contact with cement and lime

>Arch. J. Derm. u. Syph. 178:1, 1938

BRINE BOILS

skin irritation from contact with calcium chloride used as a freezing agent in the manufacture of ice cream

>Brit. Med. J. 1:364, 1960

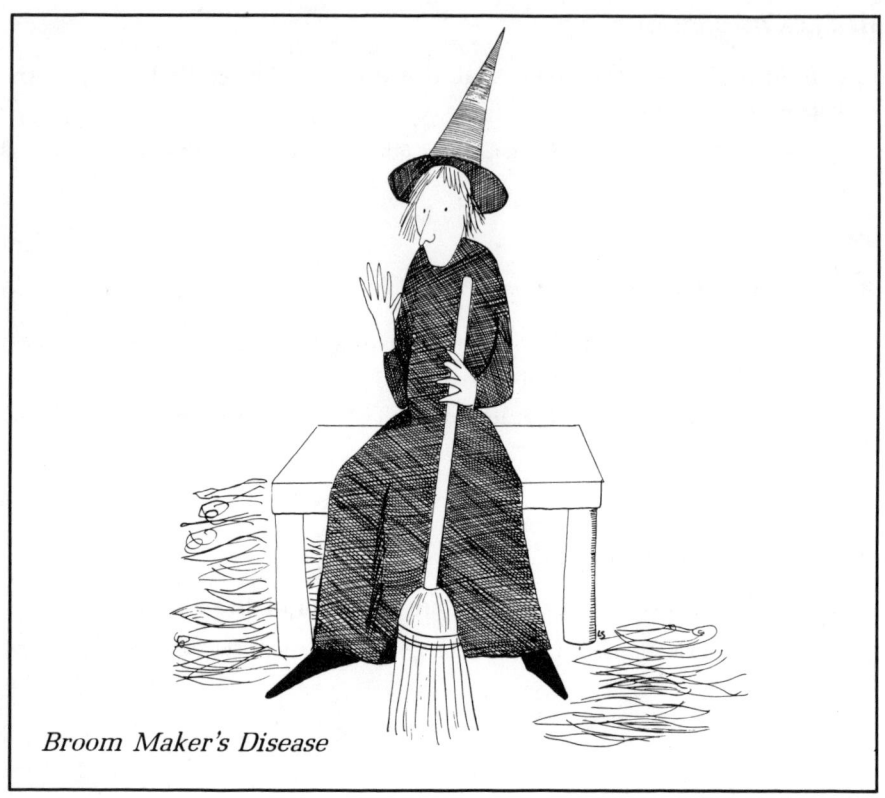
Broom Maker's Disease

BROOM MAKER'S DISEASE

mechanical irritation of the skin by broom corn dust *Sorghum vulgare*

> Schwartz, L. Occupational Diseases of the Skin. Phila.: Lea & Febiger, 1957

BROWN LUNG

BYSSINOSIS

> original source not identified

BUDGERIGAR FANCIERS' LUNG

BIRD BREEDERS' LUNG

> Hunter, D. The Diseases of Occupations. 5th ed. London: The English Univ. Press Ltd., 1975

Builders' Phthisis

chronic pulmonary disease among millstone builders caused by the inhalation of silica dust

Brit. Med. J. 1:864, 1878

Bulb Fingers

tingling, tenderness and redness of the fingertips of workers handling tulip, hyacinth, onion and garlic bulbs

Brit. Med. J. 2:1773, 1960

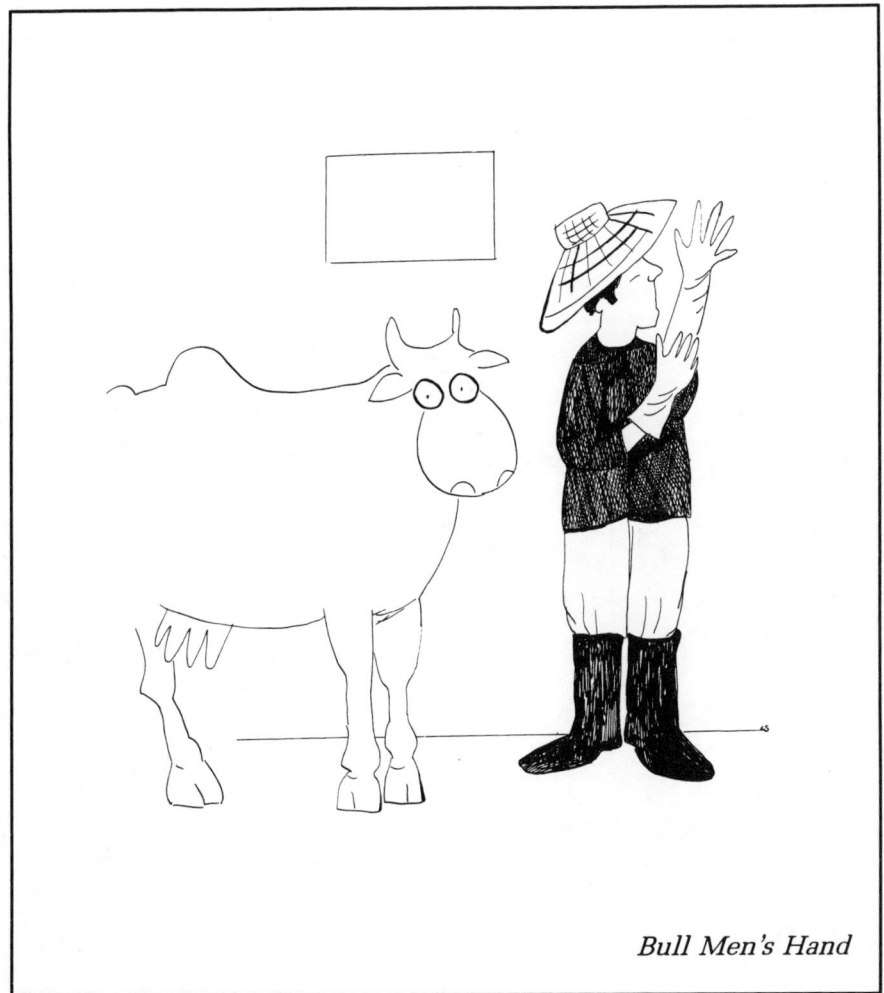

Bull Men's Hand

TRADE DISEASES

Bull Men's Hand

numbness and pain in the index and middle fingers among artificial inseminators of cattle due to the constricting effect of the rubber glove and sleeve worn for this purpose

J. Irish Med. Assoc. 67:102, 1974

Bumper Fracture

crushing injury and fracture of a leg from being struck by an automobile bumper

N. Eng. J. Med. 201:989, 1929

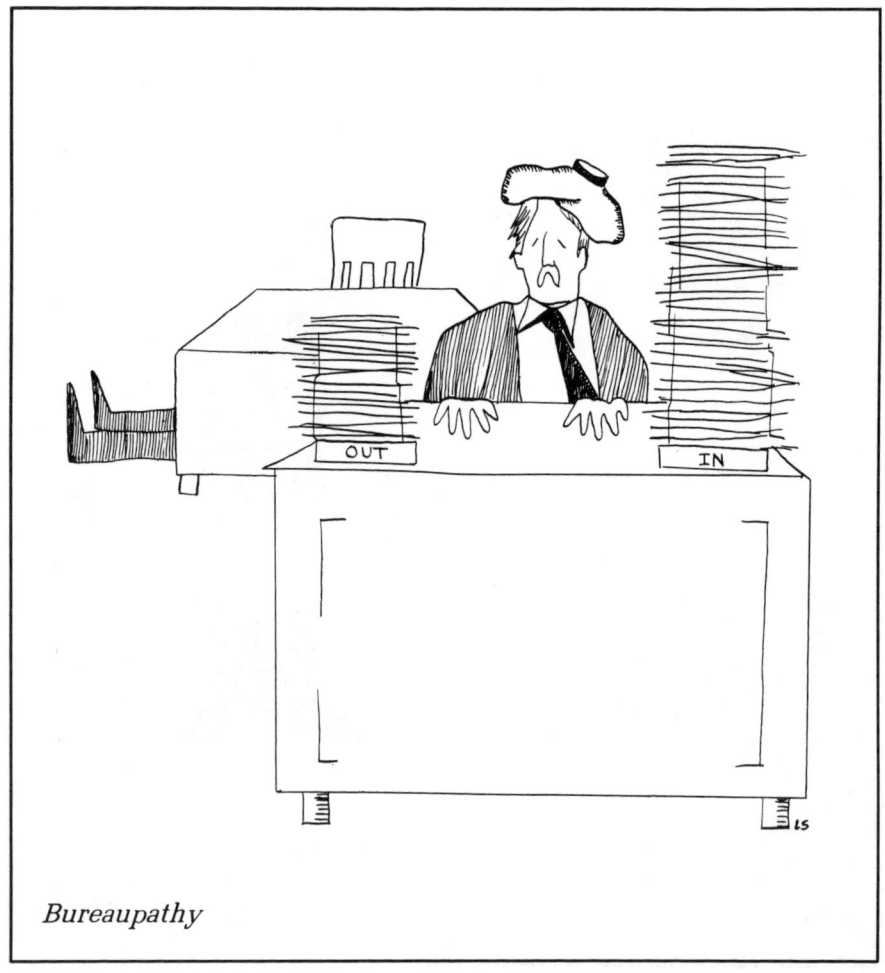

Bureaupathy

Bunches

irritable, inflammed swellings of the skin seen in coal miners due to the presence of the larvae of hookworm

Brit. Med. J. 1:611, 1904

Bureaupathy

headache, fatigue, lassitude and other psychosomatic symptoms among office workers

Euromed. 11:22, 1971

Burnishers' Eczema

skin irritation in metal burnishers presumably due to skin contact with alcohol, pyridine or turpentine

Zentrlbl. f. Gewerbehyg. 9:203, 1921

Butchers' Dermatitis

irritation of the hands of butchers, meat inspectors and veterinarians

J. Ind. Hyg. 13:233, 1931

hand irritation in slaughterhouse workers and meat inspectors caused by the digestive action of pancreatic enzymes

Cont. Derm. 2:61, 1976

Butchers' Pemphigus

eruption of watery blisters on the skin among those handling animals and animal products

Brit. J. Derm. 8:157, 1896

Butcher's Thigh

accidental stabbing of the thigh from careless use of a butcher knife with injury to the blood vessels

Brit. Med. J. 2:1309, 1957

Butchers' Tubercle

tuberculosis of the skin seen in butchers and contracted from infected meat products

>Hunter, D. The Diseases of Occupations. 5th ed. London: The English Univ. Press Ltd., 1975

Butcher's Wart

inflammatory skin lesion following accidental inoculation with the bovine tubercle bacillus from infected meat

>Brit. J. Derm. 51:166, 1939

Button Maker's Chorea

see OCCUPATIONAL NEUROSIS

>Dorland's Medical Dictionary. 25th ed. Phila.: W. B. Saunders, 1974

Byssinosis

respiratory disease affecting workers exposed to cotton dust, characterized by chest tightness, cough, shortness of breath and disability

>Traite d'hygiene publique 7:171, 1877

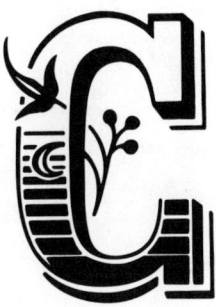

Cabinet Makers' Callosities

hand calluses corresponding to pressure points of the tools used by cabinet makers

> Hunter, D. The Diseases of Occupations. 5th ed. London: The English Univ. Press Ltd., 1975

Cabinet Maker's Cramp

see OCCUPATIONAL NEUROSIS

> Hunter, D. The Diseases of Occupations. 5th ed. London: The English Univ. Press Ltd., 1975

Cable Rash

acneiform eruption of the skin of workers installing or handling flameproof cables made from chlorinated naphthalenes

> JAMA 122:158, 1943

Caisson Disease

decompression sickness among men who work inside submerged watertight enclosures

Brit. & Foreign Med. Chir. Rev. 234, 1875

Camel Itch

dermatitis of the arms, legs and chests of camel caretakers caused by the camel mite

Lancet 2:679, 1829

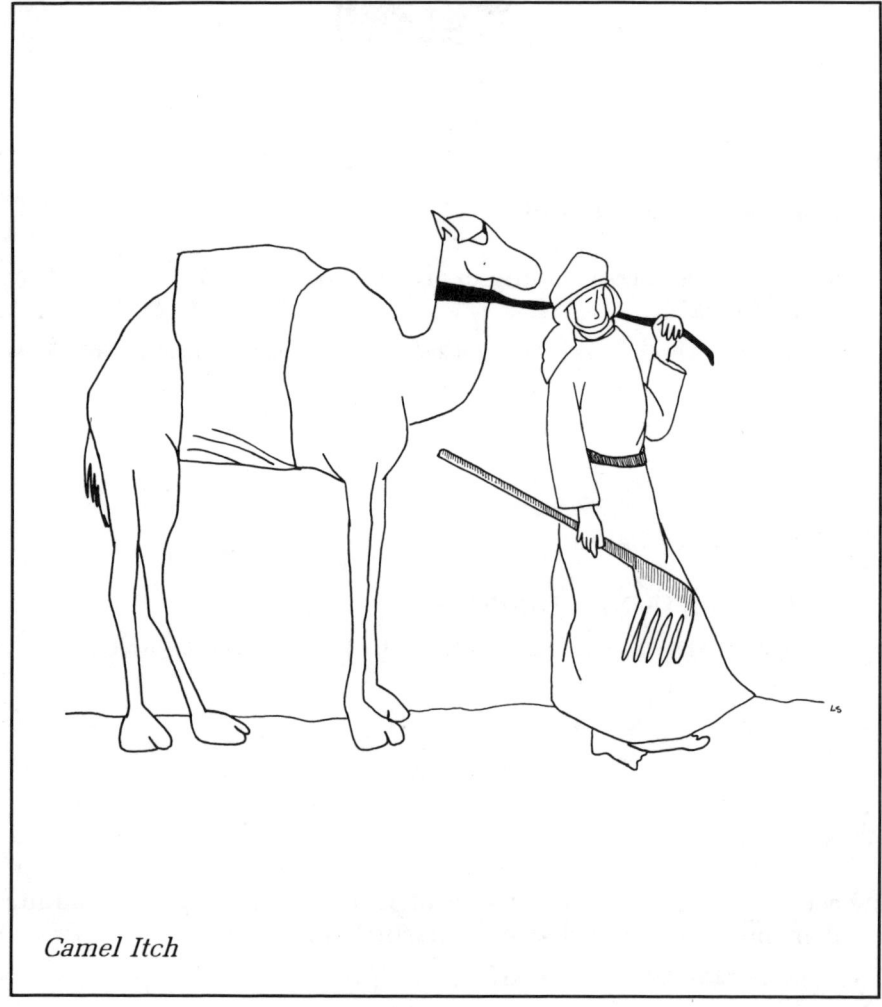

Camel Itch

Camp Diarrhea

gastroenteritis among troops caused by unsanitary conditions and dietary changes

Bost. Med. & Surg. J. 67:103, 1862

Camp Diseases

pneumonia, measles, mumps and meningitis occurring among troops mobilized for camp maneuvers

JAMA 30:1423, 1898

Camp Eyes

impaired vision from poor nutrition among prisoners of war

original source not identified

Camp Fever

typhoid fever in Civil War camps

JAMA 30:1359, 1898

Camp Jaundice

insomnia, headache, malaise, nausea, abdominal pain and jaundice affecting soldiers during WWI

Lancet 1:681, 1916

Camp Vertigo

vertigo, headache and unsteady gait seen in prisoners of war and believed due to malnutrition

JAMA 132:665 1946

Cane Cutters' Cramps

heat cramps affecting cane-field workers

Merck Manual. 9th ed. N.J.: Merck & Co., 1956

Cane Cutters' Tenosynovitis

inflammation of the forearm tendon sheaths in canefield workers

Nineteenth Ann. Rept. Med. Dept. United Fruit Co., 1930

Carders' Asthma

respiratory disease (BYSSINOSIS) affecting cardroom workers exposed to cotton dust

Hunter, D. The Diseases of Occupations. 5th ed. London: The English Univ. Press Ltd., 1975

Cardroom Workers' Asthma

CARDERS' ASTHMA

Lancet 2:366, 1933

Carpenter's Dermatitis

irritation of the hands and forearms from irritants and sensitizers common to the carpentry trade

Brit. Med. J. 2:190, 1951

Carpenter's Disease

head, neck and chest pain, shortness of breath and nervousness alleged to overuse of the upper extremities

Brit. Med. J. 2:289, 1874

Carpenter's Hands

permanent finger deformities resulting from mechanical factors in the grasping of tools

<small>Billich. München. Med. Wchnschr. 74:1941, 1927</small>

Carpet Layer's Knee

inflammation of the bursa in front of the kneecap caused by pushing the carpet-stretching block with the knee

<small>ILO Encyclopedia of Occupational Health and Safety, N.Y.: McGraw Hill, 1972</small>

Carrot Poisoning

mercurial intoxication in hat makers exposed to mercurial nitrate used to "carrot" (treat) the fur

<small>Rpt. Bd. Hlth., Connect. 6:299, 1888</small>

Cataracta Electrica

cataract development in the eye following an electrical shock

<small>Acta. Ophth. 17:460, 1939</small>

Caterpillar Dermatitis

skin irritation among gardners and forestry workers caused by contact with the nettling hairs of caterpillars

<small>Ann. Derm. Syph., Paris 9:35, 1949</small>

Cavalry Bone

formation of bone in the muscle of the inner thigh from years of horseback riding

<small>Billings Nat. Med. Dict., 1890</small>

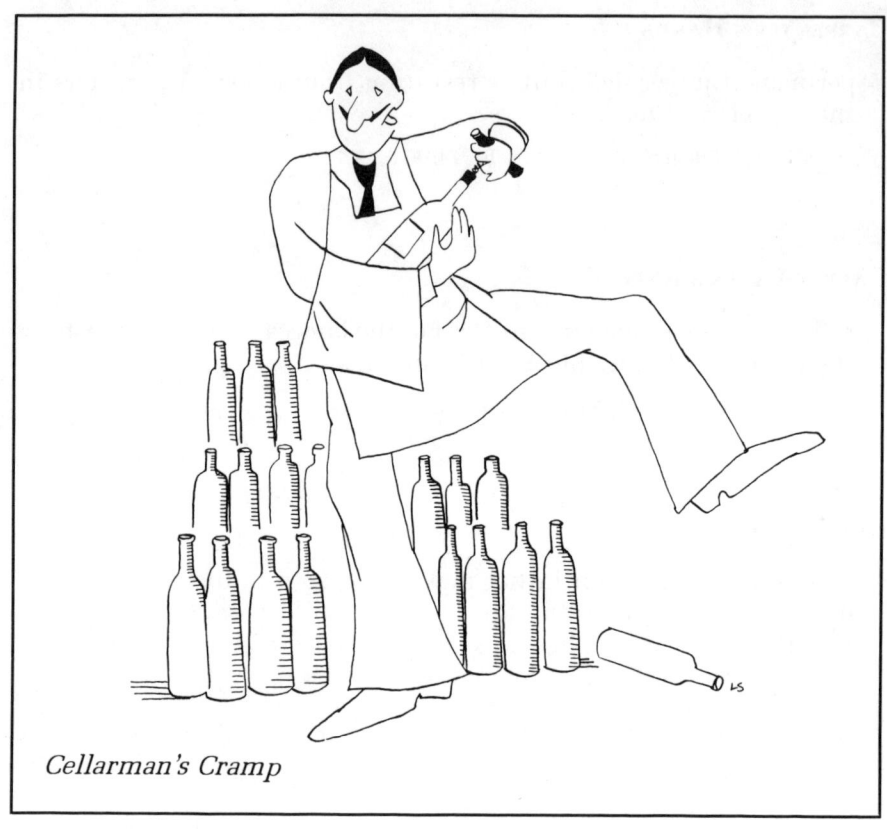
Cellarman's Cramp

CAVALRYMAN'S LEG
CAVALRY BONE

Oliver, T. Dangerous Trades. London: J. Murray, 1902

CAVALRYMAN'S OSTEOMA
CAVALRY BONE

Dorland's Medical Dictionary. 25th ed. Phila.: W. B. Saunders, 1974

CAVE DISEASE

systemic fungus infection *(histoplasmosis)* contracted by "pot-holing" in limestone caves where the fungus grows on bat guano

Lancet 1:1149, 1963

Cave Sickness

upper respiratory symptoms associated with chills, fever, cough, chest pain and weight loss seen among visitors to abandoned mines

Am. J. Pub. Hlth. 38:1521, 1948

Celery Itch

red, blistery rash affecting the hands, wrists and forearms of celery pickers, believed due to celery oil

Brit. J. Derm. 45:301, 1933

Cellarman's Cramp

occupational cramp from opening champagne bottles

Lancet 2:333, 1886

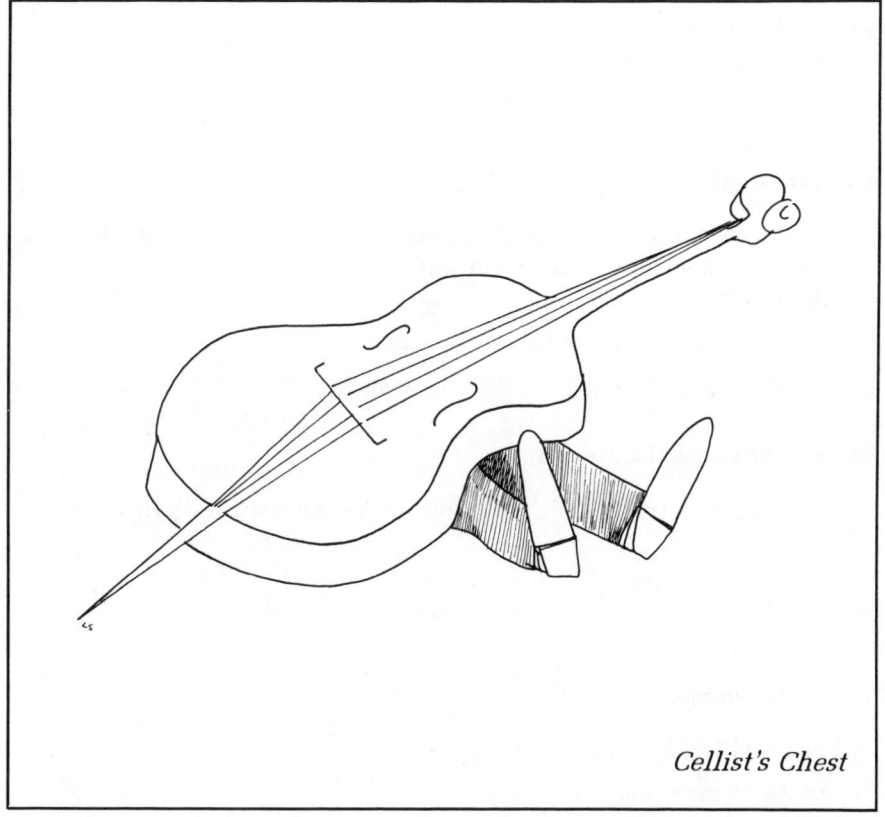

Cellist's Chest

Cellist's Chest

discomfort of the front of the chest caused by pressure of the instrument

N. Eng. J. Med. 266:348, 1962

Cellist's Cramp

see OCCUPATIONAL NEUROSIS

Singer, K. Diseases of the Musical Profession. (tr. by W. Lakond, Greensburg, N.Y., 1932)

Cello Scrotum

skin irritation of the scrotum from contact with and pressure from the cello body

Brit. Med. J. 2:335, 1974

Cementers' Itch

skin disease among cement finishers, packers and bag cleaners caused by mechanical abrasion and chemical irritation from Portland cement

Bull. de l'Acad. de Med. p. 902, 20 Oct. 1925

Cement Workers' Dermatitis

sensitivity reaction of cement workers to potassium dichromate in Portland cement

O. Hosp. 41:495, 1952

Cement Workers' Itch

CEMENTERS' ITCH

JAMA 106:2255, 1936

Chaff Cutter's Lung

allergic inflammatory response of the lungs to grain husk chaff

Brit. Med. J. 1:705, 1889

Chain Makers' Cataract

cataracts in workers who hand forge chains resulting from prolonged exposure of the eye to infrared radiation

Brit. Med. J. 1:393, 1949

Chalicosis Pulmonum

chronic lung disease in mill workers from the inhalation of stone dust generated by crushing and grinding gold-bearing quartzite

JAMA 34:70, 1900

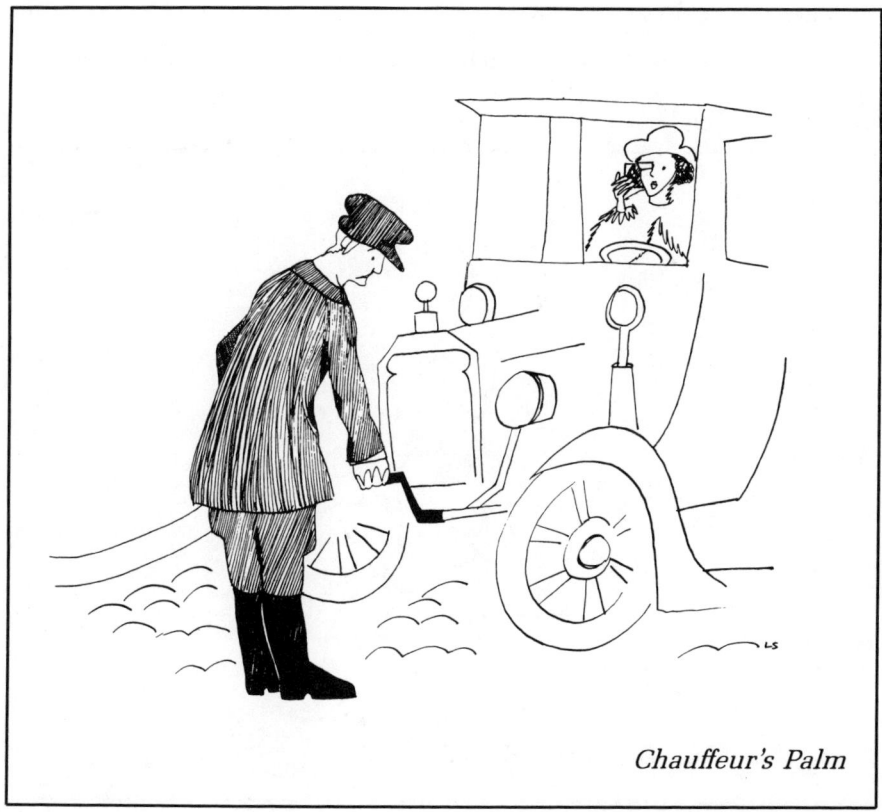

Chauffeur's Palm

TRADE DISEASES

Change Of Shift Syndrome

loss of appetite, insomnia and constipation related to the rotation of work shifts

Lancet 2:449, 1944

Charley Horse

stiffness of the legs and arms from their overuse in playing basketball

Lancet 1:799, 1914

Chauffeur's Fracture

fracture of the forearm occurring because of an engine backfire while the chauffeur is hand cranking the motor (compare PROPELLER FRACTURE)

Lancet 1:962, 1904

fracture of the fifth metacarpal of the hand from the same cause

Lancet 1:902, 1906

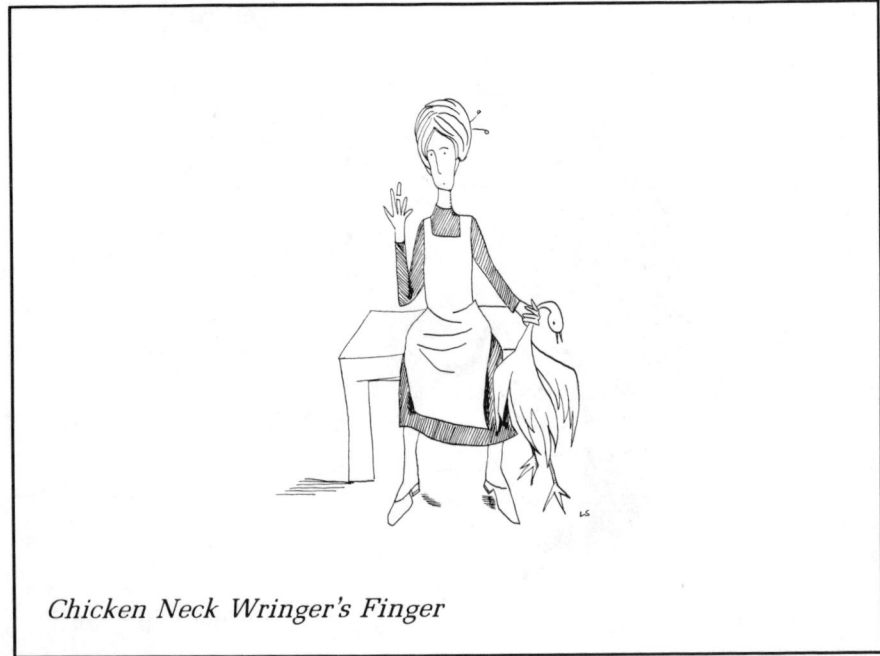

Chicken Neck Wringer's Finger

Chauffeur's Knee

bursitis in the knee from the strain produced by long periods of driving

N.Y. Med. J. 102:1195, 1916

Chauffeur's Palm

anticipated fibrosis of the palm of the hand among those who hand-crank automobile engines

Brit. Med. J. 2:305, 1923

Checkitis

pilot anxiety prior to check-rides for determining flying status eligibility (compare TESTITIS)

Av. Sp. Environ. Med. 46:1407, 1975

Cheese Washer's Asthma
CHEESE WASHER'S LUNG

Schweiz. Med. Wochen. 100:1108, 1970

Cheese Washer's Disease
CHEESE WASHER'S LUNG

Ann. Int. Med. 78:606, 1973

Cheese Washer's Lung

allergic inflammatory response of the lungs to cheese mold *Penicillium casei* inhaled while washing off aging cheeses

Schweiz. Med. Wochn. 99:872, 1969

Cheese Worker's Itch

itchy skin lesions of the hands and forearms caused by contact with the cheese fly *Piophila casei*

> Schwartz, L. Occupational Diseases of the Skin. Phila.: Lea & Febiger, 1957

Chicken Neck Wringer's Finger

partial dislocation and arthritis of the middle finger joint from continued use of this digit to dislocate checken necks for slaughtering

> Brit. Med. J. 1:47, 1955

Chicken Pickers' Dermatitis

skin irritation of the hands and forearms of fowl handlers caused by scabies or fowl mites

> JAMA 132:894, 1946

Chiclero's Ulcer

chronic ulceration of the outer ear caused by a protozoa *Phebotomus cruciatus?*, peculiar to chewing gum latex collectors (chicleros) in British Honduras

> Brit. Med. J. 1:299, 1959

Chili Grinders' Disease

eye and nose irritation, loss of appetite and nausea occurring in workers who process red peppers

> Brit. J. Ind. Med. 24:162, 1967

Chimney Sweep's Cancer

cancer of the scrotum from exposure to soot while cleaning chimneys

> Pott P. Chirurgical observations relative to . . ., the cancer of the scrotum, . . . etc. London: Hawes, Clark & Collings, 1775

Chloracne

skin eruption among chlorine gas workers

Munch. Med. Wschr. 46:278, 1899

Chlorine Acne

acne-like eruption of the skin among workers handling chlorinated naphthalenes

Paris Med. p. 62, January, 1926

pustular acne of the face, neck, ears and forearms in workers exposed to hydrochloric acid

Bull. Soc. Franc. de Derm. et Syph. p. 33, July, 1925

Chokes

decompression sickness in divers manifested by chest pain, shortness of breath, cough and unconsciousness

Northumberland and Dublin Med. J. p. 8, 1899

Chorditis Tuberosa

vocal cord nodule found in singers and public speakers caused by a faulty method of using the voice

New Eng. Med. Month. 10:313, 1891

Choristers' Heart

cardiac enlargement, palpitation and chest pain seen in choir youths as a result of the extreme physiologic demands of singing

Lancet 2:1136, 1905

Chrome Cripples

workers disabled by sensitivity to chromium compounds

Med. J. Austral. 2:720, 1975

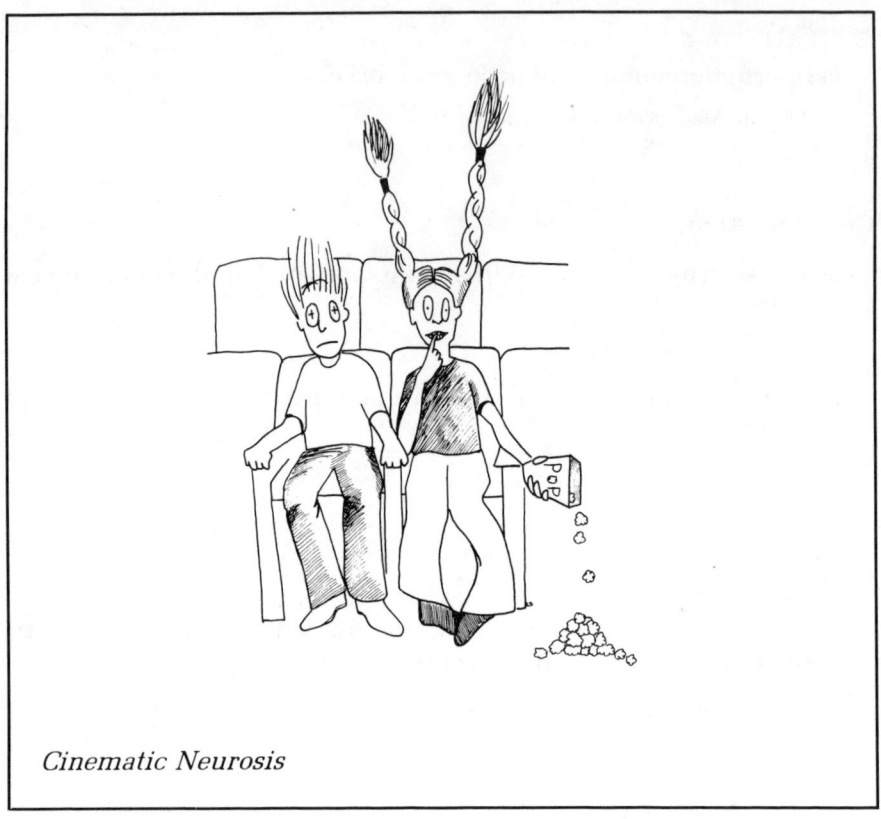
Cinematic Neurosis

CHROME HOLES

    ulceration of the hands in chromate workers brought about by the penetration of chromate through skin cuts or abrasions

        Edinburgh Med. J. 26:134, 1827

CHROME SORE

    CHROME HOLES

        Ann. Surg. 63:155, 1916

CIGARETTE ROLLER'S CRAMP

    see OCCUPATIONAL NEUROSIS

        JAMA 23:804, 1894

Cigar Maker's Cramp

see OCCUPATIONAL NEUROSIS

Brit. Med J. 2:165, 1890

Cigar Roller's Neuritis

see OCCUPATIONAL NEUROSIS

original source not identified

Cinema Eye

irritation of the eyes of performers caused by the bright camera lights (compare KLIEG EYE)

JAMA 80:1792, 1923

Cinema Fatigue

eyestrain caused by glare, flicker and an increased demand on the muscles which move the eyes

Lancet 2:744, 1919

Cinematic Neurosis

traumatic neurosis precipitated by movies with strong emotional effects such as "Jaws," "The Exorcist," etc.

J. Nerv. Ment. Dis. 161:43, 1975

Circadian Dysrhythmia

fatigue, tenseness and irritability resulting from rapid transition through multiple time zones as occurs in jet flights (compare JET LAG)

Mod. Med. 38:37, 1970

Clam Digger Itch

CLAM DIGGERS' DERMATITIS

AMA Arch. Derm. & Syph. 66:367, 1952

Clam Diggers' Dermatitis

itching and hives of the upper extremities noted in clam diggers caused by contact with flukes *Schistosome circariae* in the water

AMA Arch. Derm. & Syph. 66:367, 1952

Clarionet Player's Cramp

see OCCUPATIONAL NEUROSIS

Hunter, D. The diseases of Occupations. 5th ed. London: The English Univ. Press Ltd., 1975

Clay Shoveler's Disease

CLAY SHOVELER'S FRACTURE

International Classification of Diseases. 8th rev. USDHEW Pub. Hlth. Serv. Pub. No. 1963, 1968

Clay Shoveler's Fracture

fracture of a prominence of one of the vertebral bodies in the neck or upper back sustained while digging with a long handled shovel

J. Bone & Joint. Surg. 22:63, 1940

Clergyman's Bursitis

inflammation of the bursa in front of the kneecap from prolonged kneeling

Hunter, D. The Diseases of Occupations. 5th ed. London: The English Univ. Press Ltd., 1975

Clergyman's Sore Throat

chronic laryngitis from prolonged use of the voice (compare MINISTER'S AIL)

Lancet 2:258, 1844

Clergyman's Throat

CLERGYMAN'S SORE THROAT

Bost. Med. & Surg. J. 23:3, 1840

Coachman's Bursitis

inflammation of a bursa in the buttocks area caused by pressure and jarring from riding a coach seat

original source not identified

Coachman's Cramp

see OCCUPATIONAL NEUROSIS

Brit. Med. J. 1:11, 1886

Coal Miners' Dermatitis

coal dust tattooing of the skin occurring in coal miners (compare COLLIERS' STRIPES)

Brit. J. Derm. 52:129, 1940

Coal Miner's Elbow

inflammation of the elbow bursa from repetitive trauma (compare BEAT ELBOW)

International Classification of Diseases. 8th rev. USDHEW Pub. Hlth. Serv. Pub. No. 1963, 1968

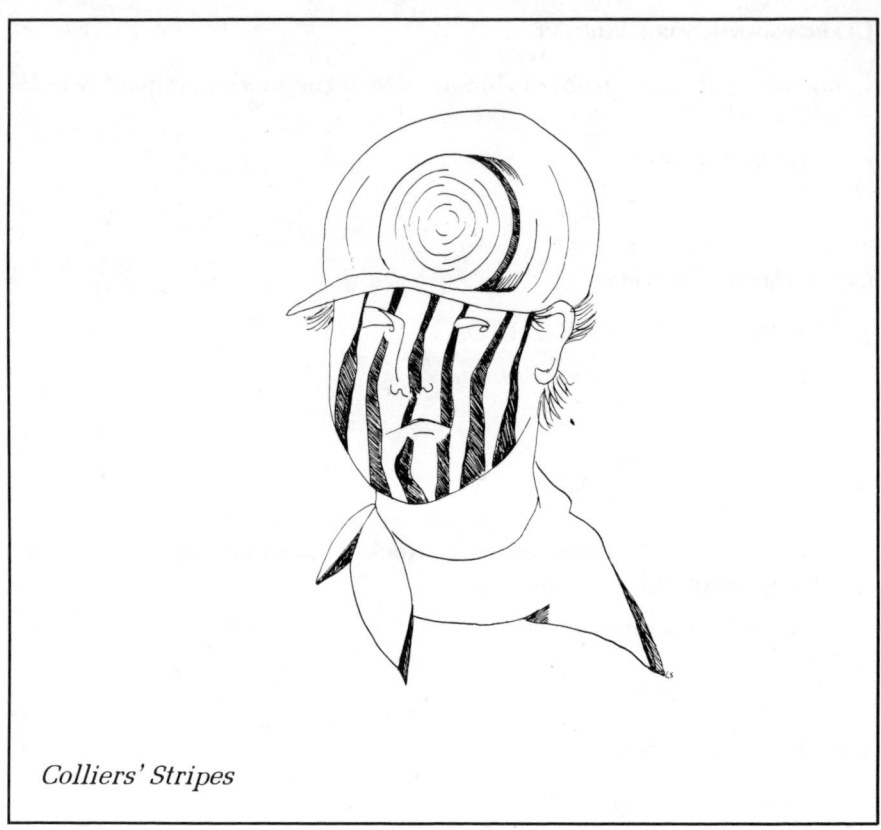

Colliers' Stripes

Coal Miner's Lung

COAL WORKERS' PNEUMOCONIOSIS

International Classification of Diseases. 8th rev. USDHEW Pub. Hlth. Serv. Pub. No. 1963, 1968

Coal Miners' Melanosis

chronic lung disease among coal workers (compare BLACK LUNG)

Edinb. Med. J. 36:389, 1831

Coal Workers' Pneumoconiosis

chronic lung disease among coal workers

original source not identified

Cobblers' Chest

hollow deformity at the base of the breast bone of shoemakers caused by pressure of the last against the chest

> Thackrah, C. T. The Effects of Arts, Trades and Professions On Health and Longevity. London: Longman, 1832

Coffee Worker's Disease

allergic inflammatory response of the lungs to inhaled coffee dust

> original source not identified

Coffee Worker's Lung

COFFEE WORKER'S DISEASE

> Thorax 25:399, 1970

Colliers' Anthracosis

COAL WORKERS' PNEUMOCONIOSIS

> Hunter, D. The Diseases of Occupations. 5th ed. London: The English Univ. Press Ltd., 1975

Colliers' Asthma

COAL WORKERS' PNEUMOCONIOSIS

> International Classification of Diseases. 8th rev. USDHEW Pub. Hlth. Serv. Pub. No. 1963, 1968

Colliers' Black Spit

chronic lung disease among coal miners characterized by the production of black sputum

> Brit. Med. J. 2:271, 1876

Colliers' Lung

COAL WORKERS' PNEUMOCONIOSIS

>International Classification of Diseases. 8th rev. USDHEW Pub. Hlth. Serv. Pub. No. 1963, 1968

Colliers' Phthisis

chronic lung disease of coal miners

>Watson, T. Lect. Prin. & Pract. Physic. ed. 5, 1871

Colliers' Stripes

light blue-grey linear and irregularly shaped marks on the face, forearms and hands of miners caused by coal dust tattooing of the skin (compare COAL MINERS' DERMATITIS)

>Brit. J. Derm. 52:129, 1940

Colliers' Tuberculosis

silicotuberculosis among coal miners

>International Classification of Diseases. 8th rev. USDHEW Pub. Hlth. Serv. Pub. No. 1963, 1968

Combat Fatigue

COMBAT NEUROSIS

>original source not identified

Combat Neurosis

anxiety, obsession, phobia, depression and other nervous reactions associated with the stresses of war

>Naval Med. Bull. 41:923, 1943

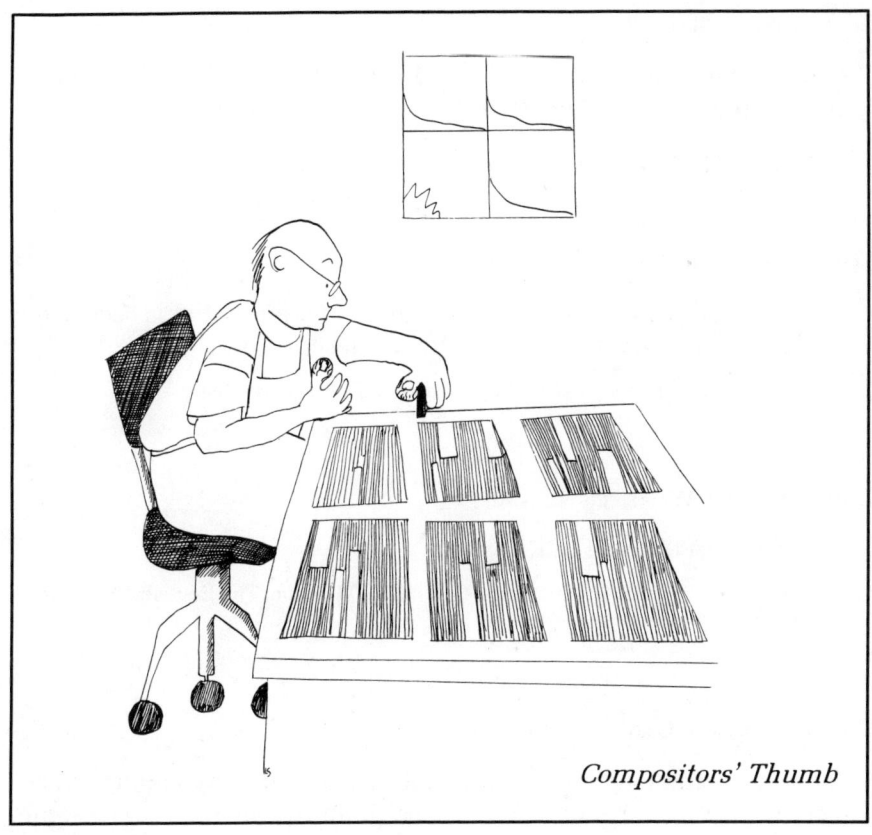
Compositors' Thumb

Comber's Fever
BYSSINOSIS from hemp dust created by combing the fibers
>Hunter, D. The Diseases of Occupations. 5th ed. London: The English Univ. Press Ltd., 1975

Compensation Neurosis
conversion hysteria following an occupational injury
>Ross, T. A. The Common Neuroses. London: Arnold, 1937

Compositor's Cramp
see OCCUPATIONAL NEUROSIS
>Lancet 2:709, 1864

TRADE DISEASES

Compositors' Thumb

painful cracking of the thumb and finger of compositors, aggravated in cold weather by skin dryness

Lancet 1:436, 1870

Compressed Air Illness

joint pains, tightness in the chest, convulsions and collapse occurring when deep-sea divers return to the surface too quickly

Snell, E. H. Compressed Air Illness. London: H. K. Lewis, 1896

Comptometer Worker's Cramp

see OCCUPATIONAL NEUROSIS

Hunter, D. The Diseases of Occupations. 5th ed. London: The English Univ. Press Ltd., 1975

Concentration Camp Syndrome

fatigue, depression, emotional instability and anxiety among survivors of WWII concentration camps (inability to forget gruesome experiences)

World Wide Abst. 7(9):17, 1964

Concussion Blindness

functional blindness due to violent explosions of shells, bombs and hand grenades

Lancet 1:15, 1916

Conditioning Dermatitis

mechanical irritation of the fingers of those handling cotton thread in the conditioning cellars of cotton mills

Lancet 1:404, 1916

Confectioners' Paronychia

inflammation of the fingernail beds of sugar workers caused by contact with corrosives and dirt

Brit. Med. J. 1:575, 1913

Conga Drummer's Pigmenturia

red-black discoloration of the urine caused by severe hand trauma associated with beating a conga drum (compare KARATE MYOGLOBINURIA)

Ann. Int. Med. 80:727, 1974

Conveyer Belt Shoulder

shoulder bursitis caused by repeated jolts in removing objects from an overhead conveyer

ILO Encyclopedia of Occupational Health and Safety. N.Y.: McGraw Hill, 1972

Coolie Itch

hookworm disease occurring among coolies employed on plantations

Brit. Med. J. 1:224, 1902

Copper Colic

headache, chills, fever and generalized aching following the inhalation of metal fumes by copper workers (compare BRASS FOUNDER'S AGUE)

Lancet 2:233, 1830

loss of appetite, thirst, abdominal pain and diarrhea due to copper intoxication in copper workers

Dana, S. L. Lead Diseases: A Treatise from the French of L. Tanquerel des Planches. Boston: Tappan, 1850

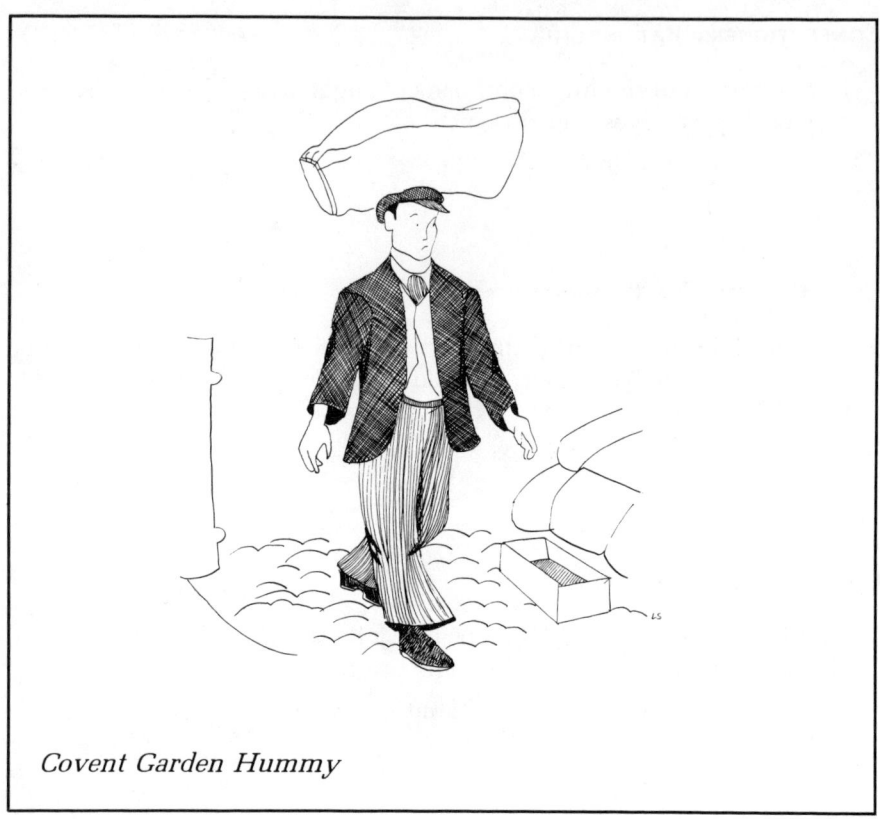

Covent Garden Hummy

COPPERMEN'S CHEST

    bronchitis and pulmonary fibrosis among copper smelters

        Lancet 1:1126, 1887

COPRA ITCH

    eruption of the extremities and trunk of workers handling copra due to scabies

        Brit. Med. J. 2:1208, 1912

CORNET PLAYER'S CRAMP

    see OCCUPATIONAL NEUROSIS

        Lancet 1:995, 1893

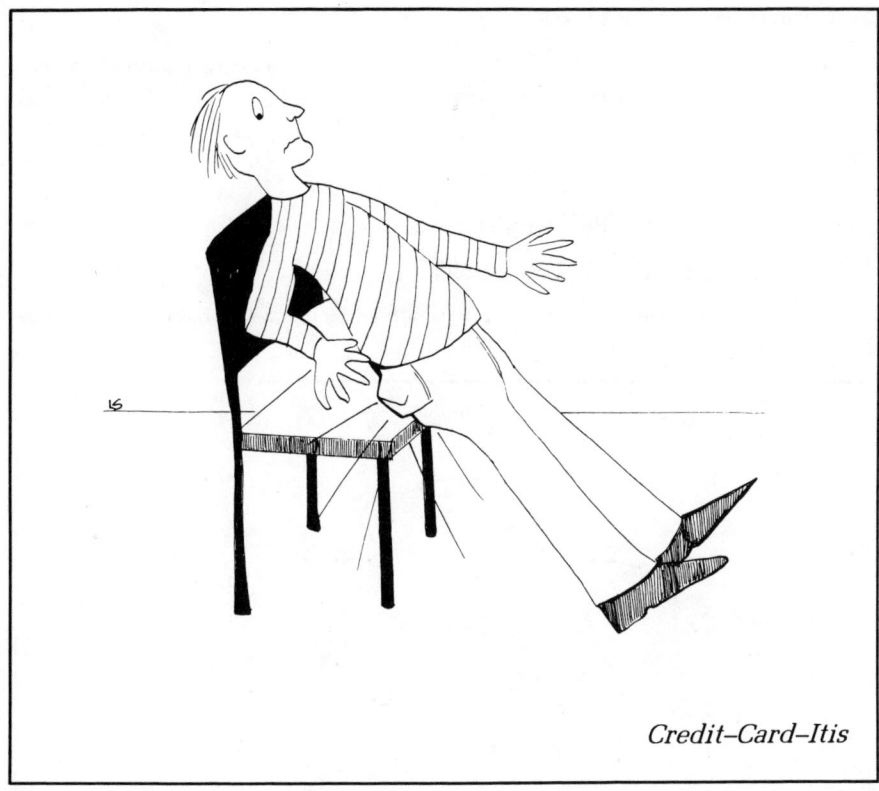

Credit–Card–Itis

Corn Itch

contact dermatitis of the hands of workers engaged in corn processing and canning

JAMA 123:124, 1943

Cornpicker Hand

multiple injuries to a hand caught in a mechanical cornpicker

J. Bone & Joint Surg. 36A:21, 1954

Cornpickers' Pupil

dilated pupils in workers who harvest corn due to jimson weed dust containing stramonium

J. Iowa St. Med. Soc. 61:475, 1971

TRADE DISEASES

Corundum Smelters' Lung

pulmonary fibrosis with shortness of breath and cough seen in workers who manufacture corundum

Ind. Hyg. & Occup. Med. 6:339, 1952

Corundum Workers' Pneumoconiosis
CORUNDUM SMELTERS' LUNG

Hunter, D. The Diseases of Occupations. 5th ed. London: The English Univ. Press Ltd., 1975

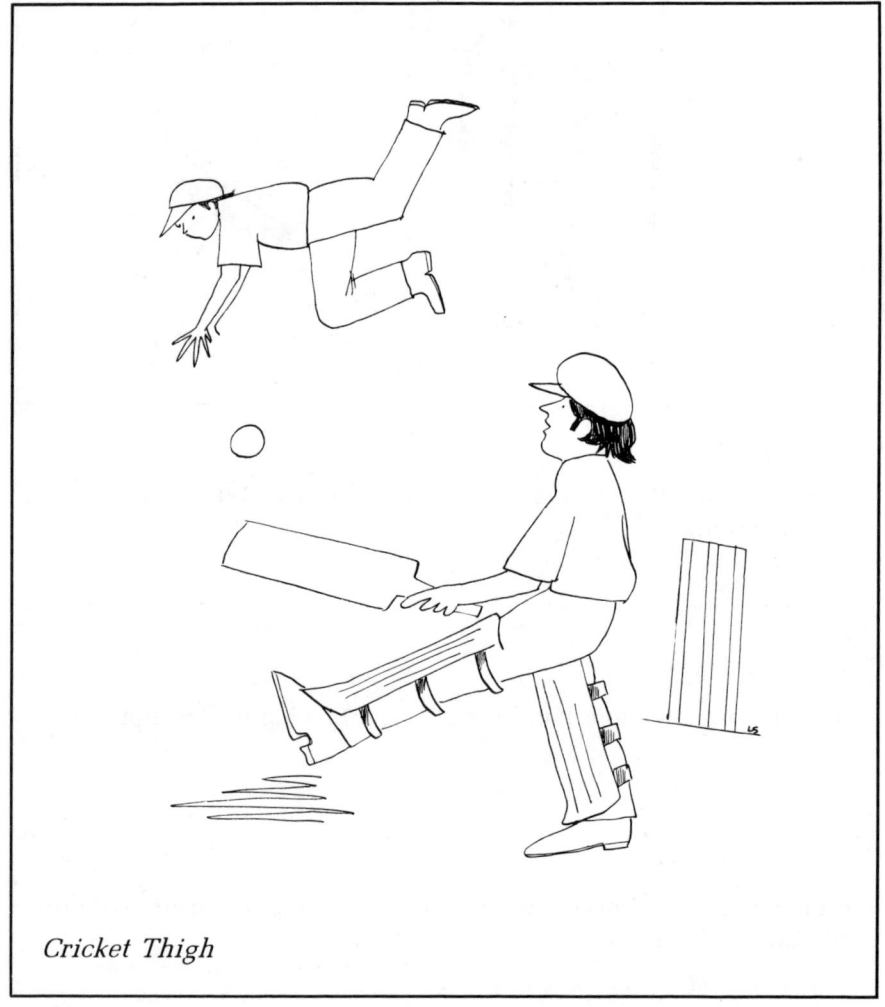

Cricket Thigh

Cotton Carders' Asthma

BYSSINOSIS among those employed in cotton carding

Lancet 2:648, 1863

Cotton Dust Disease

BYSSINOSIS

London Med. Phys. J. 39:464, 1818

Cotton Grinders' Asthma

BYSSINOSIS among workers engaged in cleaning and grinding the teeth of cotton carding equipment

Lancet 2:648, 1863

Cotton Mill Asthma

BYSSINOSIS

Ind. Med. & Surg. 30:95, 1961

Cotton Mill Fever

chills, nausea and vomiting, headache, thirst and fever affecting new workers exposed to cotton dust for the first time

original source not identified

Cotton Spinners' Cancer

skin cancer occurring in spinning machine operators from contact with spindle oil (compare MULE SPINNERS' CANCER)

Lancet 2:239, 1924

Cotton Spinners' Phthisis

chronic effects of BYSSINOSIS

Ind. Med. & Surg. 30:95, 1961

COTTON STRIPPERS' ASTHMA

BYSSINOSIS among workers who clean the teeth of the cotton carding machinery

Lancet 2:648, 1863

COTTON TWISTER'S CRAMP

see OCCUPATIONAL NEUROSIS

Hunter, D. The Diseases of Occupations. 5th ed. London: The English Univ. Press Ltd., 1975

COVENT GARDEN HUMMY

swelling over the vertex of the scalp in market garden porters

Hunter, D. The Diseases of Occupations. 5th ed. London: The English Univ. Press Ltd., 1975

COWPOX

vaccinia of the fingers from hand-milking infected cows

Zeitschr. J. Med. p. 773, 1898

CRAFT PALSY

see OCCUPATIONAL NEUROSIS

Stedman's Medical Dictionary. 23rd ed. Baltimore: William & Wilkins, 1976

CREDIT-CARD-ITIS

sciatic nerve irritation with pain over the buttock and down the thigh due to pressure from a wallet stuffed with credit cards

N. Eng. J. Med. 274:467, 1966

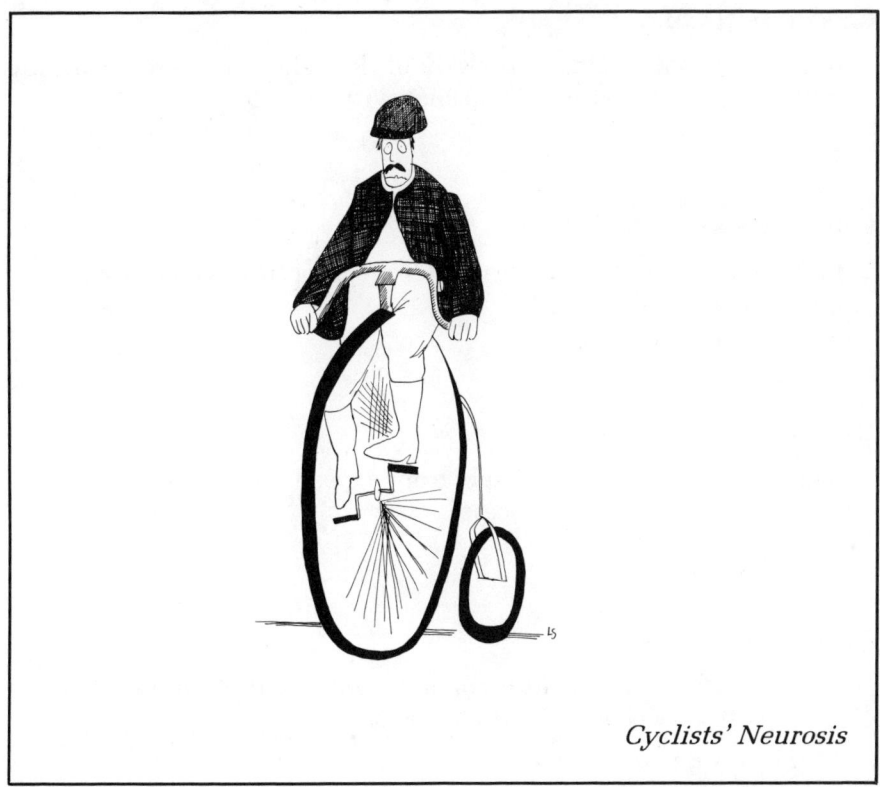

Cyclists' Neurosis

CREEPS

mild symptoms of the bends in divers (compare NIGGLES)

Lansberg, M. P. A Primer of Space Medicine. Amsterdam: Elsevier, 1960

CRICKET FINGER

disruption of the tendon to the distal end of a finger caused by a ball striking the end of the finger

Lancet 2:958, 1968

CRICKET THIGH

rupture of a portion of the thigh muscle (rectus femoris) from stress while playing cricket

Dorland's Medical Dictionary. 25th ed. Phila.: W. B. Saunders, 1974

Crocodile Hand

redness and thickening of the skin of the hands of laborers working with chestnut wood due to a sensitivity

JAMA 100:570, 1933

Crutch Palsy

nerve compression in the armpit from improper crutch use with a resultant wrist drop

Brit. Med. J. 2:825, 1876

Cyanogen Sores

hand irritation of electroplaters from exposure to potassium carbonate used in the plating process

Ann. of Surg. 63:155, 1916

Cyclists' Neurosis

pain in the scrotum and testes of males and about the anus in females from riding on poorly fitted bicycle seats

Brit. Med. J. 1:553, 1898

Cyclist's Sore Throat

dryness and inflammation of the throat from breathing road dust while bicycling

Lancet 2:95, 1898

Cyclists' Spine

indigestion and other symptoms seen in cyclists, alleged to vibratory trauma

Lancet 2:708, 1884

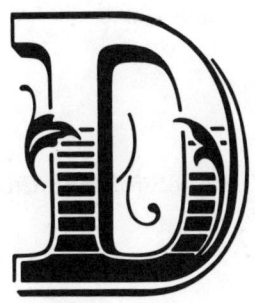

Dactylitis Discus

FRISBEE FINGER

Emerg. Med. 8:261, 1976

Dairymen's Itch

skin irritation seen among dairymen contracted from mangy cows *(Sarcoptes scabiei)*

White, R. P. The Dermatogoses or Occupational Affections of the Skin. London: H. K. Lewis, 1928

Danbury Shakes

tremor of mercury intoxication affecting felt hat workers of Danbury, Connecticut (compare HATTERS' SHAKES)

Hunter, D. The Diseases of Occupations. 5th ed. London: The English Univ. Press Ltd., 1975

Dancers' Ankle

bone spur formation in the ankle of dancers from continuous and strenuous exertion

<small>original souces not identified</small>

Dancers' Cramp

OCCUPATIONAL NEUROSIS (of ballet dancers)

<small>Brit. Med. J. 1:615, 1875</small>

Dangerous Trades

bronzing, lithography, paper staining, steam locomotive work, india rubber works, use of flammables, dry-cleaning and the aerated water trade

<small>Lancet 2:402, 1896</small>

Dashboard Dislocation

hip dislocation and/or fracture of front seat passengers involved in auto accidents

<small>Brit. Med. J. 1:903, 1938</small>

Dead Fingers

dusky discoloration of the fingers with an intolerance to cold exposure developing in workers using vibratory tools

<small>Med. Pr. 72:403, 1901</small>

Dead Hands

painful, bluish discolored hands which blanch on exposure to cold, associated with the use of vibratory tools

<small>Quart. J. Med. 5:399, 1936</small>

Deal Runner's Shoulder

bursitis over the collarbone caused by the pressure and friction of carrying timbers

> Hunter, D. The Diseases of Occupations. 5th ed. London: The English Univ. Press Ltd., 1975

Deck Ankles

swelling and aching of the ankles and feet of troop ship personnel due to unusual walking conditions

> JAMA 122:326, 1943

Deck Legs

swelling of the legs of ship passengers in tropical zones probably due to inactivity, sunburn, etc. (compare TRAVELER'S ANKLE)

> Brit. Med. J. 2:372, 1951

Decompression Sickness

joint pains, respiratory distress and central nervous system symptoms from a marked sudden decrease in barometric pressure

> Bert, P. (1878). La Pression Barometrique. Paris: Masson (tr. by Hitchcock, M. A. and F. A. Columbus, OH: College Book Co., 1943)

Degreasers' Flush

blotchy red skin in workers exposed to trichloroethylene vapors who also ingest alcohol (compare RED DISEASE)

> Arch. Environ. Hlth. 29:1, 1974

Dementia Pugilistica

degenerative brain disease of pugilists from repeated head trauma

> JAMA 210:2272, 1969

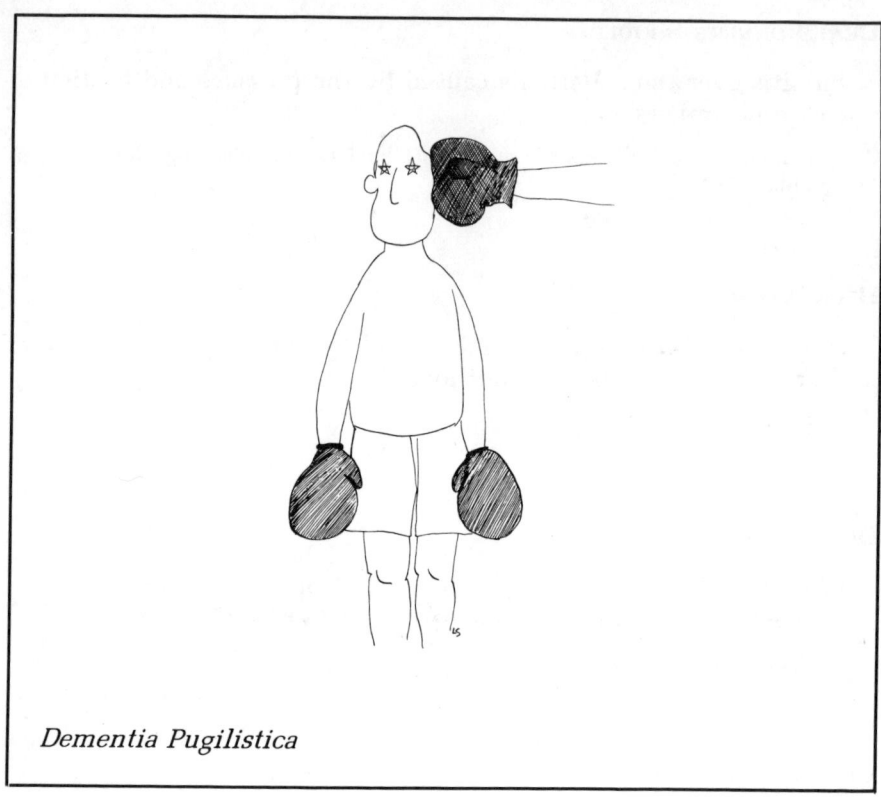

Dementia Pugilistica

DENTISTS' LEG

    leg strain and fatigue among dentists from prolonged muscular contractions in a fixed position

        Lancet 2:282, 1885

DENTIST'S NECK

    see OCCUPATIONAL NEUROSIS

        JAMA 37:934, 1901

DEPOT SORE THROAT

    malaise, fever, limb pain and sore throat incurred by navy personnel quartered in ships at harbor

        Brit. Med. J. 1:1541, 1898

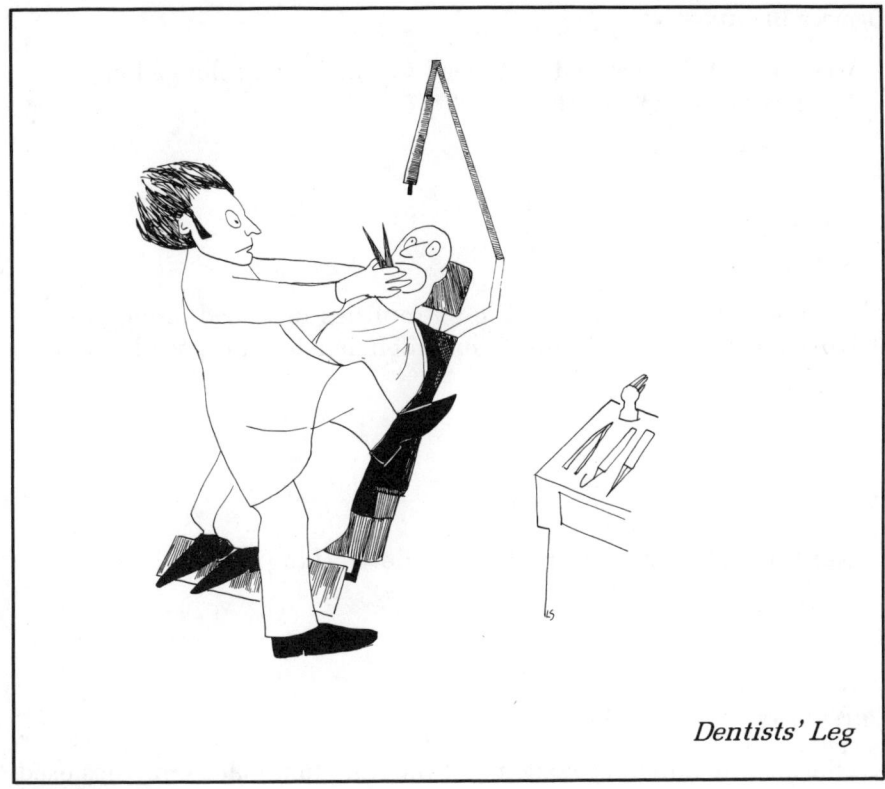

Dentists' Leg

DERBYSHIRE DROOP

impotence among Derbyshire farm workers who had been exposed to agricultural chemicals

New Sci. 72:22, 1976

DERMATOSIS INDUSTRIALIS

any occupational skin irritation

Brit. Med. J. 2:321, 1933

DESCENT SICKNESS

physiologic disturbances in pilots subjected to atmospheric pressure changes as a result of descent from altitude

Lancet 1:714, 1928

DESERT BLINDNESS

irritation of the eye and disturbed vision from prolonged exposure to ultraviolet light in the desert

Lancet 2:194, 1897

DESERT SORES

chronic skin ulceration of the extremities observed among desert troops, believed due to nutritional deficiencies and poor hygiene

Brit. Med. J. 2:96, 1942

DESK NECK

painful neck from poor posture while working over a desk

Lancet 2:1147, 1968

DETERGENT WORKER'S LUNG

allergic inflammatory response of the lung to inhaled enzymes used in detergents

Chest 61:174, 1972

DEUTSCHLANDER'S DISEASE

MARCH FRACTURE

International Classification of Diseases. 8th rev. USDHEW Pub. Hlth. Serv. Pub. No. 1963, 1968

DEVONSHIRE COLIC

lead poisoning with pronounced intestinal colic occurring in Devonshire, England, caused by the leaching of lead from pipes used for conveying cider

Med. Trans. Lond. 1:175, 1772

DHOBI ITCH

ringworm of the feet in oriental laundry workers, Dhobi is the Indian word for laundryman

Billings Nat. Med. Dict., 1890

ringworm of the arms and groin among soldiers in the tropics

Oliver, T. Dangerous Trades. London: J. Murray, 1902

DIAMOND CUTTER'S CRAMP

see OCCUPATIONAL NEUROSIS

Hunter, D. The diseases of Occupations. 5th ed. London: The English Univ. Press Ltd., 1975

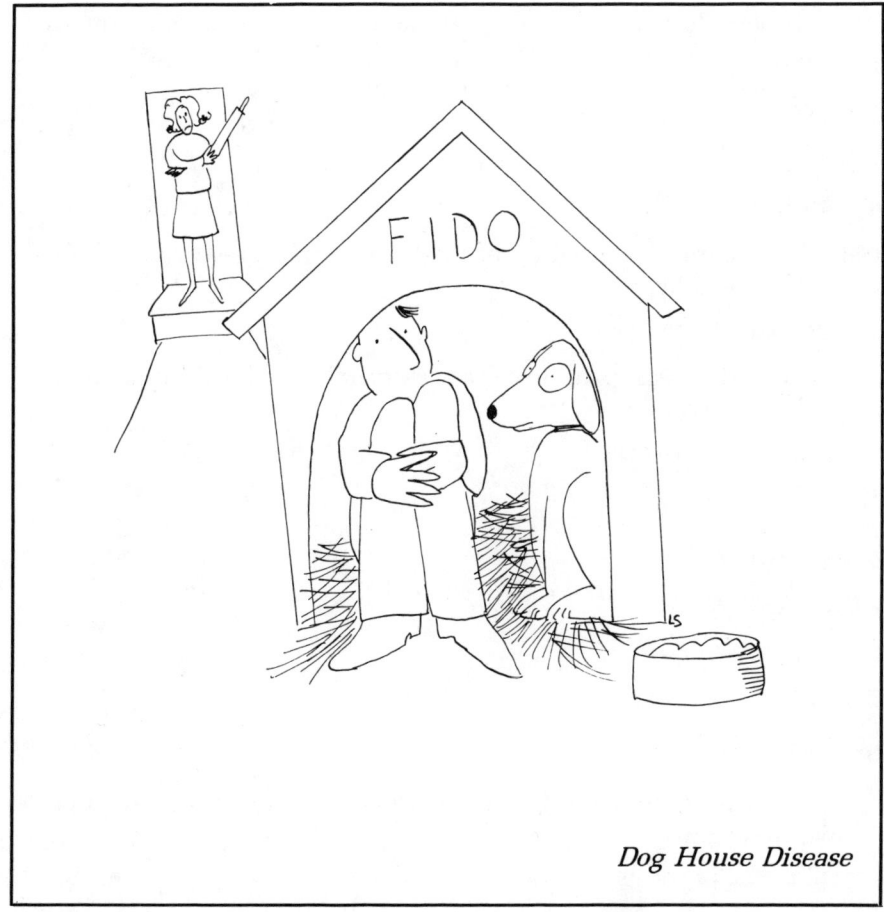

Dog House Disease

Ding String Injury

contusion or laceration of an ankle caused by the ding string (leash cord) of a surf board

N. Eng. J. Med. 295:287, 1976

Dishpan Hands

hand dermatitis from prolonged immersion in dishwater

original source not identified

Dissection Tuberculoma

skin tuberculosis incurred by pathologists and anatomists from dissecting

original source not identified

Diver's Ear

ear drum damage caused by excessive external pressure on the ear at diving depths

Brit. Med. J. 2:192, 1963

incapacitating ear pain from an external canal infection among North Sea divers

Brit. Med. J. 2:1104, 1977

Divers' Palsy

DIVERS' PARALYSIS

J. Hyg. 3:401, 1903

Divers' Paralysis

decompression sickness of divers with sensory and motor loss in the lower extremities

Brit. Med. J. 1:655, 1889

Diver's Squeeze

trauma to a diver's face when abrupt pressure changes in the helmet convert it into a "suction cup"

Occup. Med. 3:237, 1947

Divers' Vertigo

spatial disorientation in divers due to pressure changes which disturb the normal vestibular function

Emerg. Med. 10:261, 1978

Doctors' Disease

angina pectoris among doctors believed to be the result of job tension

Brit. Med. J. 1:522, 1908

Doctors' Heart Syndrome

heart disease as an occupational hazard of physicians

JAMA 88:712, 1927

Doffers' Acne

forearm eruption seen in workers who "doff" (remove) bobbins from flax spinning frames caused by contact with lubricating oils

Brit. J. Derm. 2:44, 1890

Dogger Bank Itch

skin irritation of fisherman who work the Dogger Bank of the North Sea caused by contact with the sea chervil *Alcynoidium hirsutum*

Acta Allerg. 1:40, 1948

Dog House Disease

allergic inflammatory response of the lungs to the inhalation of moldy straw particles used in dog houses

Scand. J. Resp. Dis. 52:177, 1971

Downhill Toe Jam

injury to the great toe of mountain climbers when the toe presses against the boot in going downhill

JAMA 228:24, 1974

Draft Tendon Syndrome

voluntary cutting of the flexor tendons of the index finger of the dominant hand to avoid being drafted for military service

N. Eng. J. Med. 287:549, 1972

Draper's Cramp

see OCCUPATIONAL NEUROSIS

Hunter, D. The Diseases of Occupations. 5th ed. London: The English Univ. Press Ltd., 1975

Dressmaker's Fingers

permanent contractures of the fourth and fifth fingers due to the position of the hand in sewing

Brit. Med. J. 1:637, 1879

Driver's Injury

any of the possible multiple injuries sustained by a motor vehicle operator as a result of an accident

World Wide Abst. 3(7):6, 1960

Driver's Thigh

irritation of the sciatic nerve caused by pressure from the auto seat seen in those who drive for long periods of time

Med. J. Austral. 1:265, 1932

Drummer's Cramp

see OCCUPATIONAL NEUROSIS

Singer, K. Diseases of the Musical Profession. (tr. by W. Lakond, Greensberg, N.Y., 1932)

Drummer's Neurosis

see OCCUPATIONAL NEUROSIS

Singer, K. Diseases of the Musical Profession. (tr. by W. Lakond, Greensberg, N.Y., 1932)

Drummer's Palsy

paralysis of the thumb caused by a rupture of the extensor tendon while playing a drum

JAMA 64:1138, 1915

Drummer's Thumb

rupture of the long extensor tendon from drumming

original source not identified

Drysalters' Itch

skin irritation among chemists, druggists, curers, etc. from handling numerous irritating chemicals

White, R. P. The Dermatogoses or Occupational Affections of the Skin. London: H. K. Lewis, 1928

Duck Fever

allergic inflammatory response of the lungs to the inhalation of duck proteins

Arch. des Mal. Prof. de Med. 21:67, 1960

Dustman's Bursa

swelling of the leg below the knee in men who empty dust receptacles, caused by ladder rung pressure against the leg

Brit. Med. J. 1:323, 1926

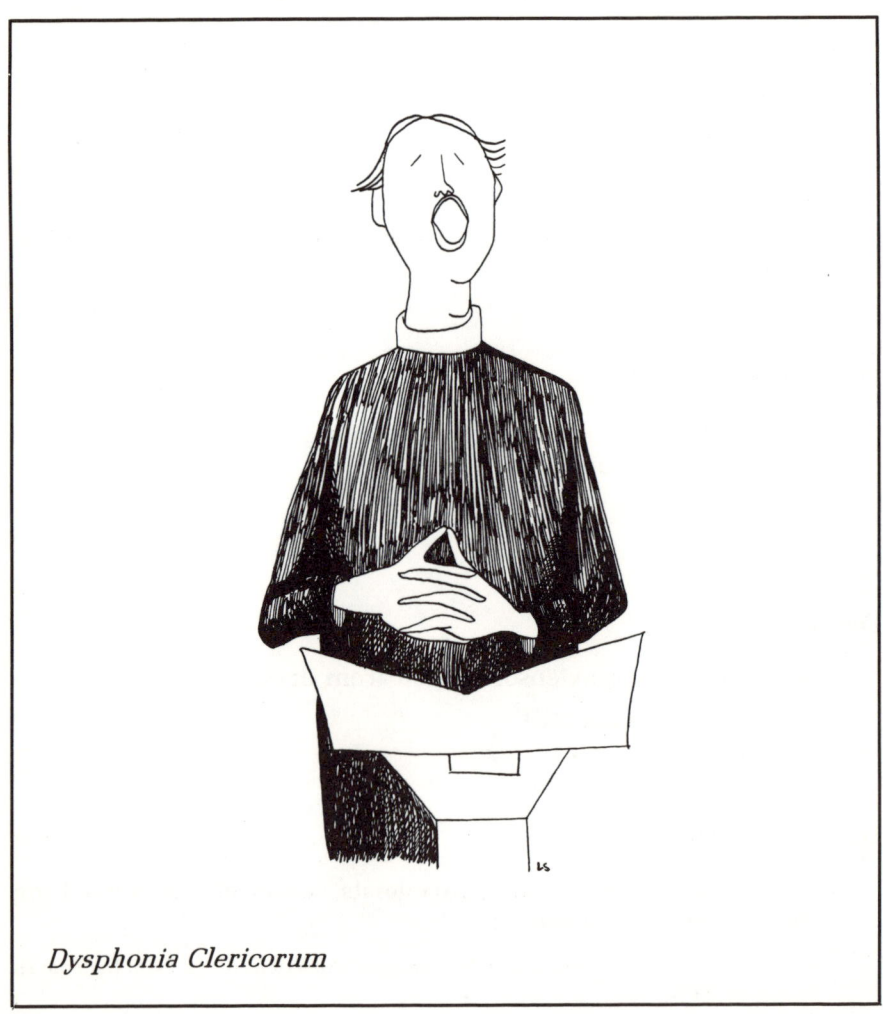

Dysphonia Clericorum

Dustman's Shoulder

swelling over the collarbone caused by pressure and friction from carrying loads of refuse and garbage

>Hunter, D. The Diseases of Occupations. 5th ed. London: The English Univ. Press Ltd., 1975

Dust Pneumonia

bronchitis and pneumonia among farmers who work in heavy concentrations of soil dust

>JAMA 153:164, 1953

Dye Workers' Cancer

bladder cancer occurring in dye workers

>Arch. Klin. Chir. 30:588, 1895

Dynamite Cephalalgia

DYNAMITE HEADACHE

>JAMA 40:1000, 1903

Dynamite Head

DYNAMITE HEADACHE

>original source not identified

Dynamite Headache

severe headache occurring among dynamite workers from the vasodilating effects of nitroglycerine

>Brit. Med. J. 2:96, 1877

DYNAMITE HEART

change in coronary blood flow to the heart in dynamite workers both during and at the cessation of exposure to nitroglycerine, with resultant cardiac symptoms

>Dorland's Medical Dictionary. 25th ed. Phila.: W. B. Saunders, 1974

DYSPHONIA CLERICORUM

CLERGYMAN'S SORE THROAT

>International Classification of Diseases. 8th rev. USDHEW Pub. Hlth. Serv. Pub. No. 1963, 1968

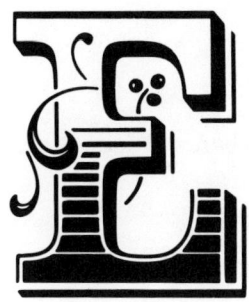

EARPHONE DERMATITIS

itching, burning, redness and swelling of the ears from sensitivity to the materials used in the manufacture of radio earphones

Arch. Derm. & Syph. 22:268, 1930

ECLIPSE BLINDNESS

loss of vision due to retinal damage caused by gazing at the sun with the naked eye

Brit. Med. J. 2:480, 1913

ECLIPSE BURNS

retinal damage to the eye from watching an eclipse

Brit. Med. J. 1:417, 1961

ECONOMY CLASS SYNDROME

venous disorders of the lower extremities as a consequence of immobility associated with air travel in the cramped economy section

Brit. Med. J. 2:1153, 1977

ECZEMA RIMOSUM

fissuring of the palm of the hands of women flax spinners caused by the use of a leather palm guard

Brit. Med. J. 2:753, 1902

EFFORT MIGRAINE

headache, visual disturbances, nausea and vomiting after strenuous physical exercise

N. Eng. J. Med. 280:1420, 1969

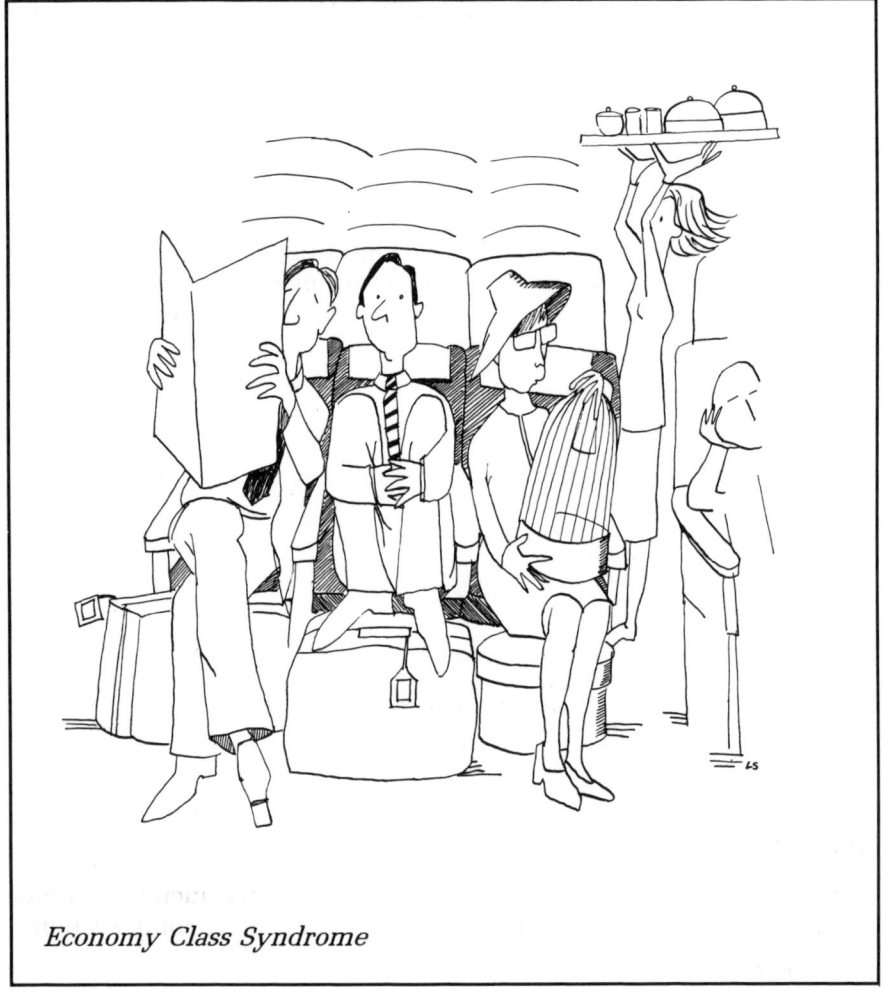

Economy Class Syndrome

Effort Syndrome

chest pain, palpitation, shortness of breath and exhaustion occurring in soldiers during WWI from numerous causes

Med. Res. Comm. Sp. Rep. Ser. No. 8, 1917

Electrical Ophthalmia

pain, tearing, light sensitivity and eyelid swelling reported to be due to working near electrical currents

Oliver, T. Dangerous Trades. London: J. Murray, 1902

Electric-Arc Welder's Eye Flash

irritation of the eye from a welder's flash characterized by pain, intolerance to light and eyelid spasm

Lancet 2:946, 1897

Electric Feet

burning and aching of the feet in malnourished prisoners of war in the Far East

Brit. Med. J. 2:260, 1946

Electric Flash Cataract

cataract following exposure of the eye to a powerful electric flash from a high voltage current

Brit. Med. J. 2:394, 1949

Electricians' Moons

balls of light seen by individuals when a current is passing through their tissues

Hunter, D. The Diseases of Occupations. 5th ed. London: The English Univ. Press Ltd., 1975

TRADE DISEASES

Electric Light Blindness

pain, tearing and eye congestion caused by exposure to ultraviolet rays generated by an electric drill

Lancet 2:194, 1897

Electric Ophthalmia

electric arc welder's conjunctivitis

U.S. Naval Med. Bull. 46:247, 1946

Electroplaters' Eczema

primary skin irritation of the hands and secondary irritation of the penis among electroplaters caused by contact with arsenical solutions

J. Cut. & Venereol. Dis. 9:294, 1891

Elevator Disease

allergic inflammatory response of the lungs of grain elevator workers caused by the grain weevil

Dorland's Medical Dictionary. 25th ed. Phila.: W. B. Saunders, 1974

Elevator "Laugh"

cough that plagues those who labor in clouds of grain dust in storage elevators

N.Y. Times 127:38, 1978

Embroiderer's Cramp

see OCCUPATIONAL NEUROSIS

Brit. Med. J. 2:165, 1890

ENAMELLER'S CRAMP

see OCCUPATIONAL NEUROSIS

> Hunter, D. The Diseases of Occupations. 5th ed. London: The English Univ. Press Ltd., 1975

ENDOSCOPIST'S EYE

herpetic eye infection contracted when effluent from an open biopsy port of an esophagoscope squirted into the operator's eye

> Gastro. Endoscopy 21:69, 1974

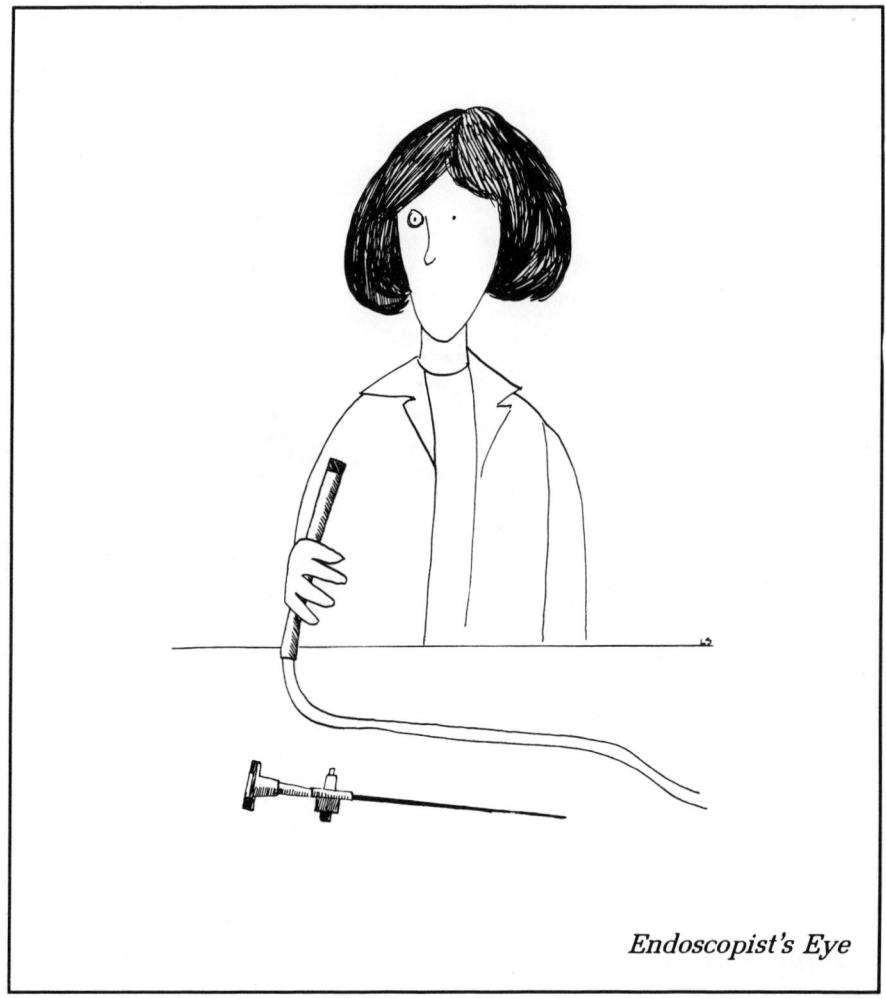

Endoscopist's Eye

Engraver's Cramp

see OCCUPATIONAL NEUROSIS

> Hunter, D. The Diseases of Occupations. 5th ed. London: The English Univ. Press Ltd., 1975

Escalator Avulsion

forceful tearing injury caused by an escalator step or comb-plate accident

> N. Eng. J. Med. 271:1310, 1964

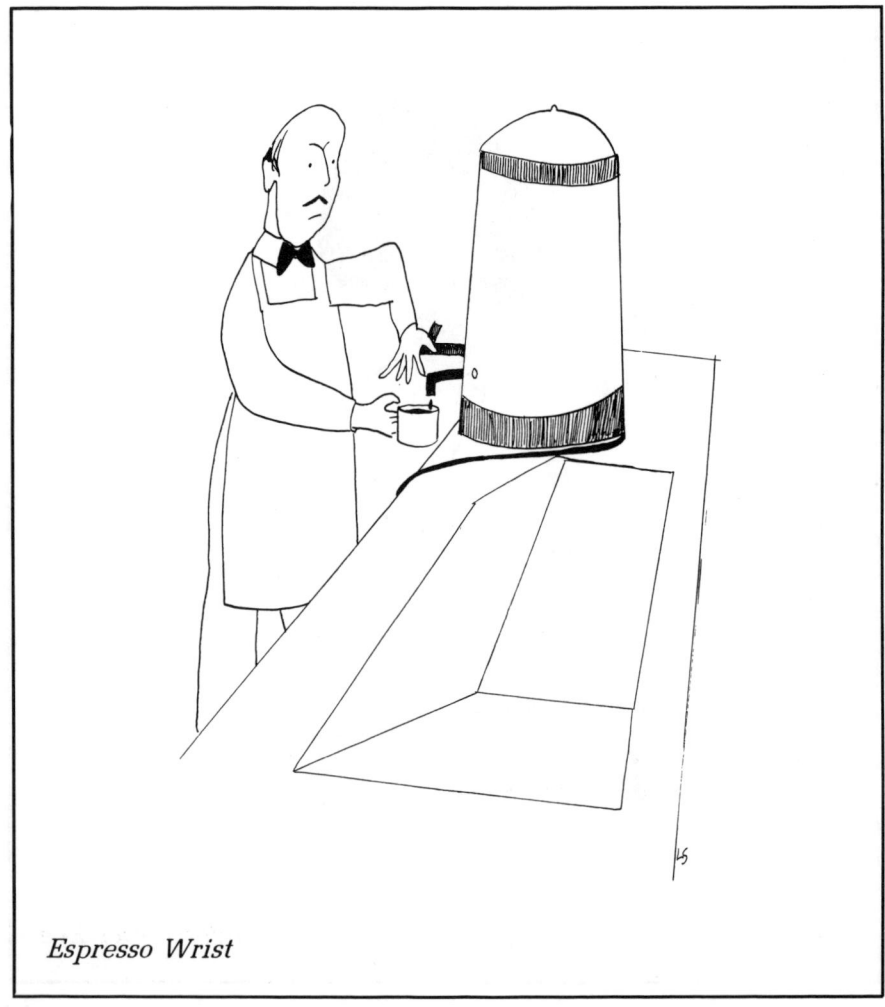

Espresso Wrist

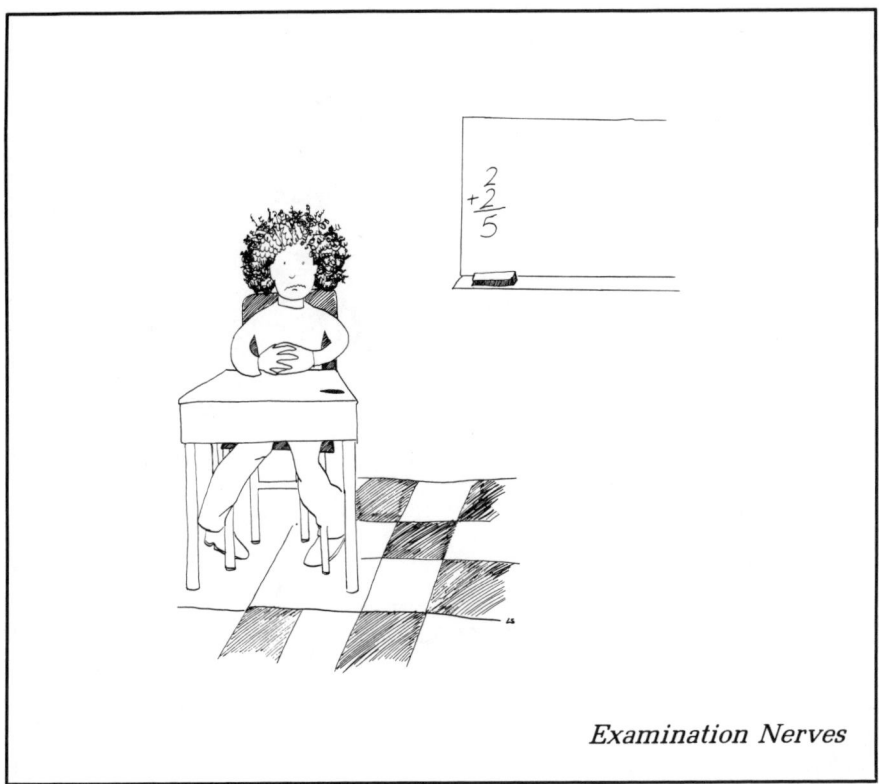

Examination Nerves

Espresso Wrist

wrist pain in espresso coffee machine operators from strong wrist motions required in making espresso coffee

JAMA 160:1532, 1956

Examination Nerves

anxiety preceeding a test or examination

Lancet 2:435, 1972

Executives' Disease

duodenal ulcers among businessmen caused by work-related tensions and frustrations

JAMA 181:31, 1962

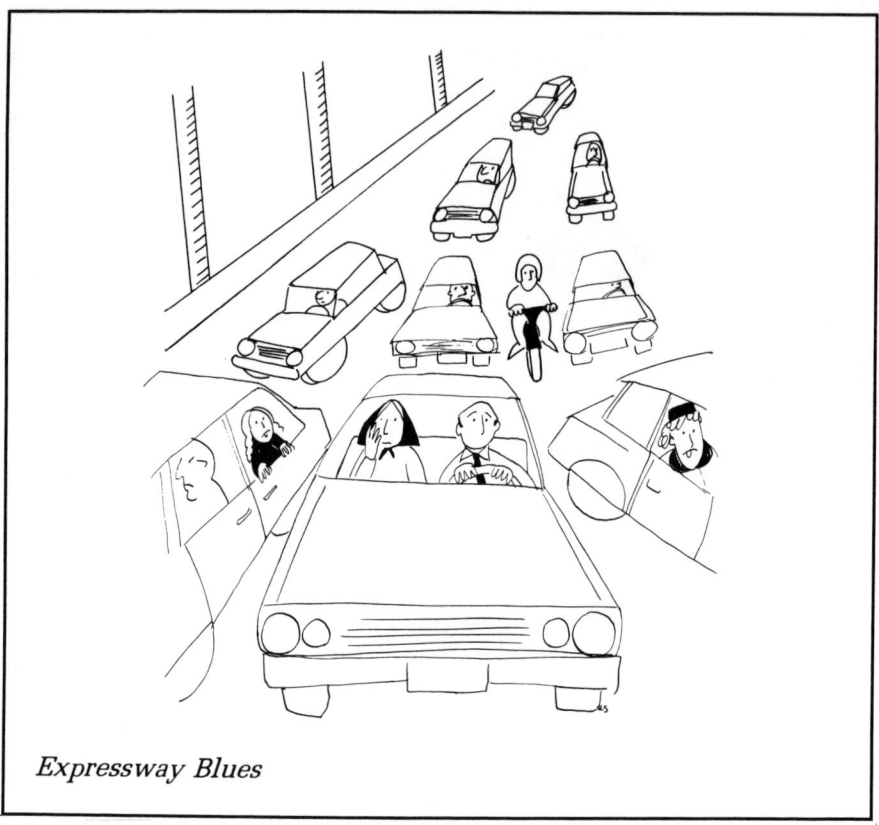

Expressway Blues

Exercise Bone
CAVALRY BONE
>Billings Nat. Med. Dict., 1890

Exercise Myoglobinuria
muscle protein in the urine after intense physical exertion
>Ann. Intern. Med. 77:77, 1972

Exertional Hemoglobinuria
red discoloration of the urine due to the excretion of hemoglobin following strenuous exercise
>Lancet 1:1136, 1965

Exhaustion Paralysis

paralysis resulting from excessive voluntary movement of a particular portion of the body to the point of failure or exhaustion

Lancet 1:573, 1889

Exhaustion Psychosis

mental disorder due to some exhausting or depressing occurrence

Dorland's Medical Dictionary. 25th ed. Phila.: W. B. Saunders, 1974

Expressway Blues

headaches noted by drivers on congested expressways attributed to exhaust fume odors and nervous tension

JAMA 185:338, 1963

Eye Flash

irritation of the eye following exposure to the ultraviolet rays from a welding arc

A Report on Electrical Accidents and Their Causes, HMSO, 1958

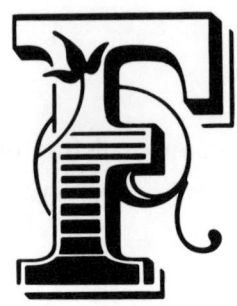

Factory Fever

typhus occurring in the overcrowded barracks used for housing child laborers in the 18th century

> Hunter, D. The Diseases of Occupations. 5th ed. London: The English Univ. Press Ltd., 1975

Byssinosis

> Brit. Med. J. 2:1069, 1948

Falling Sickness

the more than 19,000 deaths and 12 million injuries which occur in the U.S. each year due to falls

> N. Eng. J. Med. 274:107, 1966

Farmer's Lung

allergic inflammatory response of the lungs to inhaled spores *Thermoactinomyces vulgaris and Micropolyspora faeni* from moldy hay

> Brit. J. Rad. 11:378, 1938

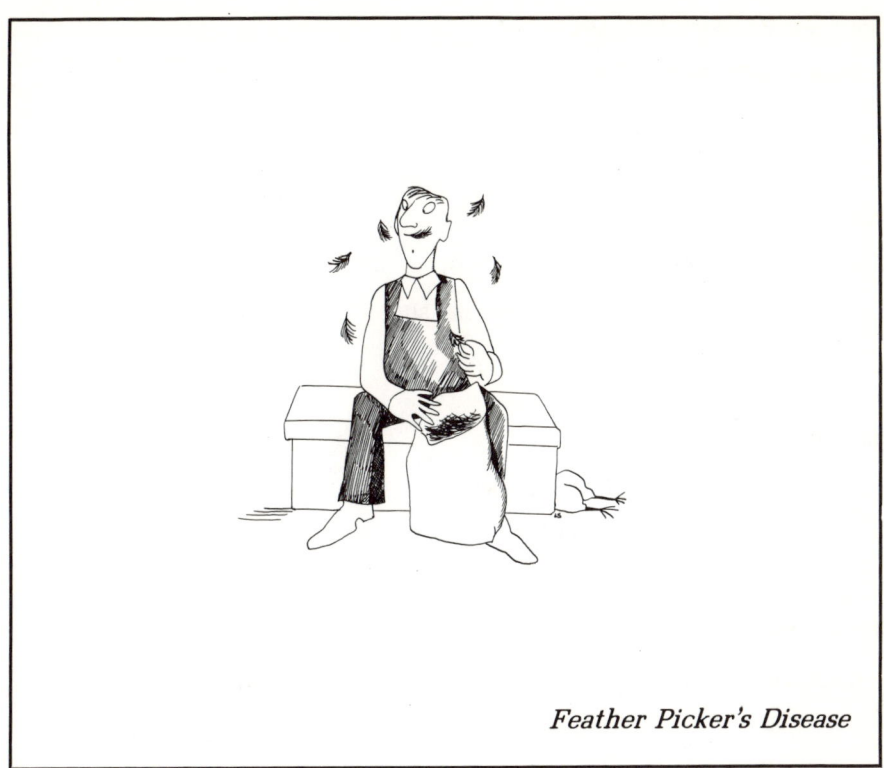

Feather Picker's Disease

Farmers' Skin

premature senility of the skin from solar radiation

JAMA 121:513, 1943

Fatigue Fracture

fracture of a bone after repeated stress (compare MARCH FRACTURE)

Stedman's Medical Dictionary. 23rd ed. Baltimore: William & Wilkins, 1976

Feather Asthma

allergic inflammatory response of the lungs to inhaled feather proteins

Thackrah, C. T. The Effects of Arts, Trades and Professions On Health and Longevity. London: Longman, 1832

FEATHER PICKER'S DISEASE
FEATHER ASTHMA
>Arch. Med. Prof. 21:67, 1959

FENCER'S CRAMP
see OCCUPATIONAL NEUROSIS
>Hunter, D. The Diseases of Occupations. 5th ed. London: The English Univ. Press Ltd., 1975

FENCER'S PUBIALGIA
strain of the inner thigh muscles
>original source not identified

FENDER FRACTURE
fracture of the leg as a result of an auto fender impact
>N. Eng. J. Med. 201:989, 1929

FERROALLOY WORKERS' DISEASE
chronic pulmonary disease in employees exposed to ferroalloy smelting fumes
>Centr. Afr. J. Med. 21:67, 1975

FERTILIZER SORES
skin irritation of the legs of rice field workers from fertilizer contact
>A Barefoot Doctor's Manual. U.S. Dept. HEW Pub. No. (NIH) 75–695, 1974

FIGHT-FOR-COMPENSATION NEUROSIS
any nervous system disorder precipitated by trauma (compare LITIGATION NEUROSIS)
>Vischer, A. L. Barbed Wire Disease. John Bale. London, 1919

FILE CUTTER'S DISEASE

lead intoxication incurred in the process of cutting files which are embedded in lead

> Brit. Med. J. 1:385, 1857

FILE CUTTERS' PARALYSIS

paralysis of the wrist and other muscles of file cutters who suffer from lead poisoning

> Hunter, D. The Diseases of Occupations. 5th ed. London: The English Univ. Press Ltd., 1975

FILE CUTTER'S PHTHISIS

PULMONARY SIDEROSIS (iron dust)

> Stedman's Medical Dictionary. 23rd ed. Baltimore: William & Wilkins, 1976

FIREBALL BLINDNESS

retinal eye damage resulting from viewing the fireball of an atomic bomb explosion

> JAMA 180:798, 1962

FIRE-EATER'S ASBESTOSIS

pulmonary asbestosis following the use of an asbestos torch in a carnival fire-eating act

> JAMA 229:23, 1974

FIREMEN'S CATARACT

cataract in those who fire pottery kilns resulting from prolonged exposure to infrared radiation

> Hunter, D. The Diseases of Occupations. 5th ed. London: The English Univ. Press Ltd., 1975

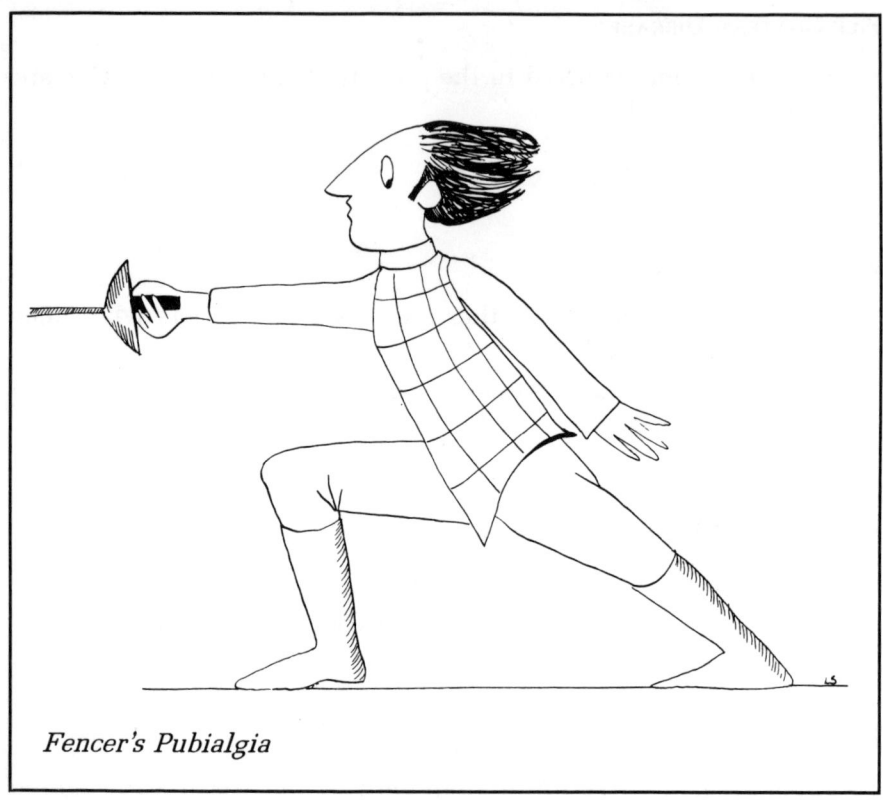

Fencer's Pubialgia

Firemen's Cramps

heat exhaustion among stokers

Proc. R. Soc. B. 95:181, 1923

Firemen's Eye

FIREMEN'S CATARACT

Hunter, D. The Diseases of Occupations. 5th ed. London: The English Univ. Press Ltd., 1975

Firemen's Frenzy

heat exhaustion among navy boiler stokers attributed to heat exposure and poor ventilation

Oliver, T. Dangerous Trades. London: J. Murray, 1902

Firemen's Lung

loss of pulmonary function in fire fighters due to chronic smoke inhalation

Lancet 1:439, 1975

Fireworks Blindness

severe eye injury resulting from accidents with fireworks

J. Ark. Med. Soc. 72:357, 1976

Fishbone Furunculosis

small boils on the fingers of fishermen following minor injuries, believed due to a staphylococcus infection

Brit. Med. J. 2:797, 1958

Fishermen's Sore

lip cancer among fishermen caused by holding a tar contaminated wooden shuttle (needle) in the mouth while repairing nets

JAMA 104:2326, 1935

Fish Filleters' Wart

viral infection of the skin among fish handlers

original source not identified

Fish Handlers' Disease

finger redness and pain in fish cannery workers caused by infection with *Erysipelothrix rhusiopathiae* (compare SEALERS' FINGER)

Arch. Derm. 14:662, 1926

Fish Porter's Bursitis

swelling over the lower neck or upper back from carrying boxes of fish

> Hunter, D. The Diseases of Occupations. 5th ed. London: The English Univ. Press Ltd., 1975

Fish Slime Disease

FISH HANDLERS' DISEASE

> Arch. Derm. 14:662, 1926

Fish Tank Granuloma

hard red nodules on the hands of fish handlers caused by *Mycobacterium marinum*

> Brit. J. Derm. 91:709, 1974

Flash Blindness

temporary loss of vision following exposure to an intense electric arc

> Hunter, D. The Diseases of Occupations. 5th ed. London: The English Univ. Press Ltd., 1975

Flash Burn

the combination of a flame burn from an arc and an electrical shock from the current

> ILO Encyclopedia of Occupational Health and Safety. NY.: McGraw Hill, 1972

Flautist's Cramp

see OCCUPATIONAL NEUROSIS

> Brit. Med. J. 1:88, 1878

Flax Dressers' Disease

shortness of breath, emaciation, noisy respiration and productive cough from prolonged exposure to flax dust

> Thackrah, C. T. The Effects of Arts, Trades and Professions On Health and Longevity. London: Longman, 1832

Flax Dressers' Phthisis

FLAX DRESSERS' DISEASE

> Stedman's Medical Dictionary. 23rd ed. Baltimore: William & Wilkins, 1976

Flax Dust Byssinosis

FLAX DRESSERS' DISEASE

> Ulster Med. J. 28:164, 1959

Flax Fever

FLAX DRESSERS' DISEASE

> Arlidge, J. T. The Hygiene, Diseases and Mortality of Occupations. London: Percival, 1892

Flax Soakers' Eczema

dermatitis of the thumb and index finger of workers who cleanse flax in water contaminated with irritating materials

> Brit. J. Derm. 1:140, 1889

Flax Workers' Eczema

skin irritation of the lower extremities of flax workers due to contact with oils used on the spinning mills

> Brit. J. Derm. 2:15, 1890

Flax Workers' Phthisis

FLAX DRESSERS' DISEASE

Brit. Med. J. 1:1097, 1894

Flicker Vertigo

dizziness produced by the rhythmic visual stimuli of rotating helicopter propellers

JAMA 170:959, 1959

Flight Blindness

visual disturbances arising from the centrifugal forces encountered in aviation

Dorland's Medical Dictionary. 25th ed. Phila.: W. B. Saunders, 1974

Flip-Flop Dermatitis

symmetrical dermatitis over the tops of the feet caused by wearing rubber "flip-flop" shoes

Brit. Med. J. 2:1431, 1965

Flock Fever

chest soreness, chills, shortness of breath and cough from the inhalation of cotton dust in the manufacture of "flock" for fabrics and wallpaper

Arlidge, J. T. The Hygiene, Diseases And Mortality of Occupations. London: Percival, 1892

Florist's Cramp

see OCCUPATIONAL NEUROSIS

Hunter, D. The Diseases of Occupations. 5th ed. London: The English Univ. Press Ltd., 1975

Flower Pickers' Dermatitis

skin irritation from working with lilies, daffodils, and narcissus

Stedman's Medical Dictionary. 23rd ed. Baltimore: William & Wilkins, 1976

Flute Player's Cramp

see OCCUPATIONAL NEUROSIS

Singer, K. Diseases of the Musical Profession. (tr. by W. Lakond, Greensberg, N.Y., 1932)

Flutter Board Dermatitis

itchy skin lesions resulting from contact with plastic flutter boards used in swimming pools

Arch. Derm. 95:667, 1967

Flying Sickness

motion sickness associated with flying

original source not identified

Flying Strain

difficulty in breathing, palpitation, headache, dizziness and weakness noted in WWI pilots and attributed to the tensions of flying and fighting

Lancet 1:714, 1928

Flying Stress

functional nervous disorders among WWII airmen

Brit. Med. J. 2:703, 1943

FOOTBALLERS' ANKLE

traumatic changes in the ankles of professional football players

Geneesk. Sport 8:37, 1975

FOOTBALLERS' FOOT

traumatic changes in the feet of professional football players

Geneesk. Sport 8:37, 1975

FOOTBALLERS' MIGRAINE

severe headache with visual field defects following head injury

Brit. Med. J. 2:326, 1972

FOOTBALL GOALKEEPER'S ELBOW

bone changes about the elbow related to game trauma

Lyon Medit. Med. 12:2093, 1976

FOOTBALL IMPETIGO

skin affection involving the face, ears and neck of football players believed to be a contagious disorder (compare SCRUMPOX)

Brit. Med. J. 1:38, 1895

FOOTBALL KEEPER'S THUMB

degenerative bone disease of the thumb following injury

J. Sports. Med. 16(2):121, 1976

FOOTBALL KNEE

damage to the knee cartilage as a result of injury in the game

Geneesk. Sport 8:21, 1975

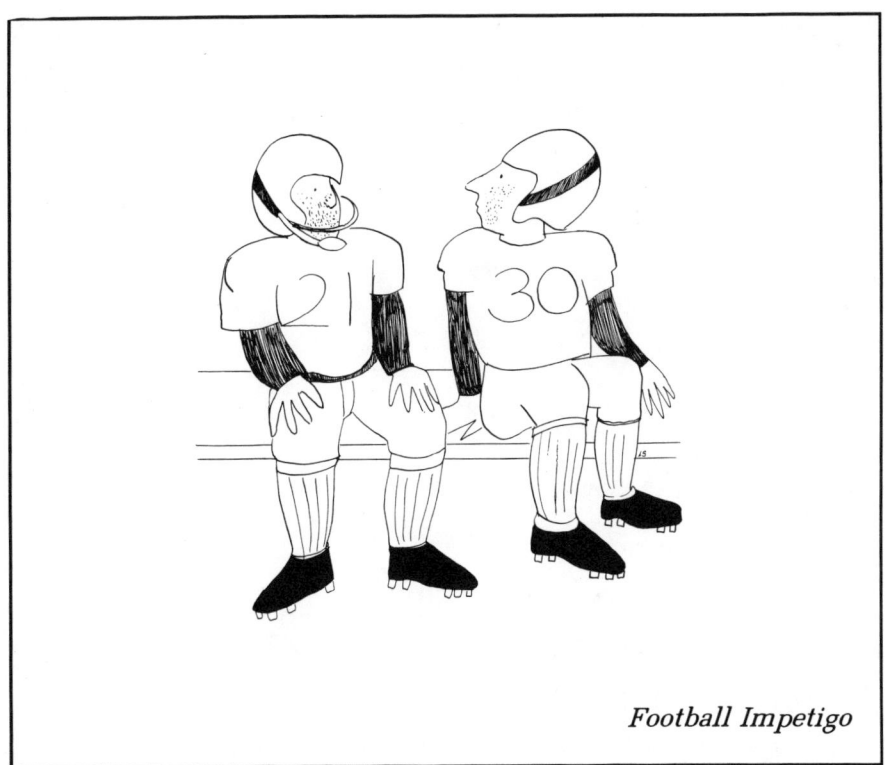

Football Impetigo

FOOT-SLOGGER'S NODULE

painful swelling over a tendon corresponding to a boot pressure point seen in military marching units

<small>Brit. Med. J. 1:193, 1945</small>

FORGE HAMMER WORKERS' CRAMPS

heat cramps among forge hammer operators

<small>Hunter, D. The Disease of Occupations. 5th ed. London: The English Univ. Press Ltd., 1975</small>

FOUNDERS' COLIC

lead colic occurring in metal casters

<small>Dana, S. L. Lead Diseases: A Treatise from the French of L. Tanquerel des Planches. Boston: Tappan, 1850</small>

FOUNDRY AGUE

headache, chills, fever, cough and sweating in foundry workers caused by the inhalation of metal fumes

Ann. Hyg. 34:222, 1845

FOUNDRY CHILLS

FOUNDRY AGUE

original source not identified

FOUNDRY FEVER

FOUNDRY AGUE

Med. Klin. 23:91, 1927

FOUNDRYMAN'S FEVER

FOUNDRY AGUE

Dorland's Medical Dictionary. 25th ed. Phila.: W. B. Saunders, 1974

FOUNDRY SHAKES

FOUNDRY AGUE

original source not identified

FOUNDRY WORKER'S CRAMPS

Heat cramps

Hunter, D. The Diseases of Occupations. 5th ed. London: The English Univ. Press Ltd., 1975

FOUNDRY WORKER'S PNEUMOCONIOSIS

deposition of iron dust in the lungs

Ind. Hyg. & Occup. Med. 10:512, 1954

Foundry Zinc Chills

FOUNDRY AGUE

Hunter, D. The Diseases of Occupations. 5th ed. London: The English Univ. Press Ltd., 1975

Fourth of July Tetanus

tetanus infection following wounds produced by fireworks and blank-pistol cartridges

Lancet 2:386, 1904

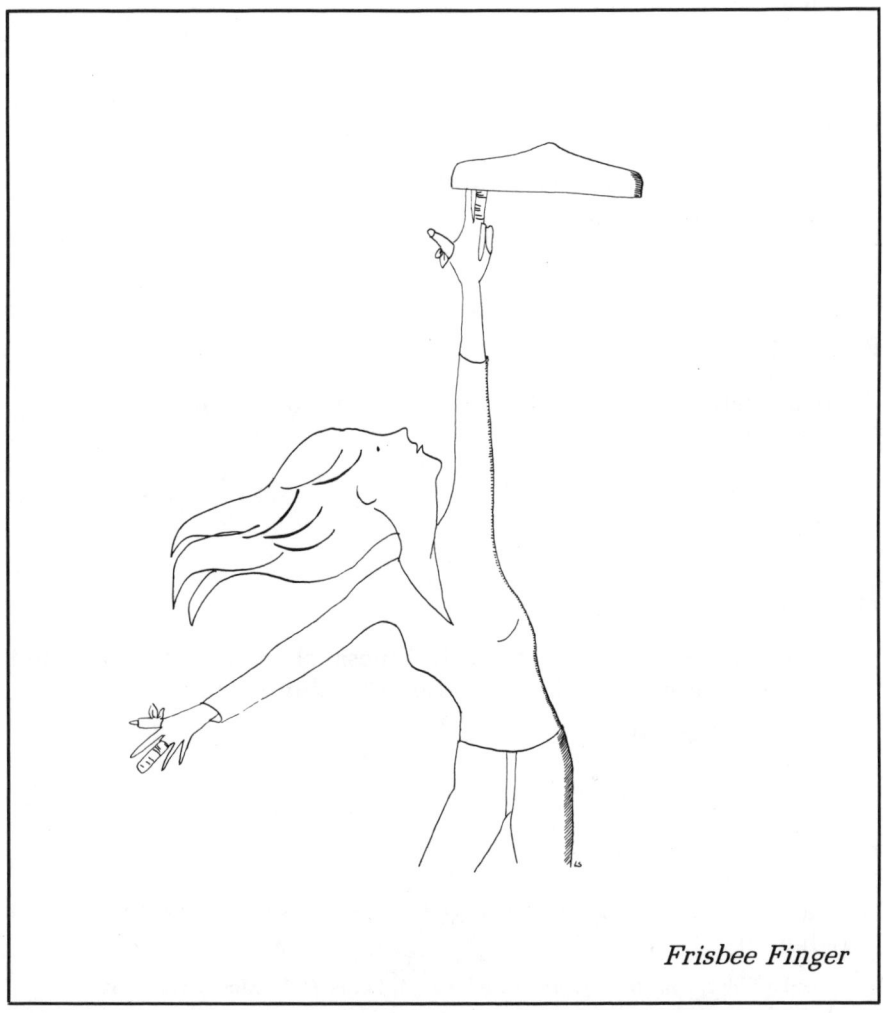

Frisbee Finger

French Millstone Maker's Lung

silicosis from the inhalation of dust while grinding and shaping millstones

Lancet 1:788, 1878

French Millstone Maker's Phthisis

FRENCH MILLSTONE MAKER'S LUNG

Brit. Med. J. 1:80, 1868

Frisbee Finger

abrasion of the finger from throwing a Frisbee disc

N. Eng. J. Med. 293:304, 1975

Frozen Meat Impetigo

inflammation of the hands of butchers and meat handlers working with frozen meats

Brit. Med. J. 1:307, 1894

Fume Fever

nausea, abdominal pain, chest tightness, shortness of breath and prostration following the inhalation of cadmium fumes

JAMA 125:229, 1944

Furnaceman's Cataract

cataract resulting from prolonged exposure of the eye to infrared radiation

Duke-Elder, System of Ophthalmology. St. Louis: C. V. Mosby Co., 1954

Furnaceman's Cramps

heat cramps

> Hunter, D. The Diseases of Occupations. 5th ed. London: The English Univ. Press Ltd., 1975

Furnace Workers' Cataract

cataract occurring among iron workers exposed to infrared radiation

> Brit. Med. J. 1:290, 1915

Furniture Polisher's Eczema

finger and knuckle irritation caused by pyridine used to denature wood alcohol

> White, R. P. The Dermatogoses or Occupational Affections of the Skin. London: H. K. Lewis, 1928

Furrier's Lung

allergic inflammatory response of the lungs to hair particles inhaled in the processing of furs

> Thorax 25:387, 1970

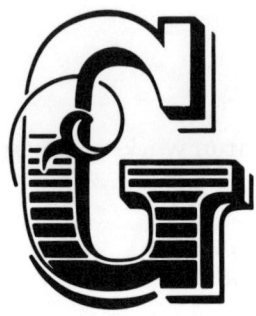

Gaiter Pain

leg pain in infantrymen associated with wearing leather gaiters

Brit. Med. J. 1:108, 1916

Galvanizers' Eczema

nickel sensitivity of the skin among metal platers sometimes associated with inflammation of the mouth and gums

Deutsche Med. Woch. 45, 1889

Galvanizer's Poisoning

metal fume fever from the inhalation of zinc fumes generated in the galvanizing process

original source not identified

Galvo

GALVANIZER'S POISONING

Brit. J. Ind. Med. 1:72, 1944

Gamekeepers' Thumb

ligament injury to the thumb of gamekeepers sustained while wringing rabbit necks

J. Bone & Joint Surg. 37B:148, 1955

Ganister Miner's Disease

pulmonary silicosis from mining ganister, a close grained mineral consisting of 95% silica

Brit. Med. J. 2:768, 1902

Gaol Distemper

GAOL FEVER

Lancet 2:705, 1894

Gaol Fever

typhus fever among prisoners and prison personnel transmitted via lice infestation

Lancet 2:705, 1894

Gardeners' Mycosis

any occupational fungus infection occurring among those who work in gardens

Derm. Vener. (Buc) 15:413, 1970

Gas Eye

irritation of the eye from hydrogen sulfide fumes occurring in artificial-silk factory workers

original source not identified

GAS EYES

itching, burning and redness of the eyes among petroleum workers caused by exposure to hydrogen sulfide fumes

Am. J. Pub. Hlth. 20:598, 1930

GAS WORKERS' EPITHELIOMA

warty growths on the hands and forearms of workers making grease from coal residue

Lancet 2:556, 1908

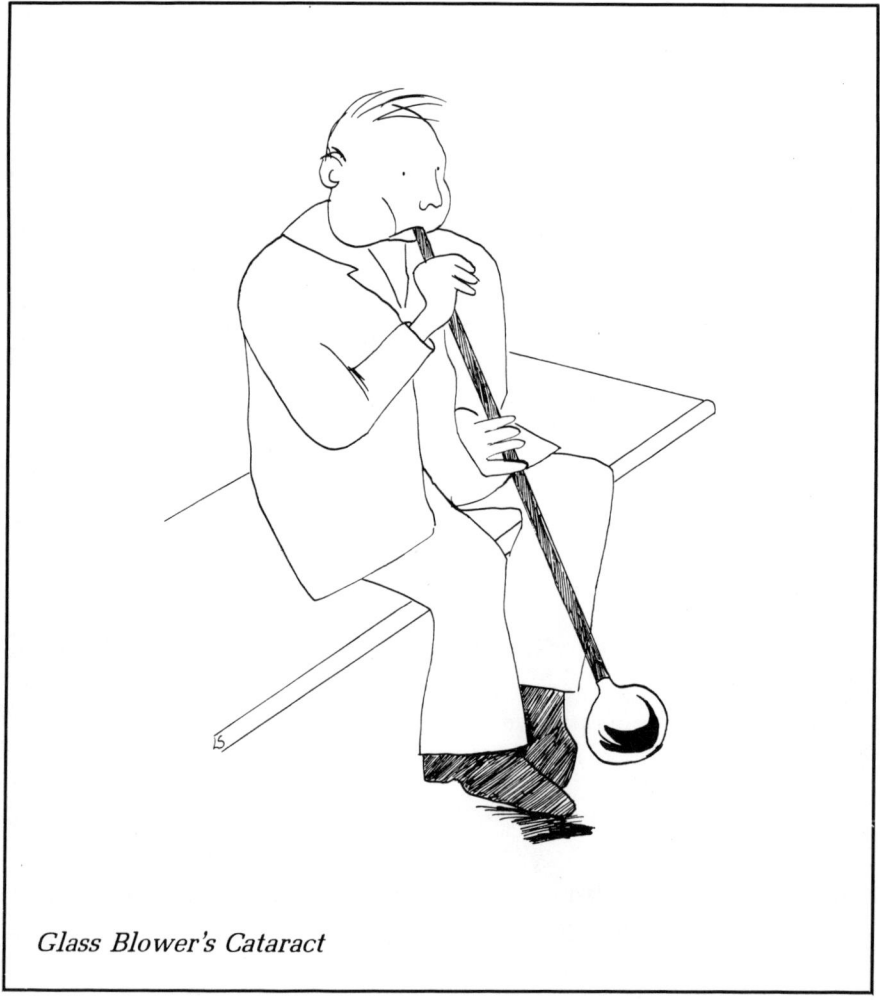

Glass Blower's Cataract

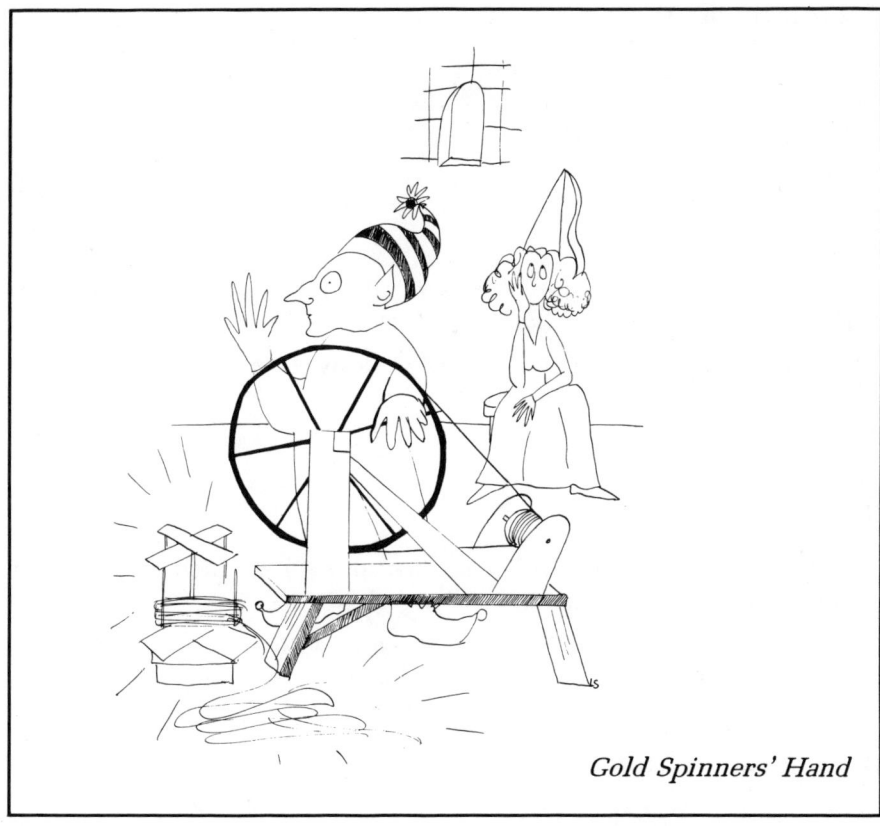
Gold Spinners' Hand

GERBIL KEEPER'S LUNG

allergic inflammatory response of the lungs to inhaled gerbil dander

Med. News 1(7), 16 May, 1977

GLASS BLOWER'S CATARACT

cataract resulting from infrared radiation from the glass furnace

Klin. Monatsbl. Augen. 24:49, 1886

GLASS BLOWERS' CRAMP

permanent flexion deformities of the fingers of glass blowers associated with a special blowpipe handhold

Lancet 1:787, 1888

Glass Blower's Disease

GLASS BLOWER'S CATARACT
original source not identified

Glass Blower's Emphysema

permanent overdistension of the air cells of the lung from the respiratory effort required in blowing glass

Arlidge, J. T. The Hygiene, Diseases And Mortality of Occupations. London: Percival, 1892

Glass Blower's Mouth

swelling of the cheeks (like mumps) due to air distention of the parotid gland as a result of blowing glass

Oliver, T. Dangerous Trades. London: J. Murray, 1902

Glass Blower's Tumor

GLASS BLOWER'S MOUTH

Deutsche Zeit. für Chir. 119:201, 1912

Glass Workers' Cataract

cataract among glass workers exposed to intense heat and light at the furnace

Brit. Med. J. 1:28, 1909

Glass Workers' Cramps

heat cramps

Hunter, D. The Diseases of Occupations. 5th ed. London: The English Univ. Press Ltd., 1975

Gold Beater's Cramp

see OCCUPATIONAL NEUROSIS

Lancet 2:328, 1890

Gold Dust Complaint

GOLD MINER'S DISEASE

Lancet 1:1678, 1902

Gold Miner's Disease

pulmonary fibrosis associated with cough, shortness of breath, tightness of chest, loss of appetite and emaciation

Lancet 1:1677, 1902

Gold Miner's Phthisis

GOLD MINER'S DISEASE

Lancet 1:1677, 1902

Gold Smelter's Cataract

cataract resulting from prolonged exposure of the eye to infrared radiation

Hunter, D. The Diseases of Occupations. 5th ed. London: The English Univ. Press Ltd., 1975

Gold Spinners' Hand

green-blue tattooing of the hands caused by penetrating small fragments of gold thread and an associated tendon inflammation occurring in workers making gold braid

Brit. J. Clin. Pract. 25:147, 1971

Golf Arm

shoulder and elbow pain with altered sensation in the thumb and index finger after prolonged golf rounds

Brit. Med. J. 1:377, 1896

Golf Back

back injury sustained when an established habitual movement is not executed properly

Lancet 1:348, 1953

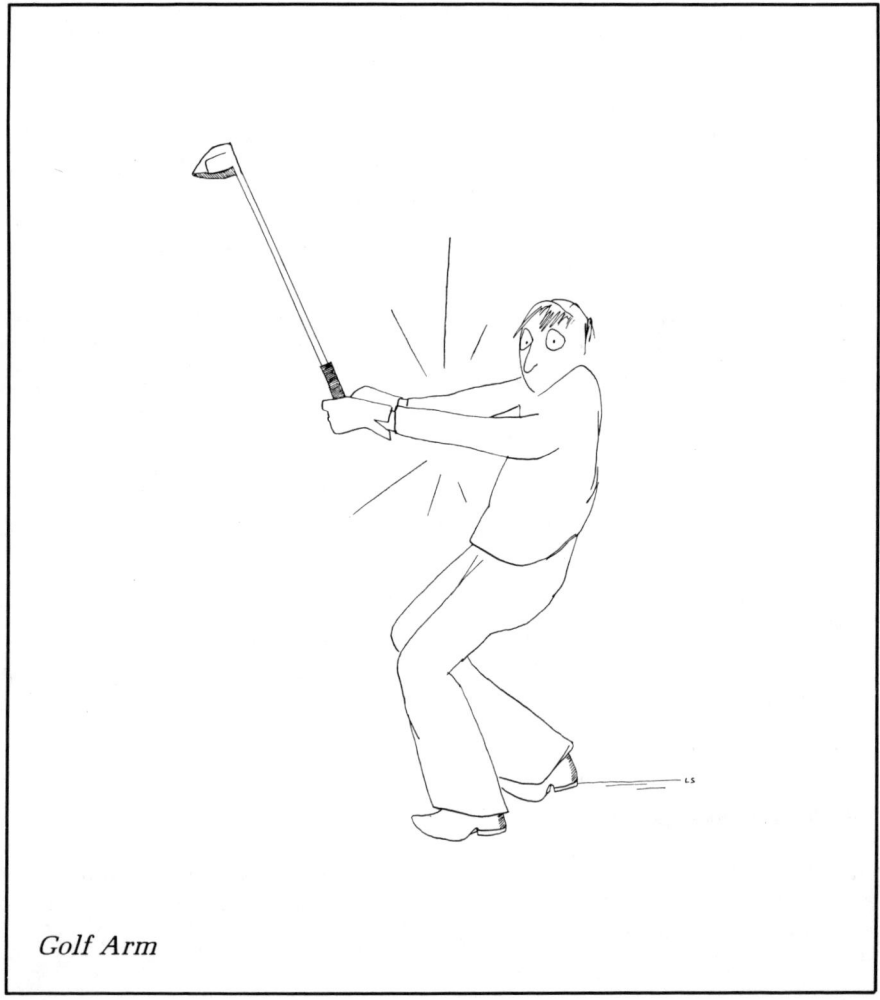

Golf Arm

Golf Course Dermatitis

skin irritation from contact with a fungicide spray (Thiram) used on the course

JAMA 188:415, 1964

Golf Elbow

pain at the outer aspect of the elbow among golfers, similar to TENNIS ELBOW

Brit. Med. J. 2:177, 1950

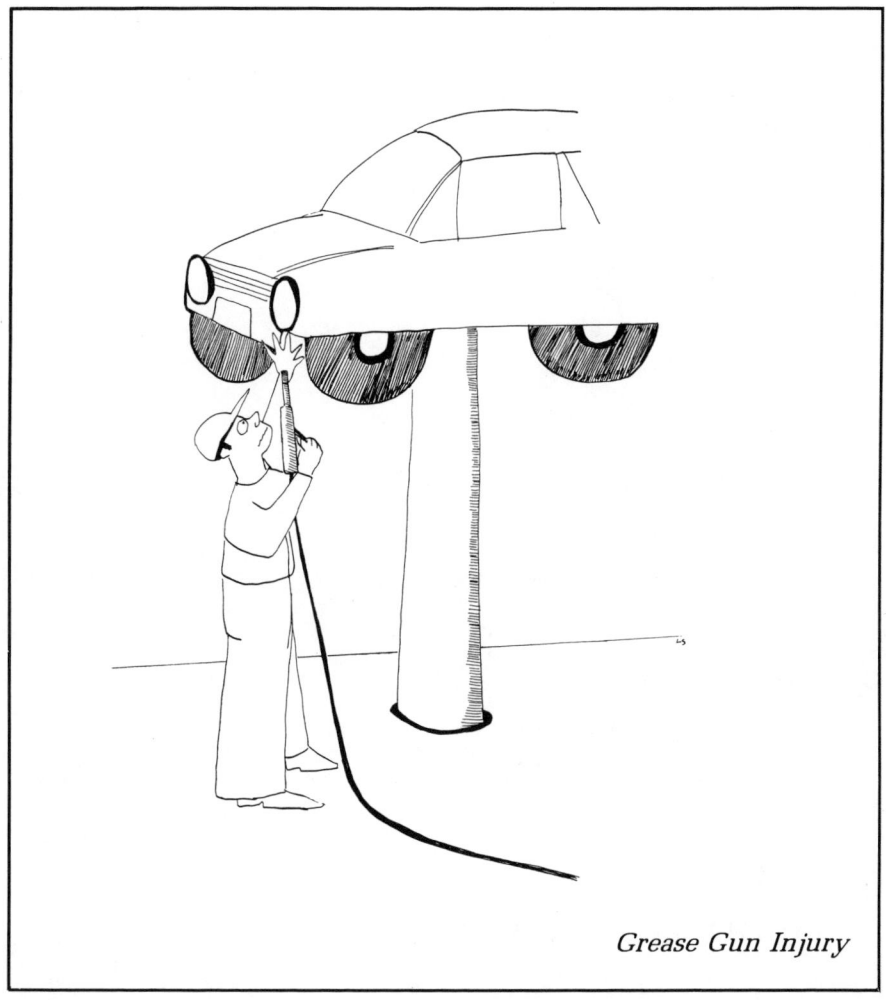

Grease Gun Injury

Golfers' Elbow

GOLF ELBOW

Brit. Med. J. 1:362, 1930

Golfer's Foot

foot pain from undue strain

Med. Rec. 89:896, 1916

Golfer's Wrist

fracture of a hand bone sustained when the hand is impinged forcefully by the end of the golf club

Brit. Med. J. 2:1622, 1977

Golf Shoulder

bursitis of the shoulder

original source not identified

Grain Handler's Asthma

allergic inflammatory response of the lungs to inhaled grain dust

original source not identified

Grain Handler's Pneumoconiosis

GRAIN HANDLER'S ASTHMA

Zenz, C. Occupational Medicine. Chicago: Yearbook Pub., 1975

Grain Porter's Fever

GRAIN HANDLER'S ASTHMA

original source not identified

Grain Threshing Catarrh

THRESHER'S LUNG

JAMA 110:1696, 1938

Granite Cutter's Ring

a callus over the top of the little finger caused by pressure from the chisel

Ind. Med. & Surg. 24:546, 1955

Granite Mason's Phthisis

GRANITE WORKER'S LUNG

Lancet 2:234, 1876

Granite Worker's Lung

chronic pulmonary disease caused by the inhalation of silica dust

International Classification of Diseases. 8th rev. USDHEW Pub. Hlth. Serv. Pub. No. 1963, 1968

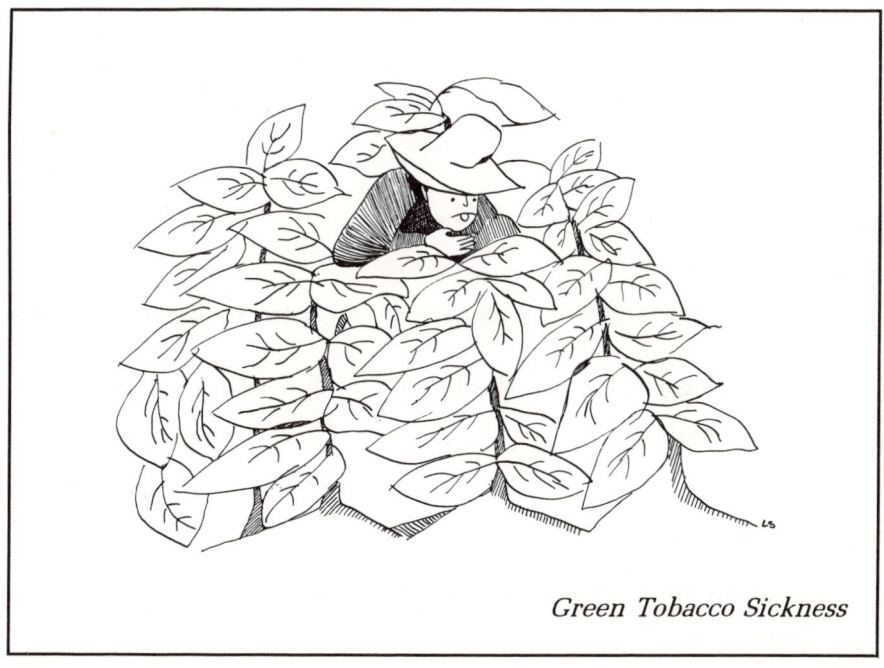

Green Tobacco Sickness

TRADE DISEASES

Grease Gun Finger

perforation of a finger (usually the index) by grease ejected from a high pressure gun nozzle

JAMA 112:907, 1939

Grease Gun Injury

accidental injection of grease beneath the skin by a grease gun (compare PRESSURE GUN INJECTION)

JAMA 125:405, 1944

Green Tobacco Sickness

headache, pallor, nausea, vomiting and prostration among workers handling uncured tobacco leaves in the field

JAMA 229:1880, 1974

Grenade Thrower's Fracture

fracture of the arm from excess exertion in tossing grenades

Dorland's Medical Dictionary. 25th ed. Phila.: W. B. Saunders, 1974

Grinders' Asthma

BYSSINOSIS

Hunter, D. The Diseases of Occupations. 5th ed. London: The English Univ. Press Ltd., 1975

deposition of iron dust in the lungs while grinding cutlery

Lancet 2:731, 1829

Grinders' Complaint

silicotuberculosis among tableware grinders

Lancet 2:408, 1841

Grinders' Consumption
GRINDERS' COMPLAINT
Bost. Med. & Surg. J. 117:198, 1887

Grinder's Dermatitis
skin irritation from contact with the lubricant sprays used in metal grinding
Ind. Hyg. Digest 11:5, 1947

Grinder's Disease
fibrotic lung disease encountered in any of the metal grinding trades
Lancet 2:234, 1876

Grinders' Lung
silicosis (compare GRINDER'S DISEASE)
International Classification of Diseases. 8th rev. USDHEW Pub. Hlth. Serv. Pub. No. 1963, 1968

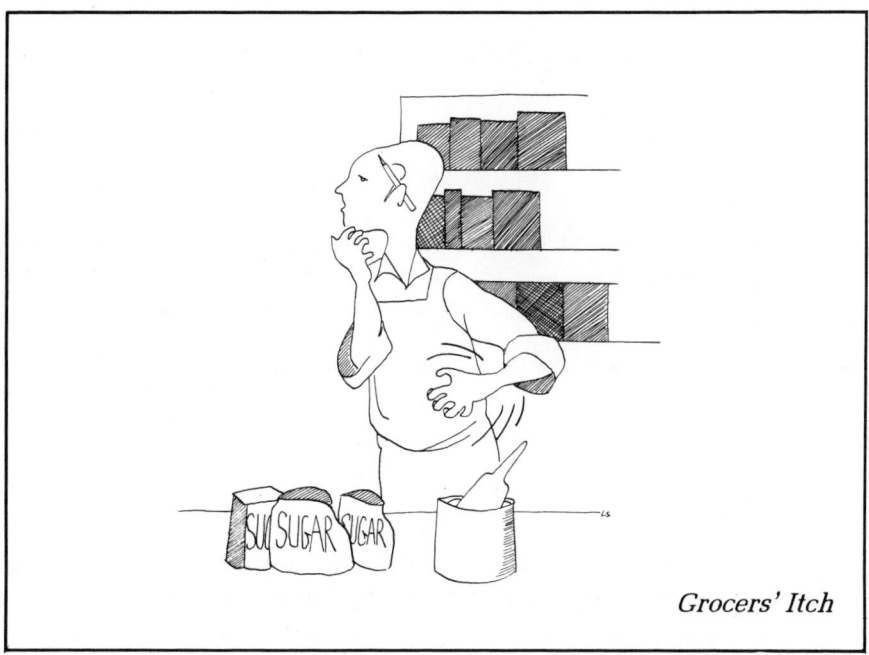

Grocers' Itch

Grinders' Phthisis

chronic bronchitis associated with cough, shortness of breath and cyanosis occurring among metal grinders

> Oliver, T. Dangerous Trades. London: J. Murray, 1902

Grinders' Rot

cough, bloody sputum, weakness, debility and heart failure among cutlers

> Brit. Med. J. 1:79, 1868

Grinders' Silicosis

silicosis in metal grinders

> Hare Juah 81:326, 1971

Grinders' Tuberculosis

silicotuberculosis

> International Classification of Diseases. 8th rev. USDHEW Pub. Hlth. Serv. Pub. No. 1963, 1968

Grocers' Itch

skin irritation caused by fruit and grain mite infestation *Glycyphagus domesticus*

> N. Eng. J. Med. 261:396, 1959

dermatitis of grocers' hands caused by prolonged contact with sugar

> Lancet 2:538, 1842

Grocery Bag Neuropathy

altered sensation and weakness of the hand caused by pressure on the radial nerve from carrying grocery bags in a clenched arm

> N. Eng. J. Med. 291:742, 1974

Guitarist's Foot Drop

paralysis of the foot by pressure on the peroneal nerve from crossing one leg over the other in order to support the guitar

Brit. Med. J. 2:669, 1974

Guitarist's Groin

inflammation of the veins caused by pressure of the guitar against the thigh

Brit. Med. J. 2:504, 1974

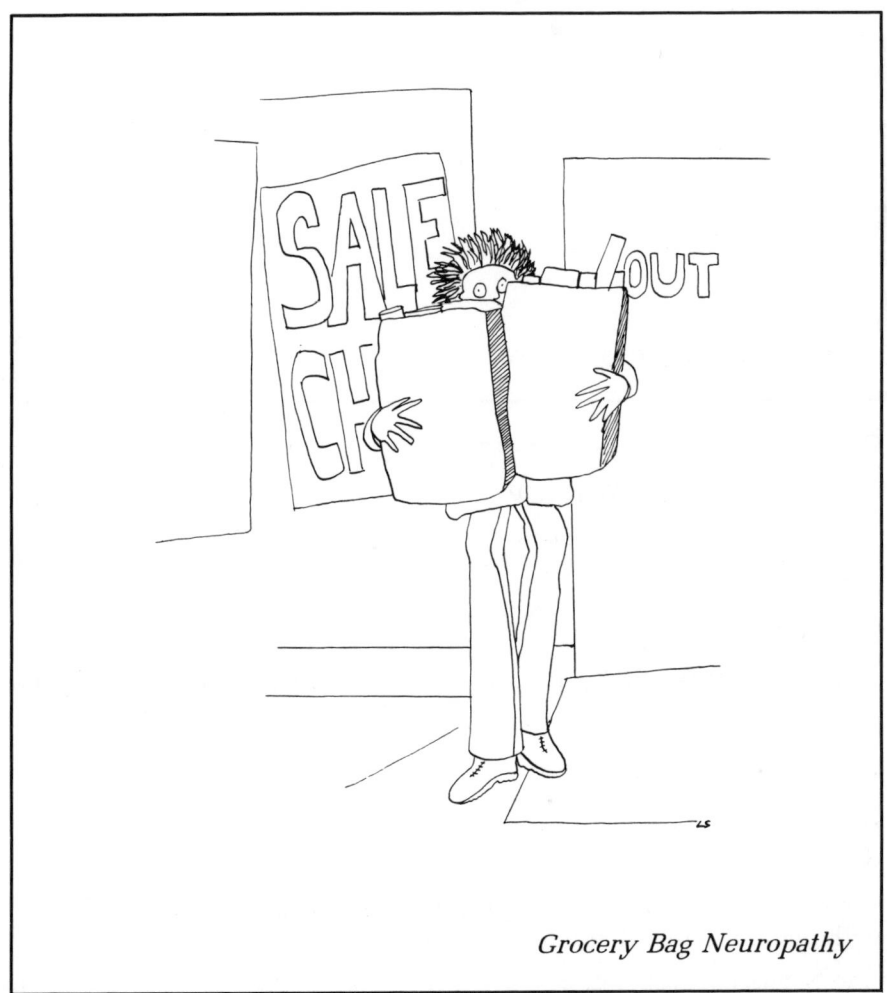

Grocery Bag Neuropathy

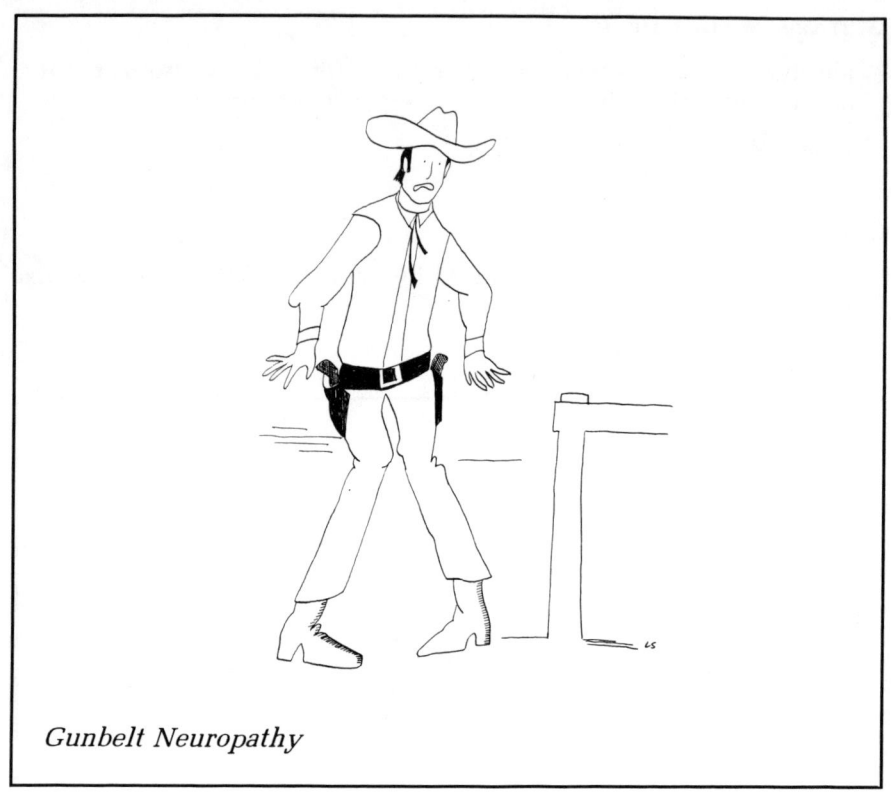

Gunbelt Neuropathy

GUITARIST'S OCCUPATIONAL PALSY

GUITARIST'S FOOT DROP

N. Eng. J. Med. 291:742, 1974

GUITAR NIPPLE

irritation of the breast from pressure of the guitar body against the chest

Brit. Med. J. 1:226, 1974

GUNBELT NEUROPATHY

altered sensation in the thigh from pressure of a gunbelt holster on the lateral femoral cutaneous nerve

N. Eng. J. Med. 291:742, 1974

Gun Deafness

hearing loss associated with ringing in the ear from exposure to the noise of naval gunfire

Lancet 2:618, 1904

Gunfighter's Wound

leg injury sustained while practicing a western-style fast draw with a handgun (compare QUICK DRAW LEG)

Ann. Surg. 157:33, 1963

Gunfire Deafness

GUN DEAFNESS

Brit. Med. J. 2:295, 1940

Gunshot Headache

headache allegedly due to the concussion effect of gunfire

Brit. Med. J. 2:1792, 1901

Gymnast's Elbow

elbow pain resulting from excessive elbow strain on the parallel bars

Encyclopedia of Sports Sciences & Medicine. N.Y.: Macmillan Co., 1971

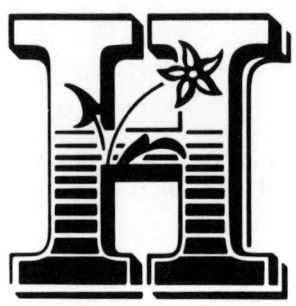

Hacklers' Disease

BYSSINOSIS from flax dust among workers exposed in the "combing" process

original source not identified

Hacklers' Lung

BYSSINOSIS from flax dust

Brit. Med. J. 2:272, 1876

Hacklers' Monday

FLAX DRESSERS' DISEASE (compare MONDAY SYNDROME)

Arch. Environ. Hlth. 14:531, 1967

Hackling Fever

FLAX DRESSERS' DISEASE

Hunter, D. The Diseases of Occupations. 5th ed. London: The English Univ. Press Ltd., 1975

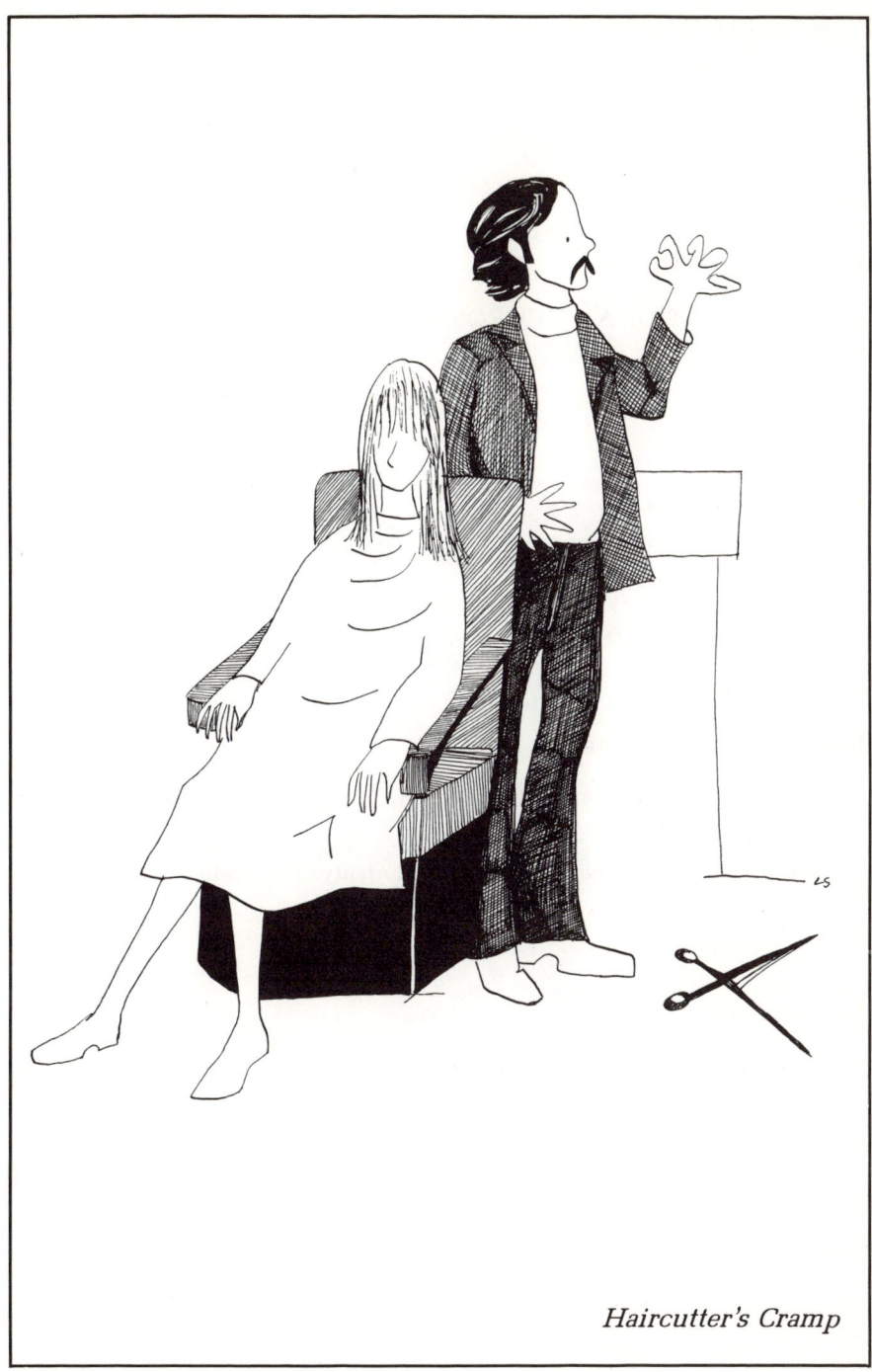

Haircutter's Cramp

TRADE DISEASES

Haircutter's Cramp

see OCCUPATIONAL NEUROSIS

> Hunter, D. The Diseases of Occupations. 5th ed. London: the English Univ. Press Ltd., 1975

Hair Dresser's Cramp

see OCCUPATIONAL NEUROSIS

> Hunter, D. The Diseases of Occupations. 5th ed. London: The English Univ. Press Ltd., 1975

Hairspray Alveolitis

allergic inflammatory response of the lungs to the inhalation of hairsprays

> Wien. Med. Wochen. 25:410, 1975

Hair Worker's Disease

anthrax infection contracted by working with animal hairs and hides

> Arlidge, J. T. The Hygiene, Diseases and Mortality of Occupations. London: Percival, 1892

Halifax Legs

rickets in malnourished children employed at the factories of Halifax, England

> Brit. Med. J. 1:671, 1879

Hammer Cramp

spasmodic jerking of the arm muscles from overuse of a hammer

> Brit. Med. J. 1:912, 1883

Hammer Hand

irritation of the pisiform hand bone from using the hand to hammer objects

Original source not identified

Hammerman's Paralysis

paralysis of the arm muscles from using sledge hammers or other heavy implements to excess

Arlidge, J. T. The Hygiene, Diseases and Mortality of Occupations. London: Percival, 1892

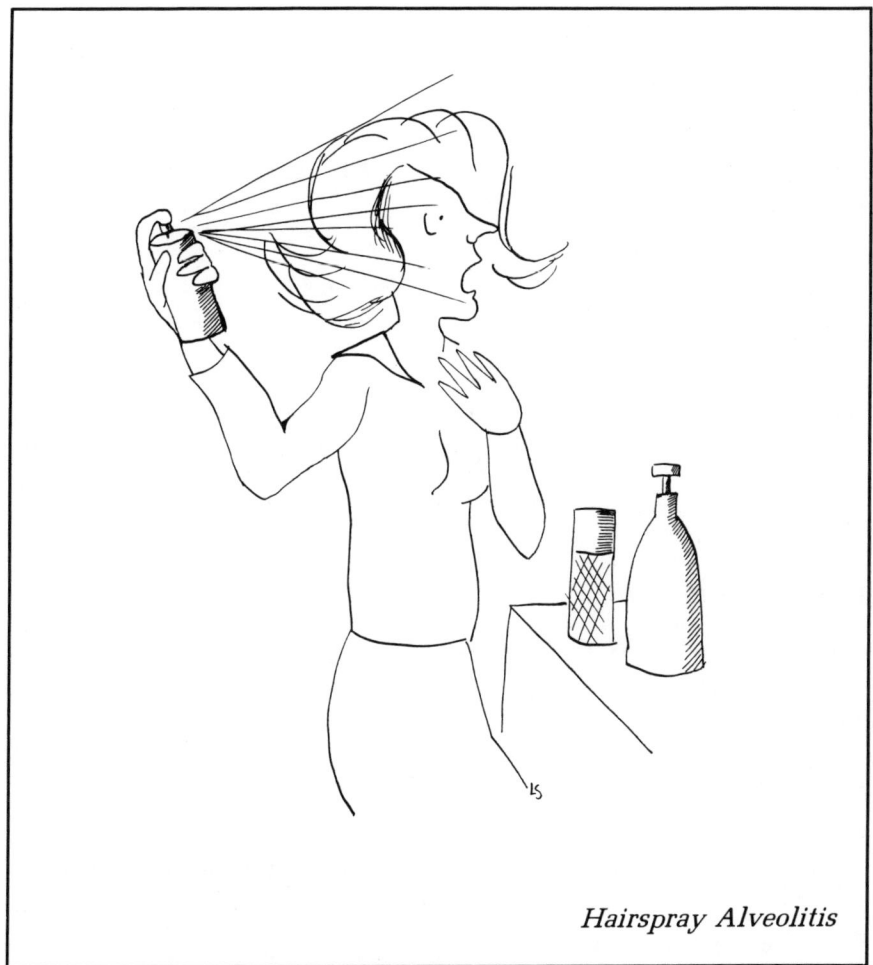

Hairspray Alveolitis

Hammerman's Cramp

see OCCUPATIONAL NEUROSIS

Lancet 2:333, 1886

Hammer Palsy

Paralysis of the wrist due to overuse of the arm in rapid, repetitive hammering

Lancet 1:427, 1869

Hammerswinger's Cramp

see OCCUPATIONAL NEUROSIS

Ann. Surg. 63:155, 1916

Hammer Syndrome

HAMMER HAND

original source not identified

Handball Palm

contusion of the palm from playing handball

Dorland's Medical Dictionary. 25th ed. Phila.: W. B. Saunders, 1974

Handicraft Spasm

see OCCUPATIONAL NEUROSIS

Dorland's Medical Dictionary. 25th ed. Phila.: W. B. Saunders, 1974

Handlebar Palsy

numbness and weakness of both hands from compression of the median and ulnar nerves by palm pressure against bicycle handlebars

N. Eng. J. Med. 292:322, 1975

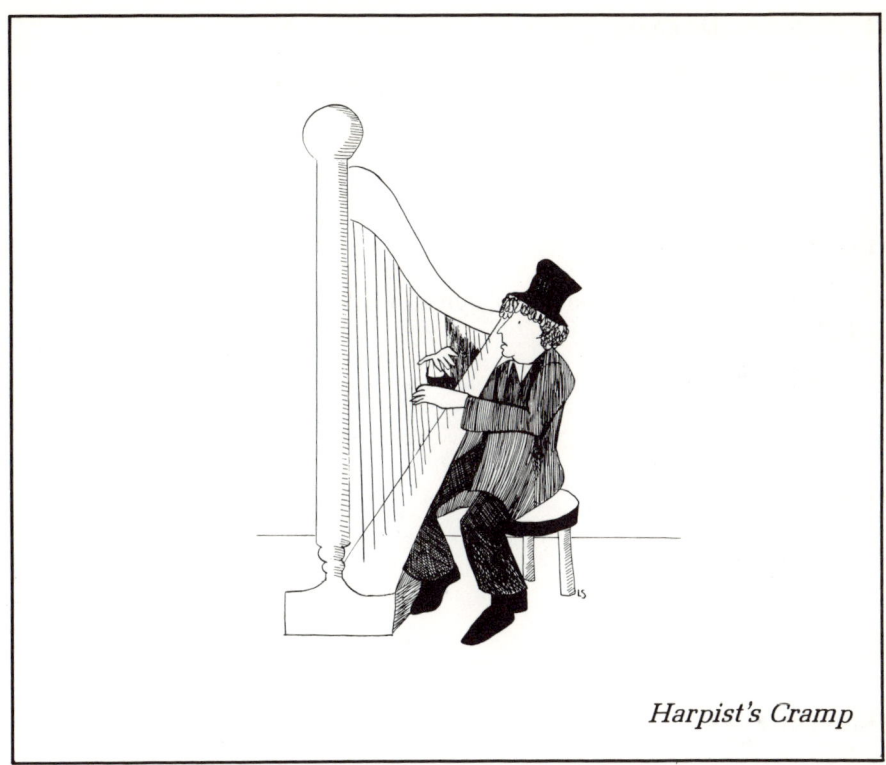

Harpist's Cramp

Hard Metal Disease

pulmonary disease of tungsten carbide workers characterized by cough, sputum production, tightness in the chest and shortness of breath

    Brit. J. Ind. Med. 19:239, 1962

Hard Metal Lung

HARD METAL DISEASE

    Brit. J. Ind. Med. 19:239, 1962

Harpist's Cramp

see OCCUPATIONAL NEUROSIS

    Hunter, D. The Diseases of Occupations. 5th ed. London: The English Univ. Press Ltd., 1975

Harvesters' Disease

dermatitis of farmers caused by the grain mite

Original source not identified

Harvesters' Keratitis

ulceration of the cornea of the eye and infection of a tear duct among field hands

Médicine (Fr) 1:210, 1920

Harvester's Lung

FARMER'S LUNG

Brit. Med. J. 2:1184, 1950

Harvest Fever

fever, redness of the eyes, stupor, vomiting, abdominal pain and diarrhea from an infectious disease, leptospirosis, contracted while working in the fields

Munsch. Med. Wchnschr. 84:481, 1937

Harvest Itch

skin irritation from contact with mite-infested crops

original source not identified

Hatters' Shakes

tremor of mercurial intoxication seen in fur-hat workers (compare DANBURY SHAKES)

Brit. Med. J. 2:402, 1901

Hatters' Sore Mouth

inflammation of the mouth associated with mercury intoxication occurring in fur-hat workers

Rpt. of Bd. of Hlth. Conn. 6:299, 1888

Hatters' Tremor

HATTERS' SHAKES

original source not identified

Haymaker's Lung

FARMER'S LUNG

Hunter, D. The Diseases of Occupations. 5th ed. London: The English Univ. Press Ltd., 1975

Heat Cataract

cataract in metal-industry workers from prolonged exposure of the eye to infrared radiation from red hot metal

Brit. Med. J. 1:392, 1949

Heat Disease

any "heat retention" disease such as heat cramps, heat exhaustion, heat stroke, etc.

Brit. Med. J. 1:621, 1937

Hedgers' Cataract

cataract of the eye following perforation of the cornea by a thorn, as occurs among hedge trimmers

Oliver, T. Dangerous Trades. London: J. Murray, 1902

Helicopter Flicker Disease

flicker dizziness or convulsion induced by the flickering effect of moving helicopter blades

Ind. Med. & Surg. 29:493, 1960

Helium Speech

high pitched, distorted speech in divers due to the helium-oxygen atmosphere used to prevent the bends

Stedman's Medical Dictionary. 23rd ed. Baltimore: William & Wilkins, 1976

Helium Tremors

decreased mental efficiency and tremors of the hands and arms seen in divers who use a helium-oxygen breathing mixture at depths over 500 feet

Underwater Physiology Subcommittee Rpt. No. 251:1, 1965

Hematite Miner's Lung

fibrotic lung disease caused by the chronic inhalation of hematite (ferric oxide)

International Classification of Diseases. 8th rev. USDHEW Pub. Hlth. Serv. Pub. No. 1963, 1968

Hemp Disease

influenza-like symptoms affecting hemp and jute textile workers

JAMA 150:1331, 1952

Hemp Worker's Disease

hemp BYSSINOSIS—cough, shortness of breath and chest tightness from hemp dust exposure

Arch. Environ. Hlth. 14:531, 1967

Herpes Gladiatorum

herpes infection among wrestlers where the virus gains access through small skin abrasions (compare WRESTLERS' HERPES)

N. Eng. J. Med. 270:979, 1964

High Altitude Decompression Sickness

DECOMPRESSION SICKNESS at flight altitudes

J. Aviat. Med. 9:172, 1938

High Altitude Disease

ALTITUDE SICKNESS

Arch. Int. Med. 59:32, 1937

High Pressure Nervous Syndrome

extremity tremors, altered brain waves and "microsleep" seen in divers exposed to high pressures of oxygen and helium

Electroenceph. Clin. Neuro. 31:383, 1971b

Hod Carriers' Shoulder

damage to the long thoracic nerve from carrying weights on the shoulder

JAMA 228:695, 1974

shoulder bursitis among hod carriers

Hunter, D. The Diseases of Occupations. 5th ed. London: The English Univ. Press Ltd., 1975

Hodmens' Shoulder

shoulder bursitis of bricklayers and hodmen

Hunter, D. The Diseases of Occupation 5th ed. London: The English Univ. Press Ltd., 1975

Holiday Expansion Syndrome

tendency to lesser productivity and greater extension of the holiday periods noted during the past decade

<small>Lancet 1:1242, 1977</small>

Holiday Heart Syndrome

irregular heart rhythms triggered by holiday "spree" drinking

<small>Sci. News 113:72, 1978</small>

Holiday Typhoid

any of the enteric diseases, including typhoid, which may affect travelers who have not taken suitable precautions

<small>Brit. Med. J. 1:515, 1970</small>

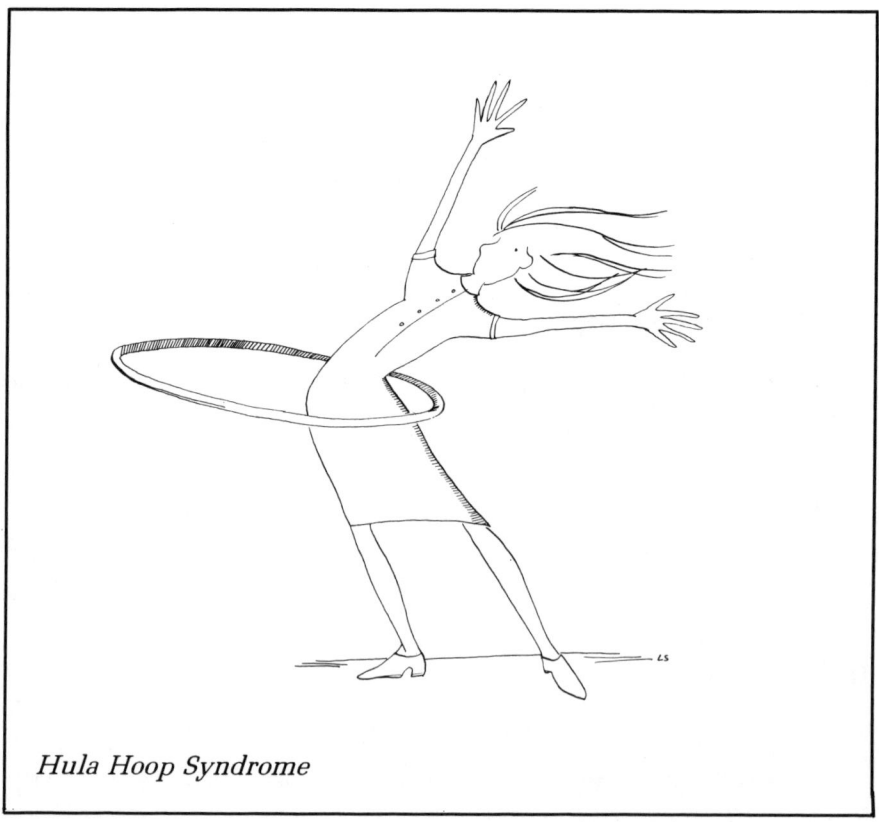

Hula Hoop Syndrome

Hollow Foot

exaggerated height of the foot arch subsequent to foot trauma

Ind. Med. & Surg. 10:126, 1941

Hong Kong Foot

ringworm of the foot seen in Oriental laundry workers

Hunter, D. The Diseases of Occupations. 5th ed. London: The English Univ. Press Ltd., 1975

Hooked Hands

GLASSBLOWER'S CRAMP

Brit. Med. J. 1:809, 1888

Hop Dermatitis

irritation of the hands, arms and face of hop pickers caused by the spine-like hairs of the plant

Lancet 2:597, 1924

Hop Eye

irritation of the eyes of hop pickers caused by the spine-like hairs of the plant

Lond. Med. Gaz. 15:112, 1834

Hop Gout

HOPPER'S GOUT

White, R. P. The Dermatogoses or Occupational Affections of the Skin. London: H. K. Lewis, 1928

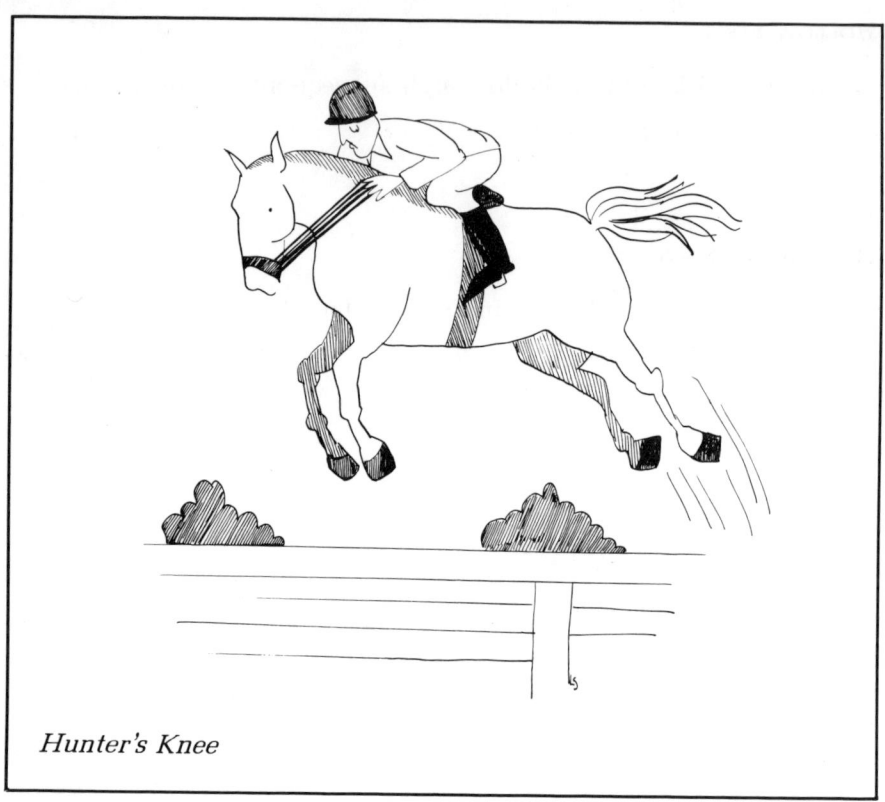
Hunter's Knee

Hoppers' Eye

inflammation, tearing and light sensitivity noted in hop pickers (compare HOP EYE)

Lancet 2:885, 1924

Hopper's Gout

mechanical irritation of the joints of the fingers, hands and wrists from picking hops

Lancet 2:885, 1924

Hop Pickers' Ophthalmia

HOP EYE

Lancet 2:531, 1893

Horn Blower's Disease

pulmonary emphysema alleged to playing wind instruments

Arch. Environ. Hlth. 12:410, 1966

Hospital Throat

throat irritation among nurses believed due to poorly ventilated infirmary wards

Oliver, T. Dangerous Trades. London: J. Murray, 1902

Hot Pants Syndrome

battery burn from a transistor battery carried in a pants pocket

JAMA 235:2082, 1976

Housemaid's Knee

inflammation of the bursa in front of the kneecap caused by pressure when doing house chores in a kneeling position

Lancet 2:381, 1825

Housewife's Dermatitis

dryness and hardness of the palms with cracking of the nail margins caused by household chemicals

Brit. Med. J. 1:401, 1947

skin irritation from detergents

Lancet 1:661, 1970

Housewife's Eczema

HOUSEWIFE'S DERMATITIS (2)

Nord. Med. 61:961, 1959

Housewife's Lime Dermatitis

eruption of the fingers and hands from contact with chloride of lime used in washing clothes

Lancet 1:599, 1925

Housewive's Eczema

hand irritation from various household items

Arch. Der. 95:487, 1967

irritant and allergic skin disease

Lancet 2:512, 1970

Housewive's Hands

skin irritation from soap, detergents and other household materials

Lancet 2:7671, 1970

Hula Hoop Dermatitis

skin irritation of the palms from contact with a hula hoop

AMA Arch. Derm. 79:590, 1959

Hula Hoop Syndrome

muscular pain in the neck and about the waist from using a hula hoop

Brit. Med. J. 2:1531, 1958

Humidifier Lung

allergic inflammatory response of the lung to the inhalation of microorganisms contaminating a ventilation system

original source not identified

Humpers' Lump

swelling over the lower neck among timber porters caused by irritation from the load

> Hunter, D. The Diseases of Occupation. 5th ed. London: The English Univ. Press Ltd., 1975

Hunter's Knee

knee pain and swelling from horseback riding in the hunt

> Brit. Med. J. 2:981, 1889

Hyperbaric Arthralgia

pain in the knees, wrist and hips with clicking noises on joint motion noted during the compression phase of deep sea diving

> Undersea Biomed. Res. 1:151, 1974

Hypothenar Hammer Syndrome

cold, painful and pale or livid fingers secondary to repetitive blunt trauma to the hands (as from using the hand to pound)

> Surg. 68:1122, 1970

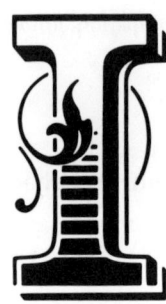

Icarus' Syndrome

any of the injuries resulting from hang gliding accidents

Brit. Med. J. 1:823, 1977

Immersion Foot

redness, swelling, blistering and hemorrhage following prolonged immersion in water

Dorland's Medical Dictionary. 25th ed. Phila.: W. B. Saunders, 1974

Immersion Hand

same symptoms as IMMERSION FOOT

International Classification of Diseases. 8th rev. USDHEW Pub. Hlth. Serv. Pub. No. 1963, 1968

Index Readers' Syndrome

fatigue, irritation of the eyes and nose, and occasional heartburn from reading many dusty volumes in uncomfortable postures in the preparation of this manuscript

author's contribution

Informational Indigestion

condition seen among physicians when the volume of new information generated by research exceeds the doctors' capacity to learn and use it

JAMA 188:40, 1964

Inhalation Fevers

pulmonary responses to inhaled foreign material; e.g. FARMERS' LUNG, BYSSINOSIS, METAL FUME FEVER and others

Lancet 1:249, 1978

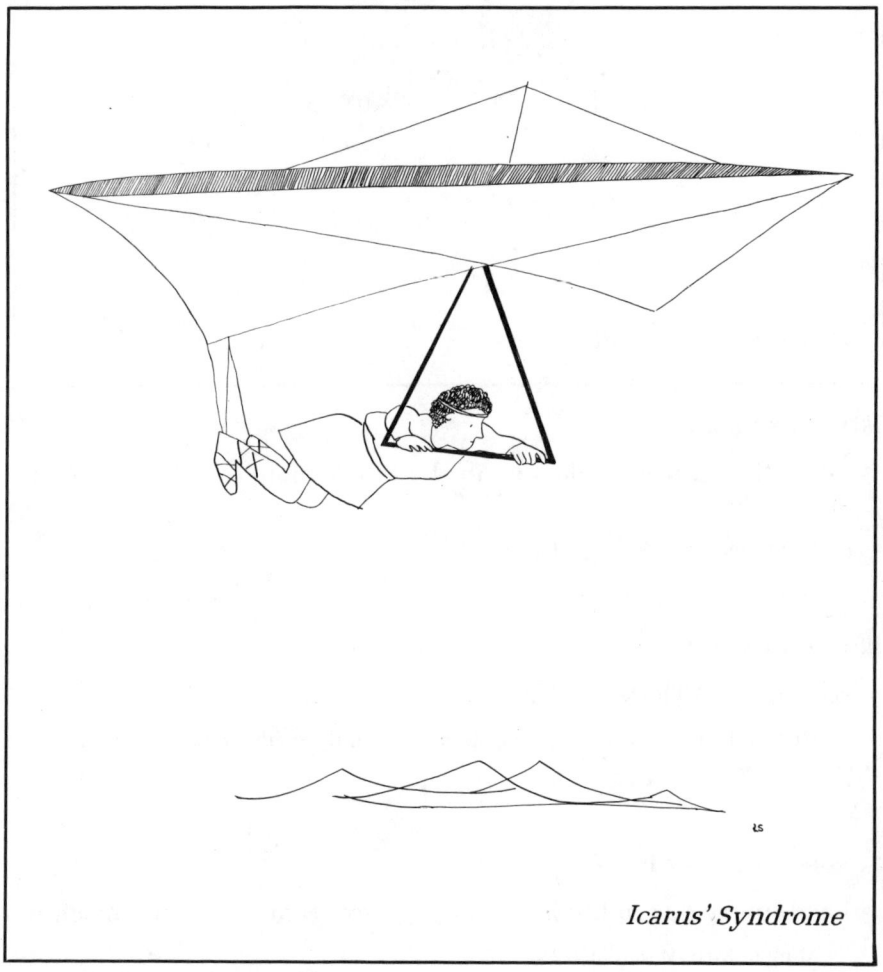

Icarus' Syndrome

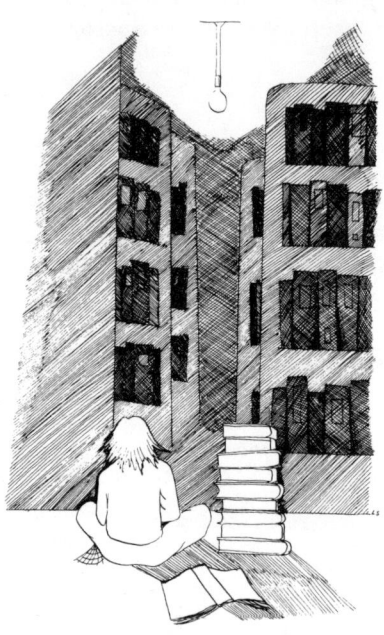
Index Readers' Syndrome

IRON DUST LUNG

deposition of iron oxide dust in the lungs, more commonly seen in arc welders

Deutsche. Med. Woch. 68:16, 1942

IRONER'S CRAMP

see OCCUPATIONAL NEUROSIS

Hunter, D. The Diseases of Occupations. 5th ed. London: The English Univ. Press Ltd., 1975

IRONING MACHINE INJURY

hand injury due to the heat and pressure from an ironing machine

Munch. Med. Wschr. 116:2185, 1974

Iron Lung

IRON DUST LUNG

Deutsche. Arch. Klin. Med. 2:116, 1867

Iron Miner's Lung

fibrotic lung disease caused by the chronic inhalation of iron and silica dusts

International Classification of Diseases. 8th rev. USDHEW Pub. Hlth. Serv. Pub. No. 1963, 1968

Iron Oxide Lung

IRON DUST LUNG

Hunter, D. The Diseases of Occupations. 5th ed. London: The English Univ. Press Ltd., 1975

Iron Puddler's Cataract

cataract resulting from prolonged exposure of the eye to infrared radiation at the iron furnace

Institutiones Chirurgicae. p. 598. Amsterdam, 1739

Iron Workers' Cramps

heat cramps in iron workers

Hunter, D. The Diseases of Occupations. 5th ed. London: The English Univ. Press Ltd., 1975

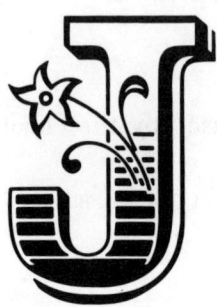

Jackhammer Arthropathy

pain and bone changes at the wrist due to the use of vibratory tools (compare RIVETER'S WRIST)

J. Occup. Med. 14:563, 1972

Jail Fever

typhus among jail prisoners due to poor hygienic conditions

Stedman's Medical Dictionary. 23rd ed. Baltimore: William & Wilkins, 1976

Jake Paralysis

paralysis of the extremities following the ingestion of a Jamaica ginger extract (beverage) contaminated with tri-ortho-cresyl phosphate

JAMA 98:298, 1932

Javelin Thrower's Elbow

pain over the inner aspect of the elbow from strain in making the throw

Encyclopedia of Sport Sci. & Med. N.Y.: Macmillan, 1971

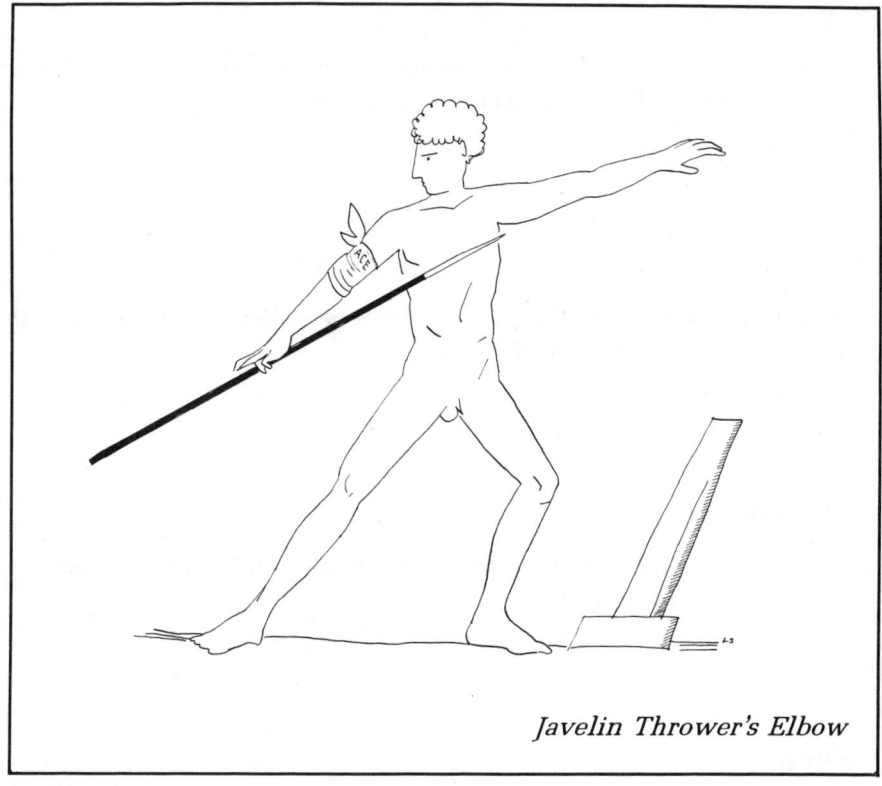

Javelin Thrower's Elbow

JEEP DISEASE

infected pilonidal cyst over the tail bone aggravated by riding in jeeps, trucks and tanks

So. Med. J. 37:103, 1944

JERK FINGER

TRIGGER FINGER

Brit. Med. J. 2:1069, 1897

JET ENGINE SICKNESS

fatigue and ear trouble among test-bed employees allegedly due to the noise and vibration of jet engines

JAMA 135:933, 1947

TRADE DISEASES

Jet Lag

disturbance of normal biologic rhythms by rapid transit across time zones (compare TRAVEL DYSRHYTHMIA)

original source not identified

Jet Tummy

abdominal swelling among airline hostesses alleged to expansion of gastrointestinal gasses at high altitudes

JAMA 185:616, 1963

Job Phobia

anxiety, depression and somatic complaints related to an overconcern about job performance

Compre. Psych. 13:251, 1972

Job Stress

physical and/or mental health impairment caused by a job

J. Occup. Med. 16:659, 1974

Jockey's Ankle

swelling over the inner aspect of the ankle from pressure caused by "riding short"; i.e. with high stirrups

J. Irish Med. Assoc. 70:282, 1977

Jogger's Heel

pain over the heel pad from striking on nonresilient surfaces in jogging

JAMA 206:2899, 1968

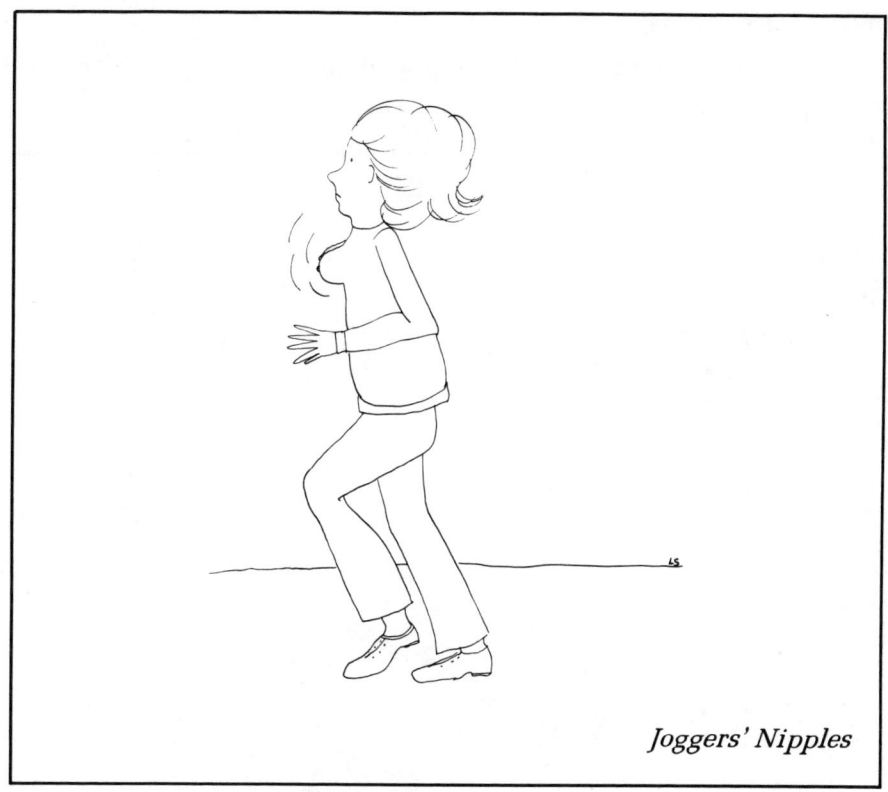

Joggers' Nipples

JOGGERS' NIPPLES

    nipple irritation among women joggers caused by shirt friction when a brassiere is not worn

        N. Eng. J. Med. 297:1127, 1977

JOGGER'S PETECHIAE

    small hemorrhages into the skin caused by the trauma of jogging

        N. Eng. J. Med. 279:109, 1968

JOINER'S HAND

    swelling at the base of the thumb and an outward deviation of the end of the little finger caused by long use of the plane

        Brit. Med. J. 1:335, 1896

Judo Man's Elbow

chronic elbow disability from repeated joint injury in judo attacks

Encyclopedia of Sport Sci. & Med. N.Y.: Macmillan, 1971

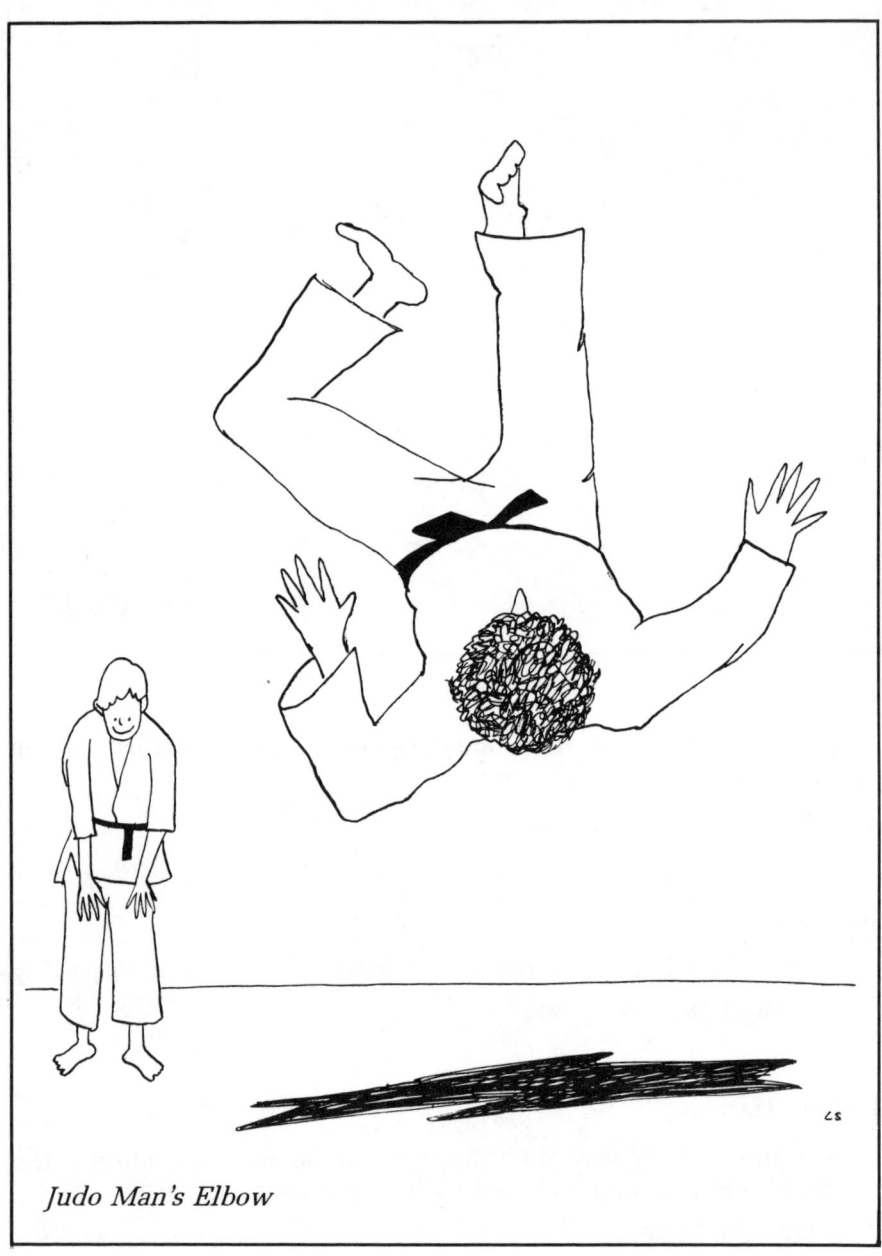

Judo Man's Elbow

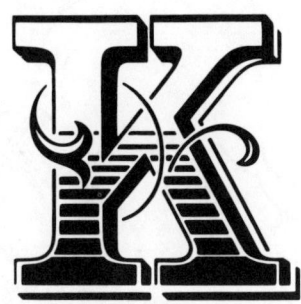

Karate Hand

marked inflammatory reaction of a hand tendon from chronic trauma

JAMA 211:1009, 1970

Karate Myoglobinuria

dark discoloration of the urine following intense karate practice (compare CONGA DRUMMER'S PIGMENTURIA)

N. Eng. J. Med. 293:941, 1975

Kieselguhr Lung

fibrotic lung disease caused by the chronic inhalation of Kieselguhr (diatomaceous earth)

ILO Encyclopedia of Occupational Health And Safety. N.Y.: McGraw Hill, 1972

Klieg Eye

irritation of the eyes of film-studio performers by bright studio lights (Kliegal electric lamps) which produce ultraviolet rays

JAMA 80:1792, 1923

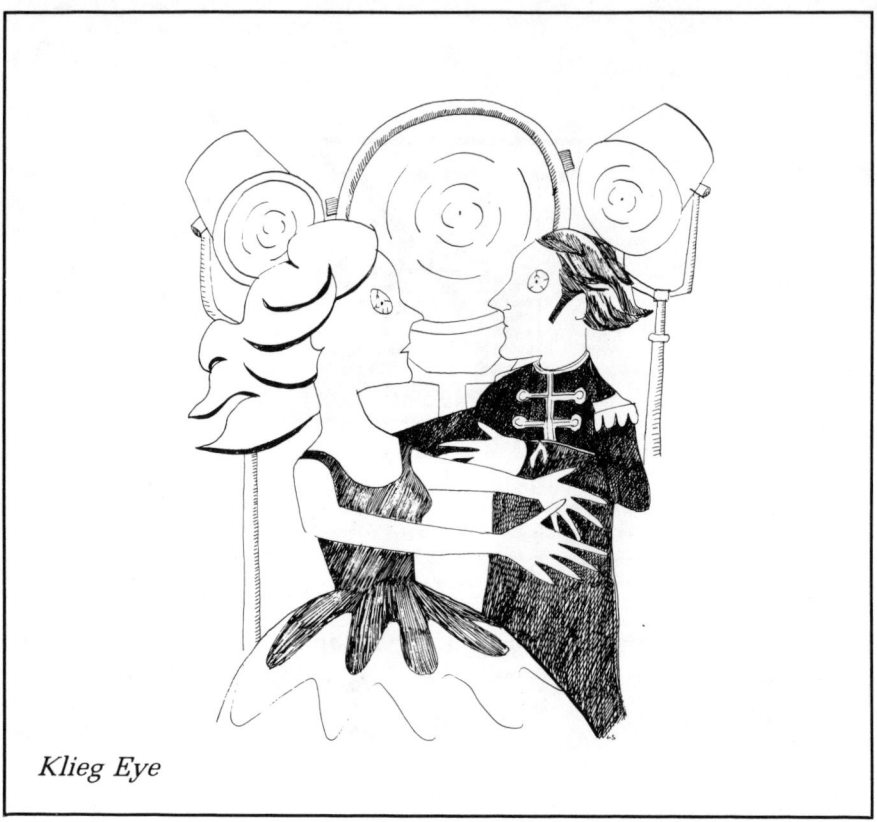

Klieg Eye

KNAPSACK PARALYSIS

    motor and sensory changes in the upper extremity from compression of the brachial nerves by the harness

        Arch. Med. 4:161, 1880

KNIFE GRINDERS' PHTHISIS

    pulmonary silicosis occurring in workers grinding knives

        Brit. Med. J. 1:768, 1889

KNIFE GRINDERS' ROT

    silicotuberculosis among knife grinders

        original source not identified

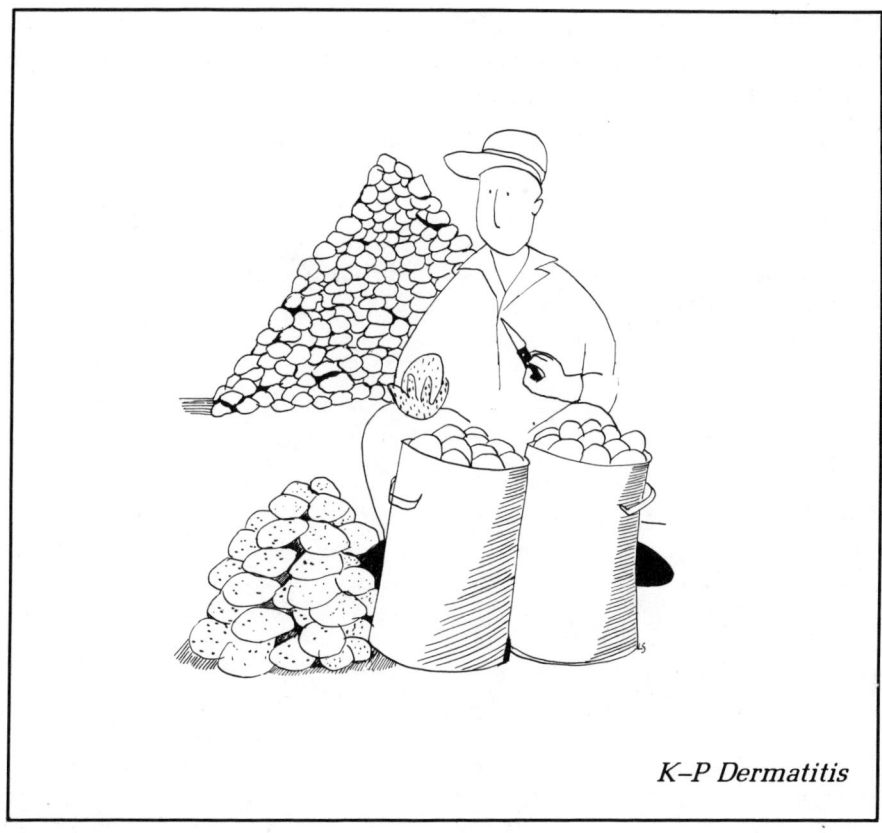

K–P Dermatitis

Knife Sharpener's Cramp

see OCCUPATIONAL NEUROSIS

Hunter, D. The Diseases of Occupations. 5th ed. London: The English Univ. Press Ltd., 1975

Knights' Disease

infection of the perianal area frequently occurring among horsemen

Dorland's Medical Dictionary. 25th ed. Phila.: W. B. Saunders, 1974

Knitter's Cramp

see OCCUPATIONAL NEUROSIS

Brit. Med. J. 1:11, 1886

Knobbies

soft tissue swellings over the knee, leg and foot of surfers following repeated trauma by the surfboard

<small>Encyclopedia of Sports Sci. & Med. N.Y.: Macmillan, 1971</small>

K-P Dermatitis

skin and nail irritation about the hands of those doing kitchen police, caused by alkaline cleansers

<small>J. Occup. Med. 10:423, 1968</small>

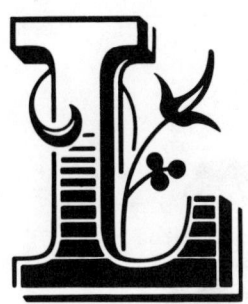

Label Lickers' Tongue

ulcers of the tongue and mouth from label gum sensitivity occurring among workers who apply labels to thread-bobbins

> Oliver, T. Dangerous Trades. London: J. Murray, 1902

Lace-Maker's Disease

near-sightedness alleged to the eyestrain of making lace

> Hunter, D. The Diseases of Occupations. 5th ed. London: The English Univ. Press Ltd., 1975

Lasters' Disease

blanching of the fingers in lasting machine operators provoked by vibration and cold (compare VWF)

> Dent. Archiv. f. Klin. Med. 187:491, 1941

Laundrymen's Itch

ringworm of the feet in Oriental laundry workers

> Schwartz, L. Occupational Diseases of the Skin. Phila.: Lea & Febiger, 1957

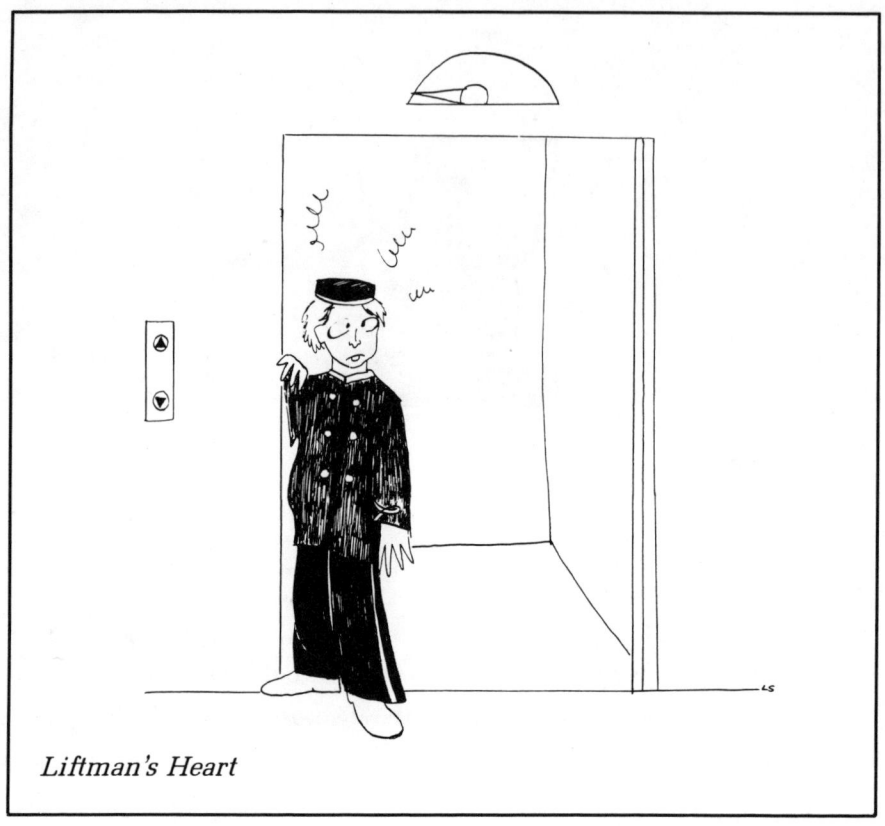

Liftman's Heart

LAWN TENNIS ARM

sprain of the forearm (pronator teres) from a backhand stroke

Lancet 2:133, 1882

LAWN TENNIS ELBOW

pain over the lateral aspect of the elbow from a chronic strain

Brit. Med. J. 2:557, 1883

LAWN TENNIS KNEE

internal damage to the knee from torsion of the joint while playing tennis

Lancet 2:179, 1883

Lawn Tennis Leg

rupture of the muscle which flexes the foot (plantaris) from tennis strain

Lancet 2:44, 1883

Lawn Tennis Wrist

wrist sprain

Lancet 2:179, 1883

Lead Line

bluish discoloration of the gums at the margin of the teeth seen in chronic lead poisoning

Lancet 1:661, 1839

Lead Miners' Lung

chronic lung disease of miners

International Classification of Diseases. 8th rev. USDHEW Pub. Hlth. Serv. Pub. 1963, 1968

Leather Buffers' Nodes

calluses over the thumbs of workers engaged in hand buffing leather

JAMA 114:571, 1940

Leather Workers' Ulcers

ulcerations of the hands of leather workers caused by chromate sensitivity

Ann. Surg. 63:155, 1916

Letter Sorter's Cramp

see OCCUPATIONAL NEUROSIS

Hunter, D. The Diseases of Occupations. 5th ed. London: The English Univ. Press Ltd., 1975

Liftman's Heart

(on elevators) "the sudden transition from the heavier air at the foot to the lighter air at the top is extremely trying to the constitution"

Bost. Med. & Surg. J. 143:513, 1900

Lightermen's Bursitis

bursitis of the hip (ischium) from repetitive friction and pressure

Hunter, D. The Diseases of Occupations. 5th ed. London: The English Univ. Press Ltd., 1975

Lightning Cataract

cataract of the eye following a lightning strike to the body

Klin. Monatsbl. Augen. 2:22, 1864

Lime Holes

skin ulcerations in workers who work with lime and lime solutions

White, R. P. The Dermatogoses or Occupational Affections of the Skin. London: H. K. Lewis, 1928

Linotypist's Cramp

see OCCUPATIONAL NEUROSIS

International Classification of Diseases. 8th rev. USDHEW Pub. Hlth. Serv. Pub. No. 1963, 1968

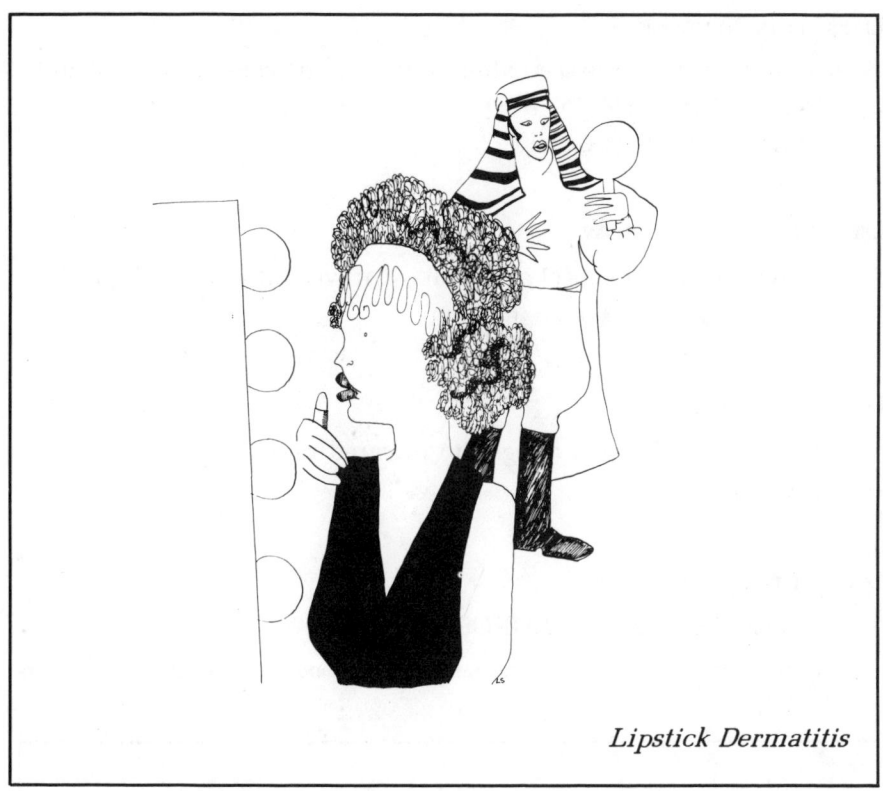

Lipstick Dermatitis

Lipstick Dermatitis

lipstick sensitivity occurring among cinema artists

<small>Gougerot H. Dermatoses Professionnelles, Librarie Maloine, Paris, 1952</small>

Listening-In Dermatitis

irritation of the ear caused by excessive contact with the telephone earpiece

<small>Derm. Wochschr. p. 999, Aug. 1924</small>

Lithographers' Dermatitis

skin irritation among lithographers caused by numerous irritants and sensitizers, including chrome compounds

<small>JAMA 169:566, 1959</small>

Litigation Neurosis

psychiatric symptoms seen after an injury and caused by legal and/or psychological factors

World Wide Abst. 6(6):20, 1963

Little Leaguers' Elbow

pain over the inner aspect of the elbow in youthful baseball pitchers

J. Bone & Joint Surg. 53A:359, 1971

Locksmith's Cancer

skin cancer of the arm alleged to infrared radiation

JAMA 85:1342, 1925

Locksmith's Cramp

see OCCUPATIONAL NEUROSIS

Hunter, D. The Diseases of Occupations. 5th ed. London: The English Univ. Press Ltd., 1975

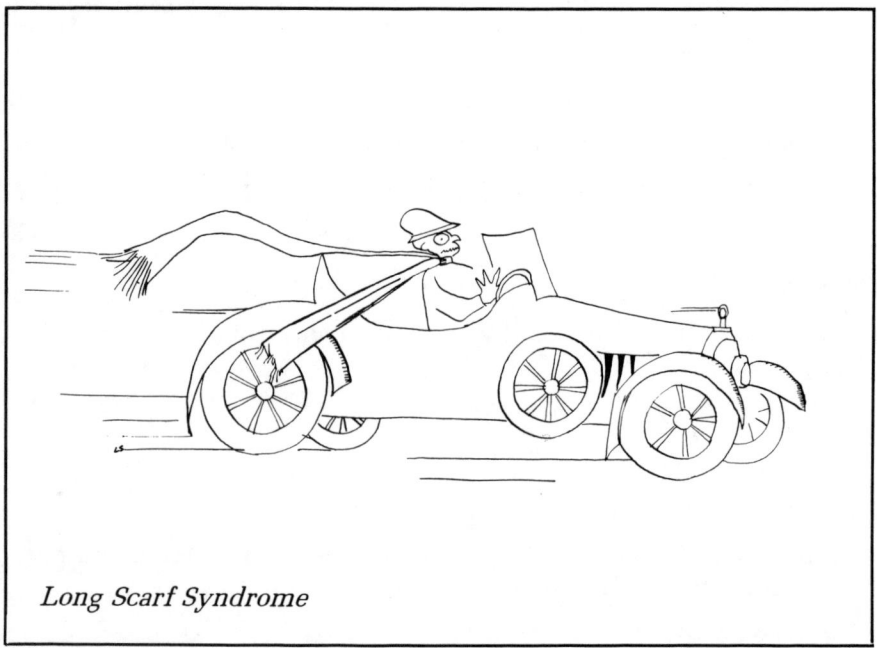

Long Scarf Syndrome

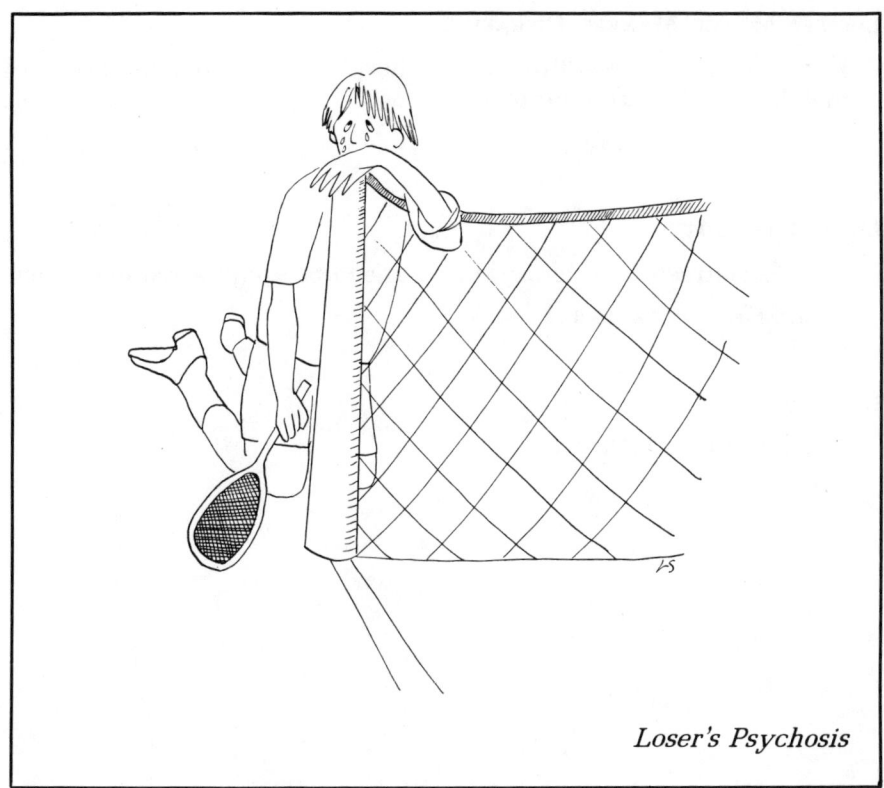

Loser's Psychosis

LONG SCARF SYNDROME

face and neck trauma occurring when scarves become entangled in moving machinery

N. Eng. J. Med. 284:734, 1971

LOSER'S PSYCHOSIS

depression associated with the loss of a squash tennis match

Encyclopedia of Sport Sci. & Med. N.Y.: Macmillan Co., 1971

LOVER'S PALSY

numbness of the forearm and hand from compression of the radial nerve at the arm level

West. J. Med. 127:303, 1977

TRADE DISEASES

LUCIFER MATCH MAKERS' DISEASE

jaw bone disease resulting from phosphorus intoxication seen in match manufacturing employees (compare PHOSSY JAW)

Brit. Med. J. 2:434, 1863

LUMBERMAN'S ITCH

scabies contracted while working in the forests or processing lumber

Brit. Med. J. 2:1004, 1888

LUNG ROT

GRINDERS' ASTHMA (2)

Brit. Med. J. 1:204, 1868

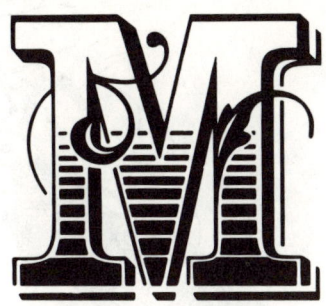

MACHINIST'S FURUNCULOSIS

skin irritation of the body surfaces exposed to cutting oils

JAMA 91:1738, 1928

MACHINIST'S TREMOR

see OCCUPATIONAL NEUROSIS

Brit. Med. J. 1:1316, 1900

MALADIE DE PLONGEURS

sea nettle stings of divers

Dorland's Medical Dictionary. 25th ed. Phila.: W. B. Saunders, 1974

MALA METALLORUM

malady of the lungs which killed the workers of the metal mines of Saxony and Bohemia in the 16th century (now considered to be due to the inhalation of radioactive dust) (compare SCHNEEBERG TUMOR)

Brit. Med. J. 1:5, 1966

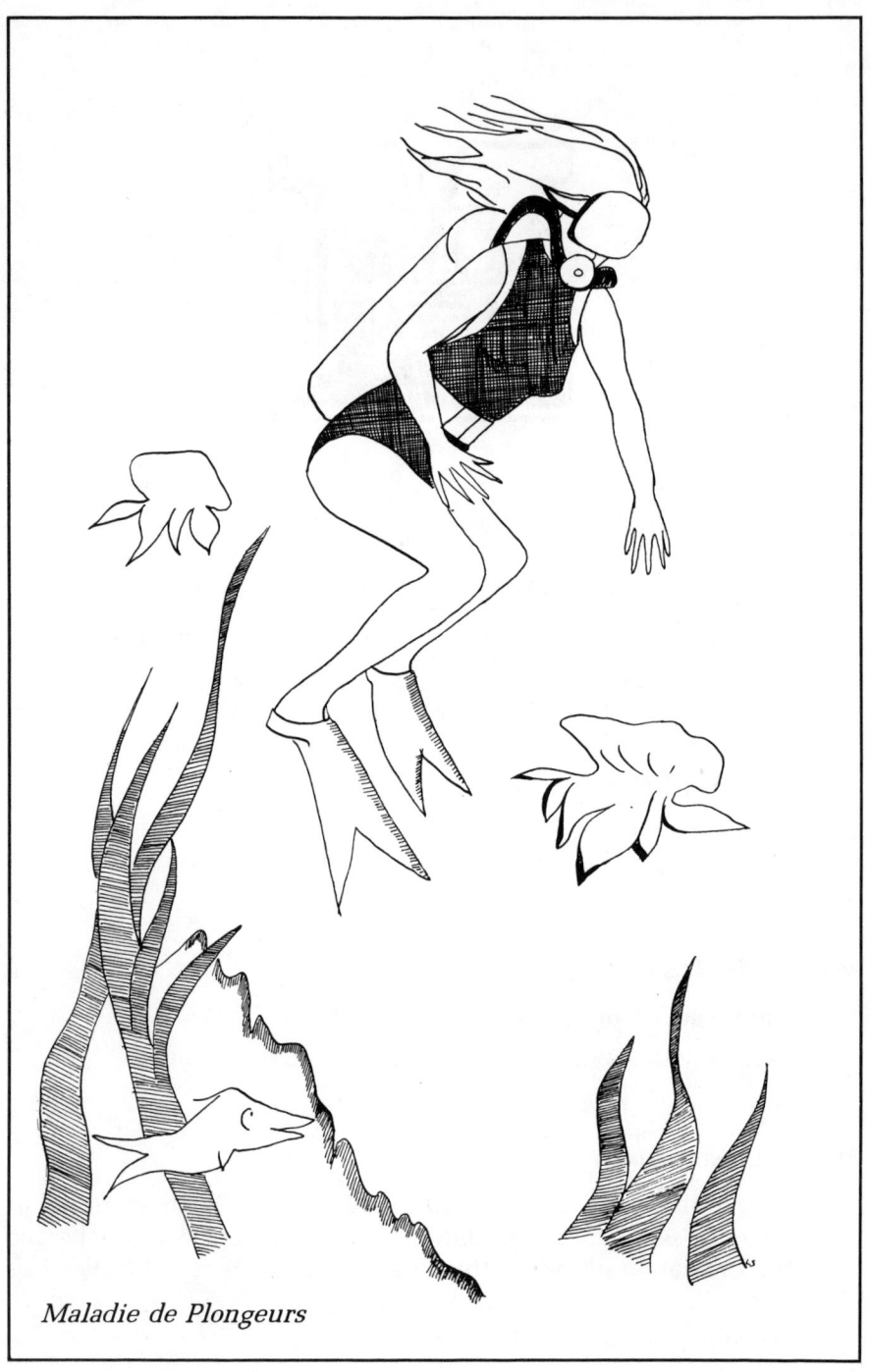
Maladie de Plongeurs

Mal de Mer

sea sickness

Dorland's Medical Dictionary. 25th ed. Phila.: W. B. Saunders, 1974

Malibu Disease

soft tissue swelling over the leg and foot caused by surfboard injury

International Classification of Diseases. 8th rev. USDHEW Pub. Hlth. Serve. Pub. No. 1963, 1968

Maltster's Itch

rash over the neck, chest and extremities from barley dust irritation while working in malting chambers

Bull. Soc. Franc Derm. et Syph. p. 17, May 1924

Malt Worker's Disease

MALT WORKER'S LUNG

original source not identified

Malt Worker's Lung

allergic inflammatory response of the lung to the inhalation of *Aspergillus clavatus* spores in contaminated barley

Morgan, W. K. C. and A. Seaton. Occupational Lung Diseases. Phila.: W. B. Saunders, 1975

Maple Bark Stripper's Disease

allergic inflammatory response of the lungs to the inhalation of *Cryptostroma corticale,* a fungus which grows beneath the bark of the tree

Morgan, W. K. C. and A. Seaton. Occupational Lung Diseases. Phila.: W. B. Saunders, 1975

MARBLE CUTTER'S PHTHISIS

fibrotic lung disease caused by the inhalation of marble dust containing silica

Dorland's Medical Dictionary. 25th ed. Phila.: W. B. Saunders, 1974

MARCH FOOT

painful foot from unusual stress such as marching

Brit. Med. J. 2:776, 1933

fracture of the foot in soldiers after prolonged marching

Hauser, E. D. W. Diseases of the Foot. Phila.: Saunders, 1939

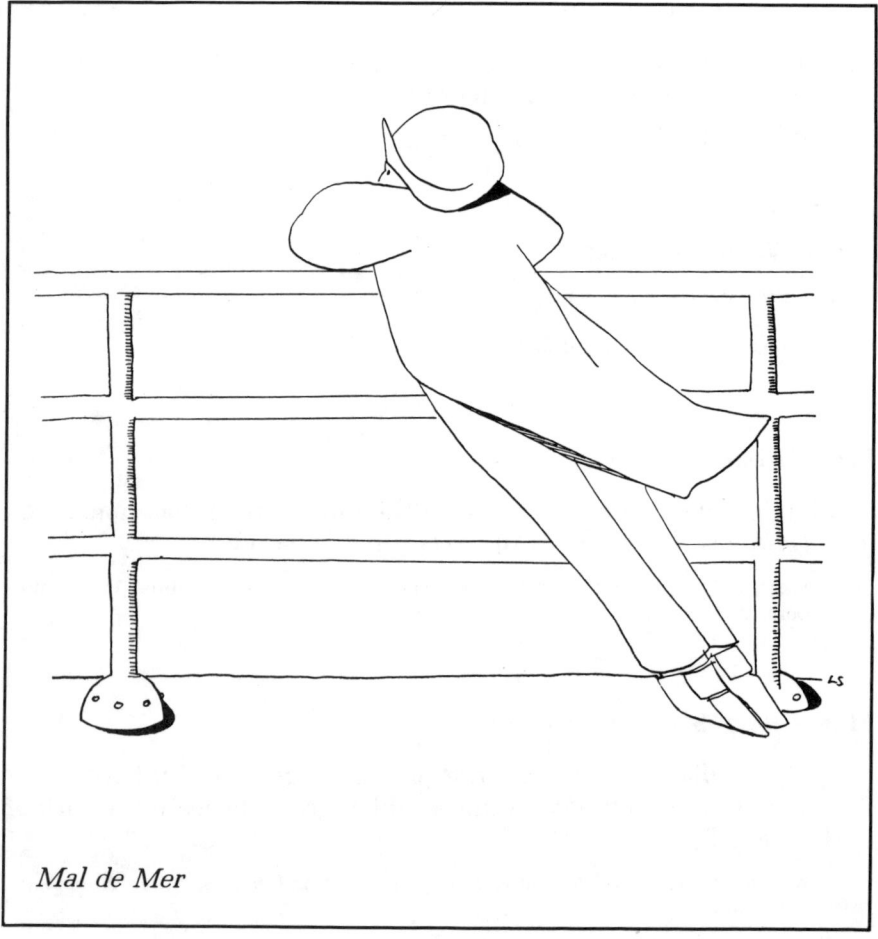

Mal de Mer

March Fracture

fracture of the thigh or leg occurring during a prolonged march

Arch. Klin. Chir., Berlin 118:530, 1921

MARCH FOOT (2) (compare FATIGUE FRACTURE)

Brit. Med. J. 2:64, 1945

March Hemoglobinuria

dark stained urine following prolonged walking or marching

Berl. Klin. Wschr. 18:691, 1881

March Tumor

inflammation and swelling of the ligaments of the foot after prolonged marching

Dorland's Medical Dictionary. 25th ed. Phila.: W. B. Saunders, 1974

Mason's Cramp

see OCCUPATIONAL NEUROSIS

Hunter, D. The Diseases of Occupations. 5th ed. London: The English Univ. Press Ltd., 1975

Mason's Disease

fibrotic lung disease caused by the chronic inhalation of silica

Lancet 1:297, 1929

Masons' Eczema

irritation of the hands of masons caused by sensitivity to bichromate in cement

Arch. f. Derm. u. Syph. 178:1, 1938

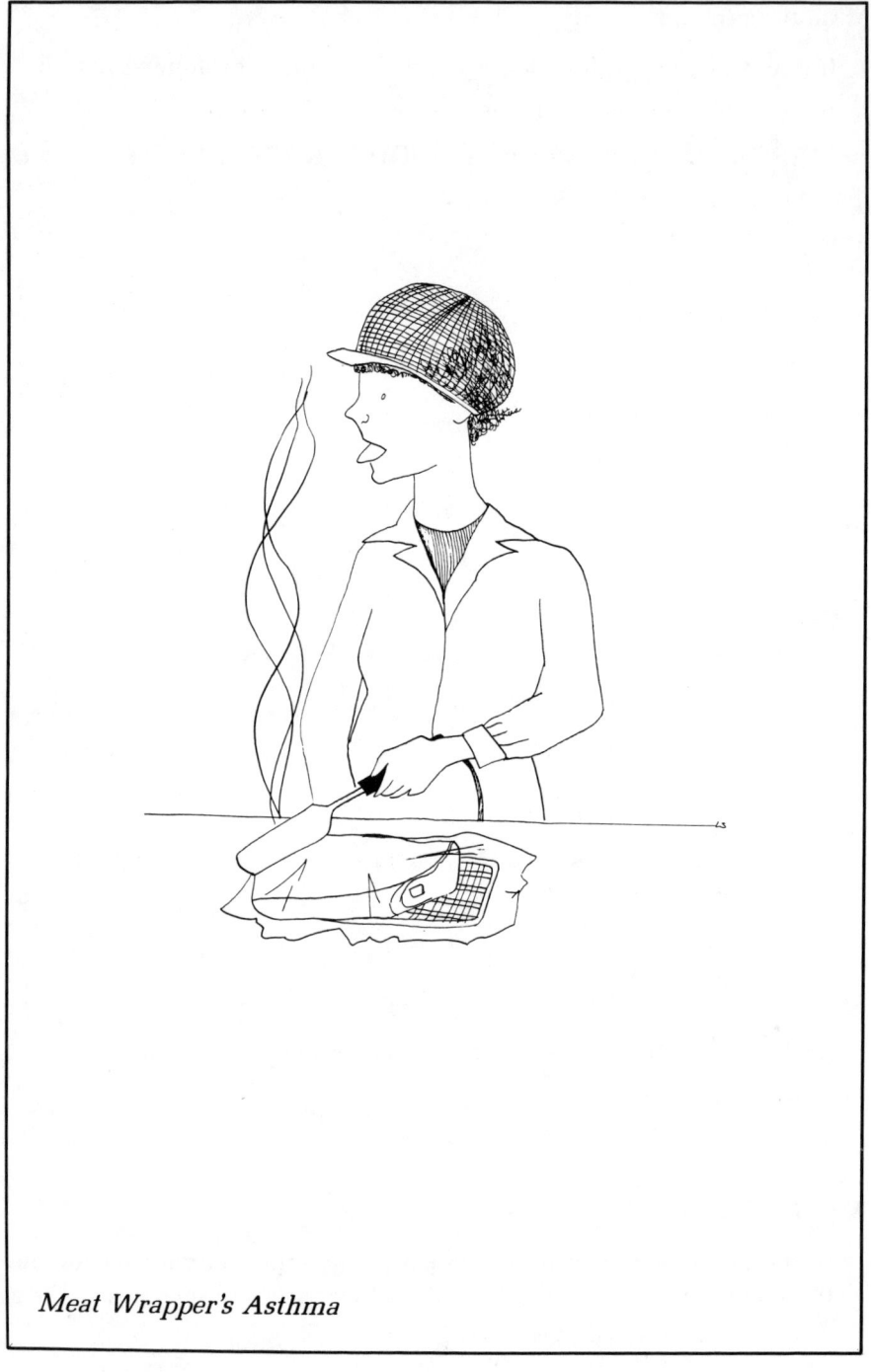

Meat Wrapper's Asthma

Mason's Lung

MASON'S DISEASE

Bost. Med. & Surg. J. 117:198, 1887

Mason's Trouble

MASON'S DISEASE

Lancet 1:364, 1841

Mattress Maker's Disease

BYSSINOSIS from exposure to cotton dust in mattress manufacturing

Brit. Med. J. 1:46, 1943

Mattress Makers' Fever

BYSSINOSIS among workers who open cotton bales, fluff the cotton and fill the mattresses

JAMA 119:1074, 1942

Meat Worker's Asthma

respiratory distress provoked by exposure to the fumes emitted by heated price labels

J. Occup. Med. 20:116, 1978

Meat Wrapper's Asthma

shortness of breath, cough and wheezing from inhaling the fumes from heated polyvinyl chloride film

JAMA 226:639, 1973

Metal Casters' Cramps

heat cramps among metal workers

> Hunter, D. The Diseases of Occupations. 5th ed. London: The English Univ. Press Ltd., 1975

Metal Fume Fever

headache, chills, fever and generalized aching following the inhalation of metal fumes (brass, copper, zinc, etc.)

> Arch. Hyg. Berl. 72:358, 1910

Metalliferous Miner's Lung

deposition of any metal dust in the lungs

> International Classification of Diseases. 8th rev. USDHEW Pub. Hlth. Serv. Pub. No. 1963, 1968

Metal Plater's Dermatitis

skin irritation due to nickel sensitivity

> Hunter, D. The Diseases of Occupations, 5th ed. London: The English Univ. Press Ltd., 1975

Metal Polisher's Disease

pulmonary silicosis

> International Classification of Diseases. 8th rev. USDHEW Pub. Hlth. Serv. Pub. No. 1963, 1968

Metal Welder's Disease

chronic disturbance of thyroid and liver function alleged to welding fumes

> Arch. Gewerbepath. Gewerbehyg. 11:179, 1941

Metal Workers' Cataract

cataract among workers handling molten metal caused by infrared radiation

Rass. Med. Indust. 26:531, 1957

Metal Worker's Cramp

see OCCUPATIONAL NEUROSIS

Hunter, D. The Diseases of Occupations. 5th ed. London: The English Univ. Press Ltd., 1975

Me-Too Syndrome

multiple worker complaints following the diagnosis of a compensable illness in one member of a group

Occup. Hlth. 29:289, 1977

Microscope Worker's Cramp

see OCCUPATIONAL NEUROSIS

Hunter, D. The Diseases of Occupations, 5th ed. London: The English Univ. Press Ltd., 1975

Microwave Cataract

cataract of the lens following exposure of the eye to microwaves

AMA Arch. Ind. Hyg. 6:512, 1952

Microwave Neurosis

irritability, fatigue, weakness and anxiety associated with exposure to microwaves (compare RADIOWAVE SICKNESS)

Psychiat. Pol. 6:111, 1972

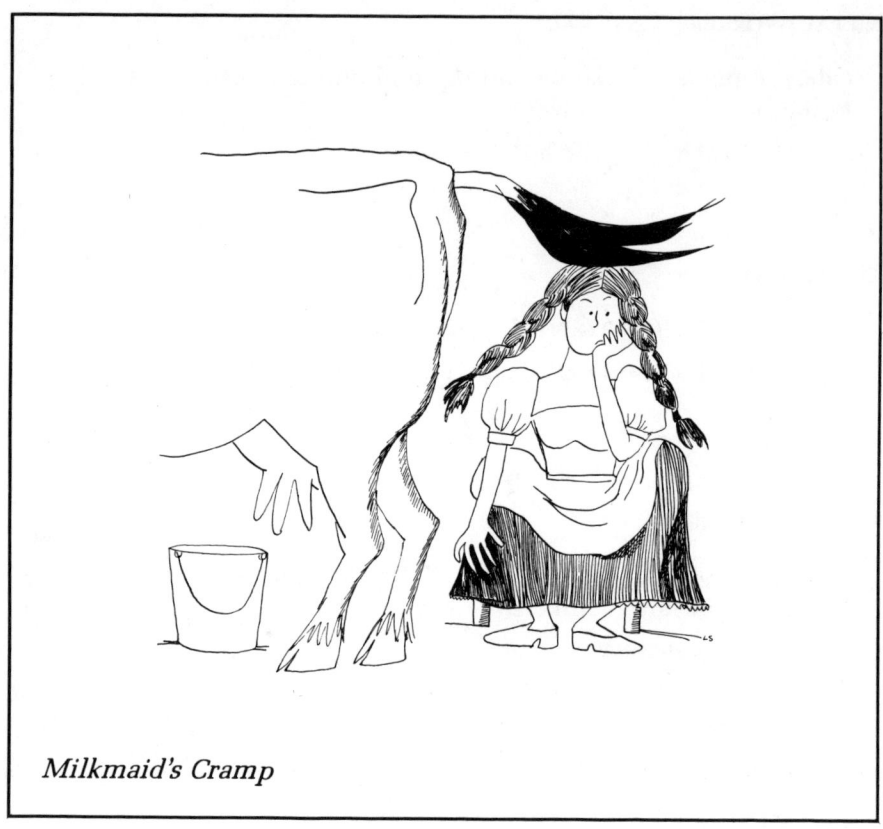
Milkmaid's Cramp

MIDWIFE'S DISEASE

    pain and swelling of the wrists and forearms from overuse of the extremities in supporting the perineum of a patient in labor

        Brit. Med. J. 1:735, 1890

MILITARY CARDITIS

    SOLDIERS' HEART

        Lancet 2:662, 1917

MILITARY FRENZY

    marked irritability exhibited by battle-fatigued soldiers

        Vischer, A. L. Barbed Wire Disease. London: John Blake, 1919

Milker's Cramp

see OCCUPATIONAL NEUROSIS

Lancet 1:585, 1875

Milkers' Felon

painful finger infection in dairy workers caused by the penetration of small hairs from the cow's udder

Zentral. für Chir. 35:841, 1908

Milker's Granuloma

small red nodules of the hand caused by penetrating hairs from the cow's udder

Deut. Zeit. Chir. 223:339, 1930

Milkers' Hands

arthritic changes of the index and middle finger joints caused by an improper milking technique

Med. Lavoro 38:81, 1947

Milker's Node

MILKER'S GRANULOMA

Derm. Wochenschr. p. 134, Feb. 1934

Milker's Nodules

MILKER'S GRANULOMA

Kanavel, A. B. Infections of the Hand. Phila.: Lea & Febiger, 1939

nodules from cowpox infection

JAMA 115:2140, 1940

Milkers' Panaritium

finger and palm irritation in dairy workers caused by penetration of small hairs from a cow's udder

Brit. J. Derm. 49:164, 1937

Milker's Spasm

occupational cramp of milkmaids

Oliver, T. Dangerous Trades. London: J. Murray, 1902

Milkers' Vaccinia

skin eruption of milkers' hands following contact with cows infected by cowpox *Variola bovinum*

Arch. f. Derm. u. Syph. 178:88, 1938

Milkers' Warts

MILKERS' VACCINIA

Brit. J. Derm. 49:164, 1937

Milkmaid's Cramp

see OCCUPATIONAL NEUROSIS

Brit. Med. J. 1:11, 1886

Miller's Asthma

allergic inflammatory response of the lungs to inhaled cereal dusts

Brit. Med. J. 1:704, 1889

Miller's Bronchitis

MILLER'S ASTHMA

original source not identified

Mill Fever

chills, nausea and vomiting, headache, thirst and fever affecting new workers exposed to cotton dust for the first time
>Brit. Med. J. 1:704, 1889

Mill Reek

lead poisoning among workers exposed to reek fumes (smelter fumes)
>Scots Mag. 16:287, 1754

Millstone Maker's Asthma

fibrotic lung disease from the inhalation of silica dust while grinding and shaping millstones
>Brit. & Foreign Med. Chir. Rev. 25:214, 1860

Millstone Maker's Lung

MILLSTONE MAKER'S ASTHMA
>Lancet 1:788, 1878

Millstone Maker's Phthisis

MILLSTONE MAKER'S ASTHMA
>Brit. Med. J. 2:485, 1865

Millstone Maker's Tuberculosis

silicotuberculosis among millstone grinders
>International Classification of Diseases. 8th rev. USDHEW Pub. Hlth. Serv. Pub. No. 1963, 1968

Mill Worker's Asthma

allergic inflammatory response of the lungs to inhalation of grain weevil protein

   Brit. J. Ind. Med. 23:149, 1966

Mill Worker's Lung

MILL WORKER'S ASTHMA

   Hunter, D. The Diseases of Occupations. 5th ed. London: The English Univ. Press Ltd., 1975

Miner's Anemia

hookworm disease contracted via unsanitary conditions in coal mines

   Arch. Physiol. Heilk. 13:528, 1854

Miners' Asthma

COAL WORKERS' PNEUMOCONIOSIS

   Brit. Med. J. 2:417, 1893

Miners' Back

back complaints of coal miners due to cold wet work conditions, constrained postures and muscular strain

   Brit. Med. J. 1:131, 1904

Miners' Bunches

irritable inflamed swellings of the skin seen in coal miners due to the presence of the larvae of hookworm

   J. Hyg. 3:95, 1903

MINER'S BURSITIS

elbow bursitis from repeated trauma (compare BEAT ELBOW)

> Hunter, D. The Diseases of Occupations. 5th ed. London: The English Univ. Press Ltd., 1975

MINERS' CACHEXIA

debility from hookworm infection in coal miners

> original source not identified

MINERS' CONSUMPTION

silicosis of coal miners

> Leifchild, J. R. Cornwall Mines p. 285, 1855

MINERS' CRAMPS

heat cramps in coal miners

> Brit. Med. J. 1:65, 1929

MINERS' DERMATITIS

skin irritation of hookworm disease among coal miners

> Hunter, D. The Diseases of Occupations. 5th ed. London: The English Univ. Press Ltd., 1975

MINERS' DISEASE

silicosis of coal miners

> Lancet 2:1253, 1906

MINERS' DYSPNEA

COAL WORKERS' PNEUMOCONIOSIS

> original source not identified

MINER'S ELBOW

bursitis over the posterior aspect of the elbow (compare BEAT ELBOW)

Lancet 2:272, 1841

MINER'S HEADACHE

headache from the gases produced by explosives

Dorland's Medical Dictionary. 25th ed. Phila.: W. B. Saunders, 1974

MINER'S ITCH

skin irritation from the dirty work and skin maceration produced by wetness in the coal mines

Brit. Med. J. 2:500, 1922

MINER'S LUNG

anthracosis of the lungs

Stedman's Medical Dictionary. 23rd ed. Baltimore: William & Wilkins, 1976

MINERS' LUNG DISEASE

silicosis in coal miners

Brit. Med. J. 1:903, 1911

MINERS' MELANOSIS

black discoloration of the lungs of coal miners

original source not identified

MINERS' NYSTAGMUS

rapid horizontal movements of the eyeballs, often associated with sensitivity to light and headache occurring in coal face mine workers

Brit. Med. J. 1:11, 1874

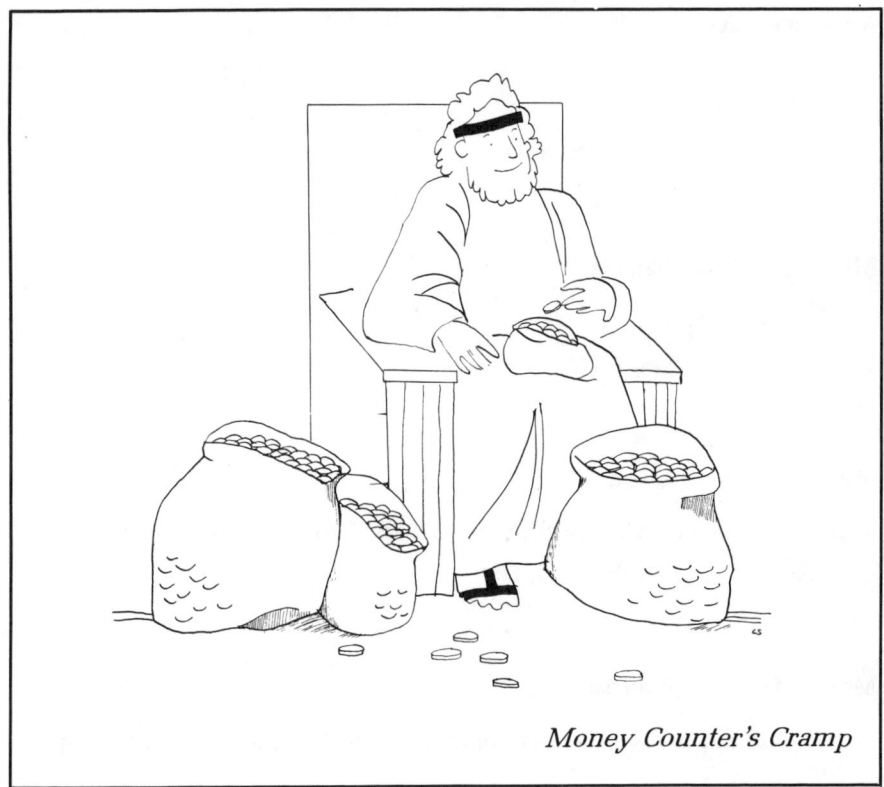

Money Counter's Cramp

MINERS' PHTHISIS

chronic pulmonary disease among miners, such as anthracosis, silicosis, chalicosis, siderosis, etc.

Brit. Med. J. 2:568, 1903

MINERS' ROT

MINERS' PHTHISIS

Allbutt's Syst. Med. 5:244, 1898

MINERS' TUBERCULOSIS

silicotuberculosis

International Classification of Diseases. 8th rev. USDHEW Pub. Hlth. Serv Pub. No. 1963, 1968

TRADE DISEASES

Minister's Ail

laryngitis from overuse of the voice (compare CLERGYMAN'S SORE THROAT)

Bost. Med. & Surg. J. 23:3, 1840

Minister's Sore Throat

MINISTER'S AIL

Bost. Med. & Surg. J. 23:3, 1840

Minute Man Disease

lead intoxication occurring in an ICBM missile silo sandblaster

Arch. Environ. Hlth. 10:801, 1965

Mold Machine Pneumonia

polymer fume fever occurring in polyurethane-foam-molding operators

J. Occup. Med. 16:481, 1974

Monday Diseases

any of the group of ailments which reach a peak on Monday; e.g. BRASS MOLDER'S AGUE, FOUNDRY FEVER, ZINC CHILLS, etc.

JAMA 183:39, 1963

Monday Fever

tendency for the chest tightness of BYSSINOSIS to be more pronounced on return to work after a week-end at home, subsiding by the following day (compare MONDAY SYNDROME, HACKLERS' MONDAY)

Brit. Med. J. 2:1069, 1948

Monday Head

nitrate-induced headache among workers in a pharmaceutical plant making a coronary artery dilator drug (compare MONDAY HEADACHE)

Brit. Med. J. 2:745, 1961

Monday Headache

nitroglycerine headache in munition workers following loss of habituation after a week-end free from exposure (compare MONDAY HEAD)

Brit. Med. J. 2:746, 1961

Monday Syndrome

chest tightness, shortness of breath, nasal irritation, cough and headache occurring on exposure to cotton, flax or hemp dust after an absence from work (compare MONDAY FEVER)

Arch. Environ. Hlth. 14:531, 1967

Monday Tightness

MONDAY SYNDROME

CMA Jour. 114:435, 1976

Money Counter's Cramp

(a most acceptable disease) see OCCUPATIONAL NEUROSIS

Hunter, D. The Diseases of Occupations. 5th ed. London: The English Univ. Press Ltd., 1975

Money Counters' Disease

skin eruption, anemia and weakness afflicting those who count bank notes, attributed to arsenic intoxication from the arsenites used in paper

N. Eng. Med. Monthly 3:46, 1883

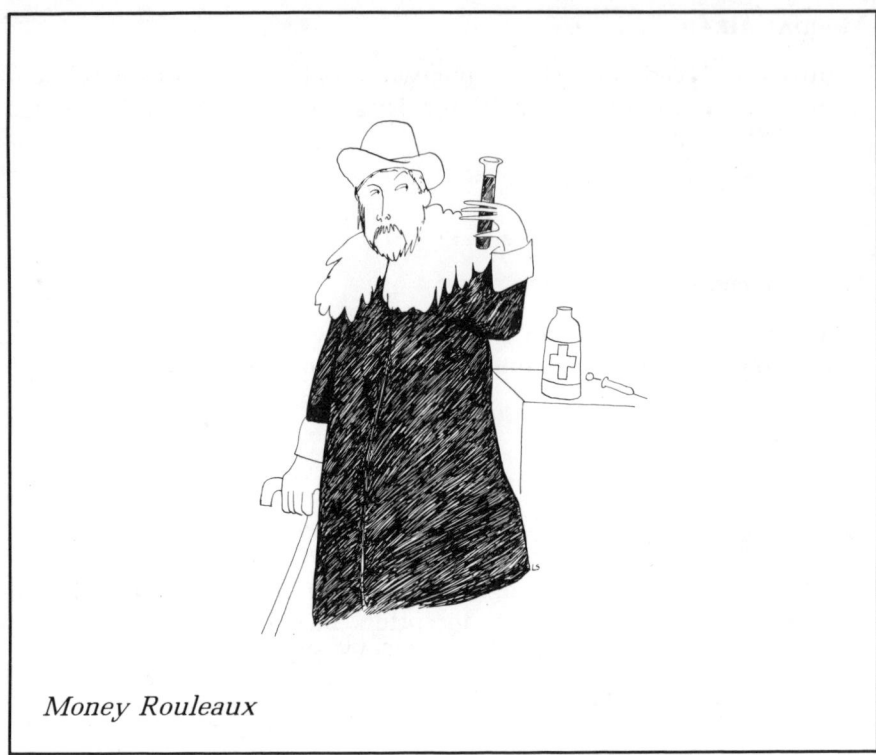

Money Rouleaux

MONEY ROULEAUX

Baron Rothschild, on having his blood examined, was told that the red blood corpuscles showed a tendency to the formation of "money rouleaux." He replied, "What is bred in the bone will out in the blood."

Bost. Med. & Surg. J. 137:327, 1897

MORBUS BRITANNICUS

heat exhaustion among sailors of British trawlers

Lancet 1:23, 1936

MOSQUITOS

skin irritation from caustic exposure in the chloralkali industry

original source not identified

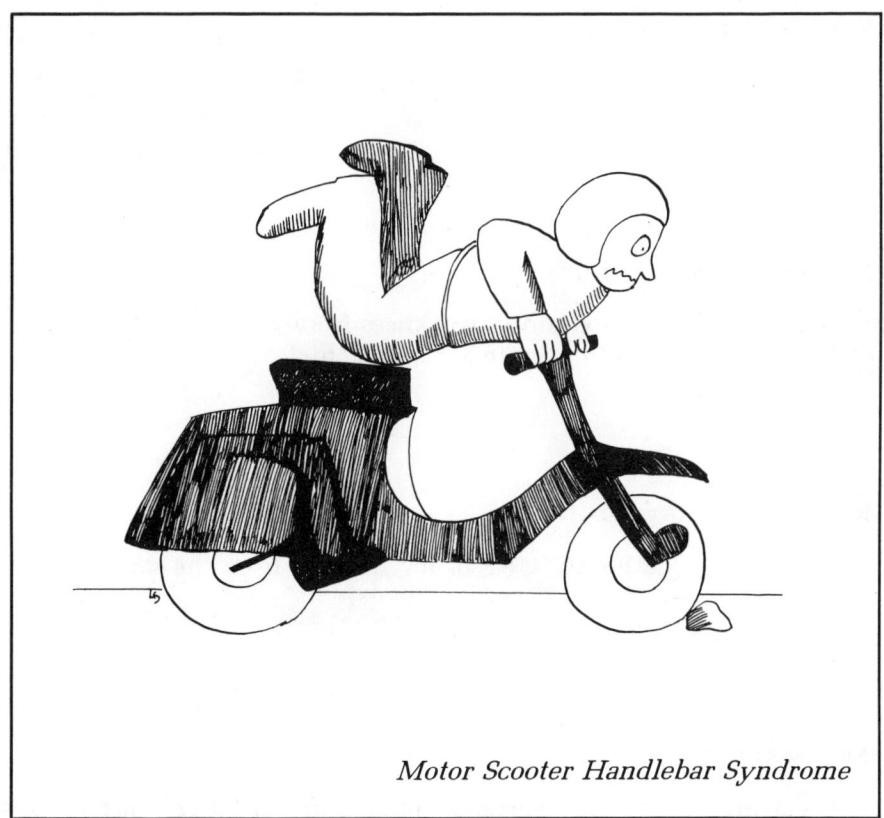

Motor Scooter Handlebar Syndrome

Mother-Of-Pearl Worker's Osteomyelitis

PEARL WORKER'S OSTEOMYELITIS

Rev. de Chir. 22:10, 1903

Motor Backache

backache and neuralgia from a poorly-fitting automobile seat

Brit. Med. J. 2:791, 1934

Motor Conjunctivitis

eye irritation caused by dust and wind exposure from riding in open cars

Brit. Med. J. 1:935, 1914

TRADE DISEASES

Motorcyclist's Ptosis

drooping and fluttering of the upper eyelid following prolonged motorcycle riding

Lancet 2:972, 1954

Motor Driver's Spine

right hip pain and extremity weakness from jarring and the muscular effort required to operate a motor vehicle

Lancet 2:23, 1906

Motorist's Fractures

CHAUFFEUR'S FRACTURE or leg fracture from the same mechanism

Lancet 1:962, 1904

Motorist's Heel

heel pain caused by local pressure plus an upward tilt of the foot used on the accelerator pedal

Brit. Med. J. 2:855, 1929

Motorist's Knee

pain and stiffness over the inner side of the knee due to poor positioning of the auto foot controls

Brit. Med. J. 2:1142, 1929

Motor Scooter Handlebar Syndrome

injury to the external iliac artery in the abdomen from impact by the motor scooter handlebar in an accident

Lancet 2:1051, 1968

Moulder's Bronchitis

fibrotic lung disease caused by the chronic inhalation of silica dust in a foundry

> International Classification of Diseases. 8th rev. USDHEW Pub. Hlth. Serv. Pub. No. 1963, 1968

Moulder's Tuberculosis

silicotuberculosis in foundry workers

> International Classification of Diseases. 8th rev. USDHEW Pub. Hlth. Serv. Pub. No. 1963, 1968

Mountain Climber's Syndrome

dizziness, nausea, shortness of breath, headache, thirst and fatigue from decreased oxygen

> original source not identified

Mountain Disease

oxygen deficiency from ascending mountains, from balloon ascents and from other high altitude activities

> Brit. Med. J. 2:873, 1881

Mountaineering Malady

ALTITUDE SICKNESS from climbing mountains

> Lancet 1:1524, 1893

Mountain Fever

altitude sickness

> Stedman's Medical Dictionary. 23rd ed. Baltimore: William & Wilkins, 1976

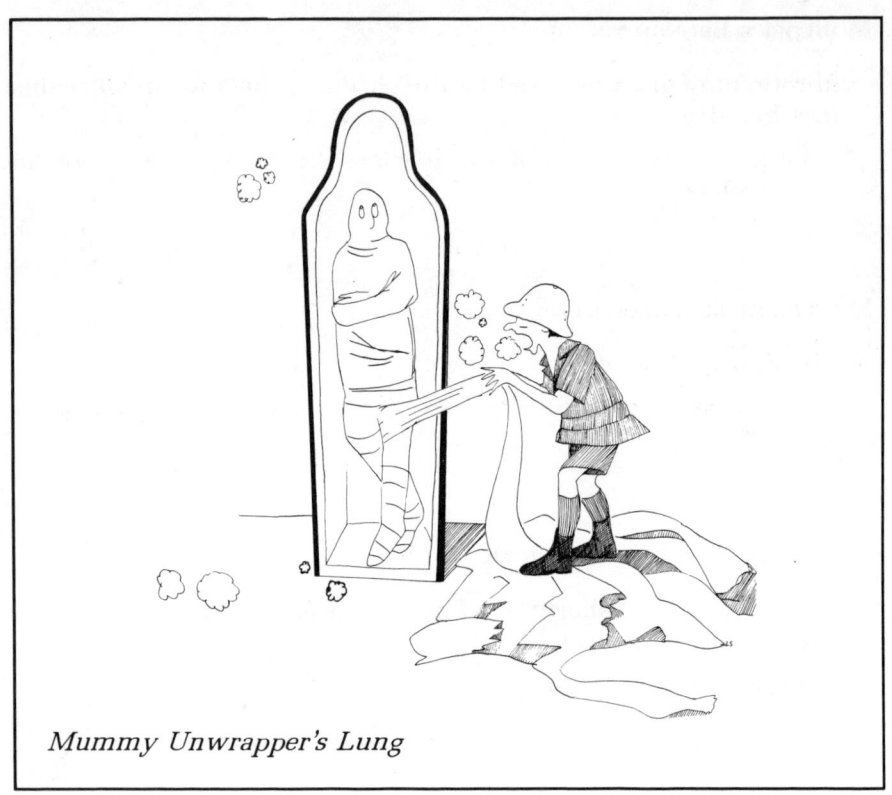
Mummy Unwrapper's Lung

MOUNTAIN SICKNESS

ALTITUDE SICKNESS

Arch. Int. Med. 59:32, 1937

MULE SPINNERS' CANCER

cancer of the scrotum among cotton mule spinners from contact with spindle oil and from pressure of the body against the spindle carriage (mule) (compare SPINNERS' CANCER)

Brit. Med. J. 2:971, 1922

MULE SPINNERS' DISEASE

MULE SPINNERS' CANCER

Brit. Med. J. 2:971, 1922

Mummy Unwrapper's Lung

allergic inflammatory response of the lungs to inhaled organic compounds contained in mummy wrappings

Sci. News. 112:296, 1977

Museum Fatigue

exhaustion associated with long museum tours

JAMA 90:1120, 1928

Mushroom Grower's Lung

MUSHROOM WORKER'S LUNG

Senr. Hop. Paris 49:3639, 1973

Mushroom Picker's Lung

MUSHROOM WORKER'S LUNG

Hunter, D. The Diseases of Occupations. 5th ed. London: The English Univ. Press Ltd., 1975

Mushroom Worker's Lung

allergic inflammatory response of the lungs to the inhalation of mushroom mold

JAMA 171:15, 1959

Mushroom Worker's Pneumonitis

MUSHROOM WORKER'S LUNG

Ann. Allergy 33:282, 1974

Musician's Cramp

see OCCUPATIONAL NEUROSIS

Bost. Med. & Surg. J. 72:156, 1865

MUSICIAN'S MOUTH

physical changes associated with playing certain instruments; i.e., a mark on the lower lip caused by compression of the lip between a reed instrument and the lower front teeth; bone absorption of the lower teeth from heavy instruments such as the saxophone; lip lesions from brass instruments with large mouthpieces; and allergic reactions to some woods

Lancet 2:1084, 1953

MUSICIAN'S NEUROSIS

see OCCUPATIONAL NEUROSIS

Singer, K. Diseases of the Musical Profession. (tr. by W. Lakond, Greensberg, N.Y., 1932)

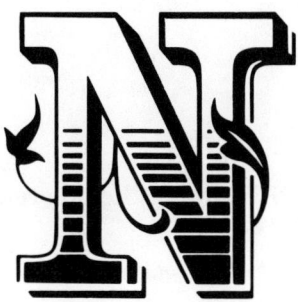

Nailers' Consumption

cough, sputum production, emaciation, chills and fever noted in nail makers due to the inhalation of fine mineral particles

Bost. Med. & Surg. J. 114:396, 1886

Nail Gun Injury

any penetrating injury produced by a nail-gun missile

J. Bone & Joint. Surg. 53A:383, 1971

Nail Maker's Cramp

see OCCUPATIONAL NEUROSIS

Lancet 2:333, 1886

Nailsmith's Cramp

see OCCUPATIONAL NEUROSIS

Brit. Med. J. 1:11, 1886

Naphtha Jag

dizziness, headache, nausea and transient excitement followed by depression from the inhalation of benzene fumes by rubber workers

JAMA 69:2039, 1917

Navvies' Disease

SHOVELER'S FRACTURE among the laborers (navvies) who work on canals and railroads

Suppl. to Occup. & Hlth. p. 7. ILO. Geneva, Oct. 1939

Needle Grinder's Siderosis

fibrotic lung disease caused by chronic inhalation of silica dust and characterized by cough, blood spitting and emaciation

Mem. Med. Soc., London 5:89, 1799

Newspaper Folder's Cramp

see OCCUPATIONAL NEUROSIS

Hunter, D. The Diseases of Occupations. 5th ed. London: The English Univ. Press Ltd., 1975

NG Head

NITROGLYCERINE HEAD

JAMA 54:793, 1910

Nickel Platers' Rash

eruption of the hands, forearms and neck of metal platers due to nickel sensitivity

Urol. & Cut. Rev. 33:606, 1929

Nickel Refiner's Itch

dermatitis caused by nickel sensitivity

Zbl. Gen. Hyg. Nr. 8 S. 185, 1908

Niggles

mild symptoms of the bends (DECOMPRESSION SICKNESS) (compare CREEPS)

original source not identified

Night Nurse's Paralysis

a condition similar to "sleep paralysis" in which one awakens to full consciousness after a terrifying dream to find that he cannot move a muscle, open his eyes or even cry out for help

Lancet 2:1324, 1954

Nitrate Head

NITROGLYCERINE HEAD

Brit. Med. J. 2:745, 1961

Nitrogen Narcosis

loss of emotional control, motor incoordination and unconsciousness among divers, caused by nitrogen intoxication

Physiol. Rev. 25:1, 1945

Nitroglycerine Head

flushing of the skin and severe headache in explosive manufacture workers due to the absorption of nitroglycerine

JAMA 54:793, 1910

Nitroglycerine Headache

headache among dynamite workers due to the vasodilating effect of nitroglycerine

>Hunter, D. The Diseases of Occupations. 5th ed. London: The English Univ. Press Ltd., 1975

Noxious Trades

trades stigmatized by poor health conditions in the late 19th century; e.g., slaughterhouses, wool scouring work, tanneries, tallow works, etc.

>Med. J. Austral. 2:1109, 1971

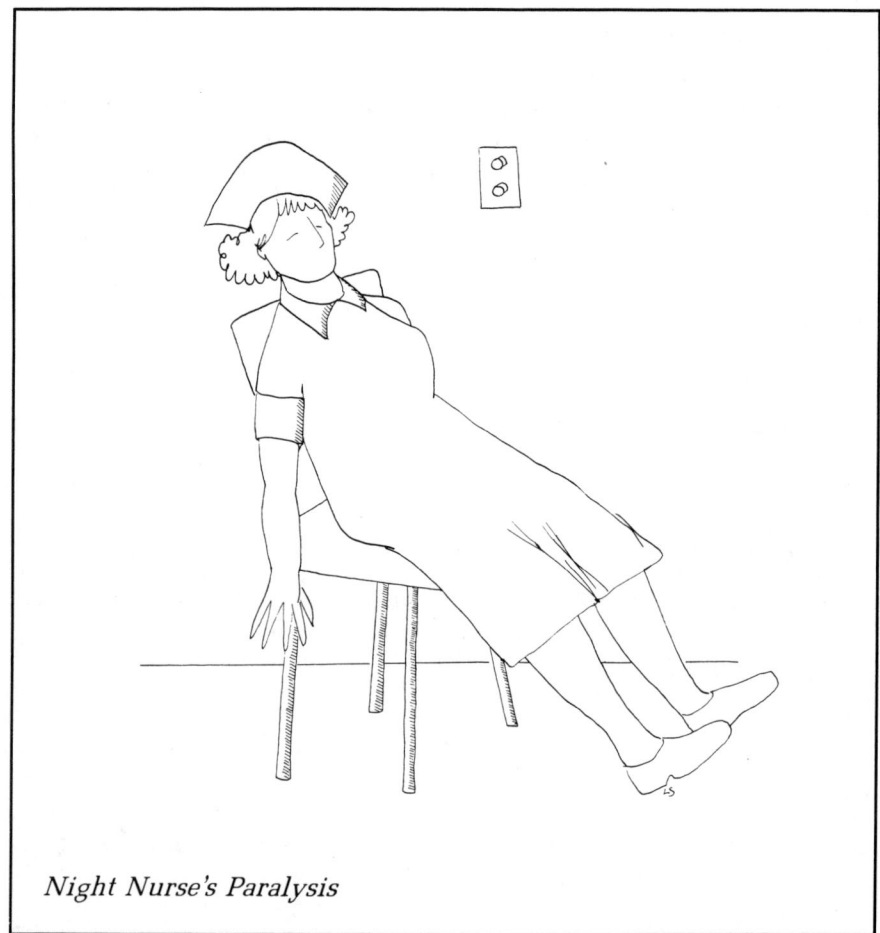

Night Nurse's Paralysis

Nun's Bursitis

swelling over the front of the knee cap from the repeated pressure and friction of kneeling.

> Hunter, D. The Diseases of Occupations. 5th ed. London: The English Univ. Press Ltd., 1975

Nun's Knee

NUN'S BURSITIS

> International Classification of Diseases. 8th rev. USDHEW Pub. Hlth. Serv. Pub. No. 1963, 1968

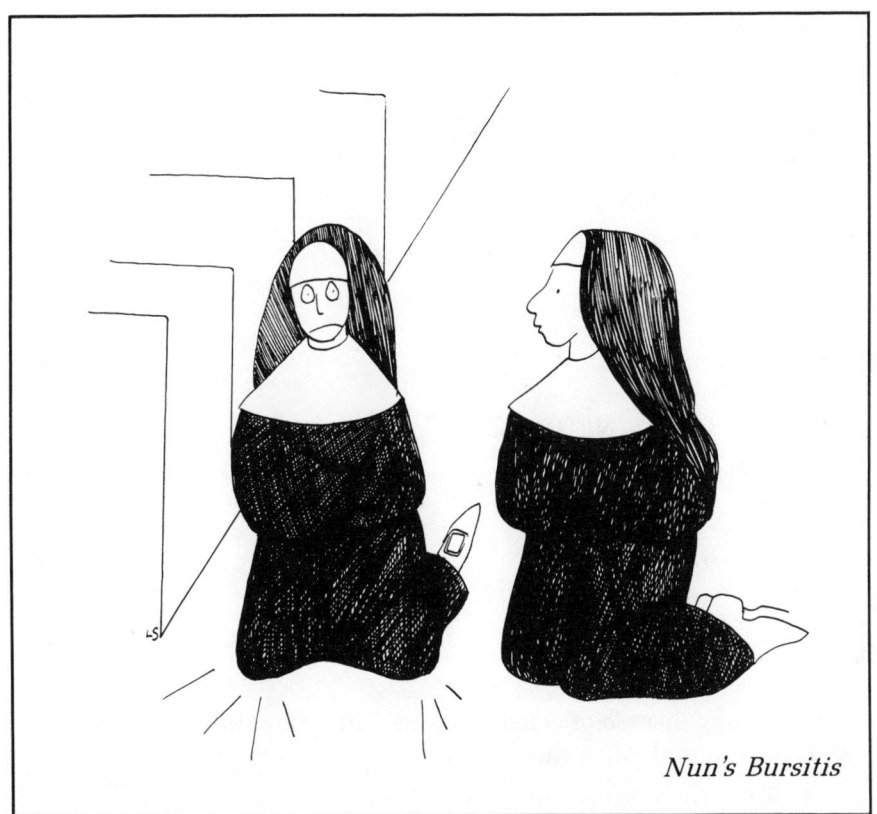

Nun's Bursitis

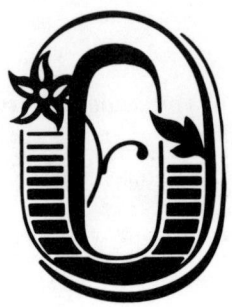

Occupational Neurosis

spasm or pain, often with a total loss of function, in a special group of muscles used for coordinated intricate movements of a particular vocation or avocation

    Brit. Med. J. 1:319, 1933

Occupational Spasm

OCCUPATIONAL NEUROSIS

    International Classification of Diseases. 8th rev. USDHEW Pub. Hlth. Serv. Pub. No. 1963, 1968

Ocher Lung

fibrotic lung disease of ocher workers caused by the chronic inhalation of iron and silica dust

    Arch. Gewerbepath. u. Gewerbehyg. 18:349, 1961

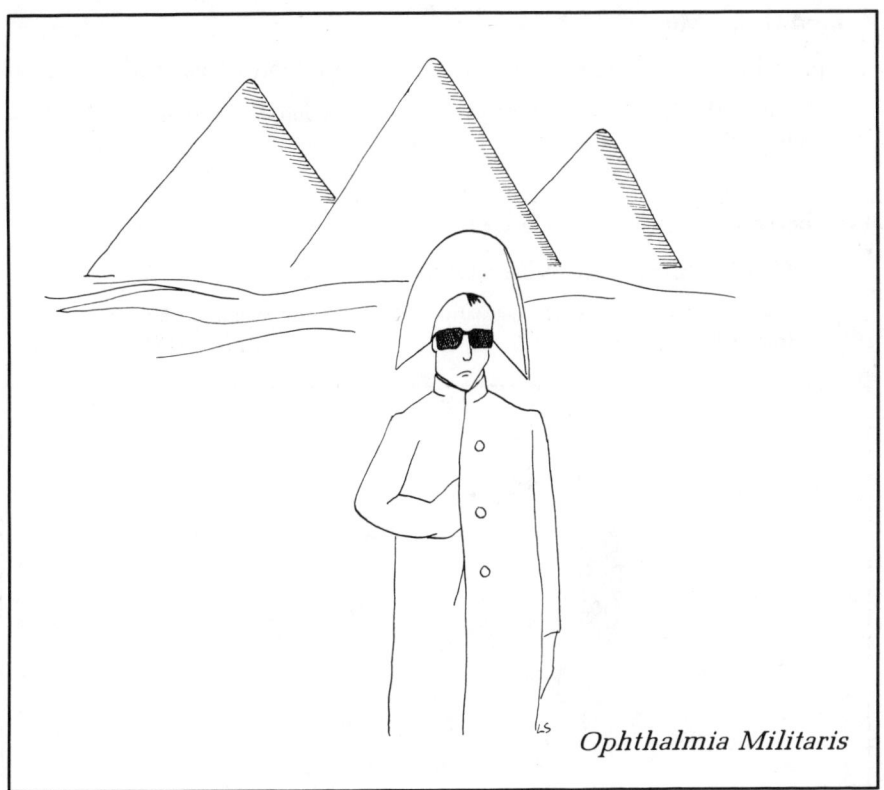
Ophthalmia Militaris

Ocher Pneumoconiosis

OCHER LUNG

Arch. f. Gewerbepath. 9:487, 1939

Oil Refiner's Dermatitis

irritation of the hair follicles from saturation with oil, sometimes followed by thickening of the horny layer of the skin

Hunter, D. The Diseases of Occupations. 5th ed. London: The English Univ. Press Ltd., 1975

Ophthalmia Electrica

eye irritation from exposure to a welding arc

USN Med. Bull. 46:247, 1946

OPHTHALMIA MILITARIS

epidemic eye disease which afflicted Napoleon's Egyptian troops

Hunter, D. The Diseases of Occupations. 5th ed. London: The English Univ. Press Ltd., 1975

ORCHESTRA CONDUCTOR'S CRAMP

see OCCUPATIONAL NEUROSIS

Hunter, D. The Diseases of Occupations. 5th ed. London: The English Univ. Press Ltd., 1975

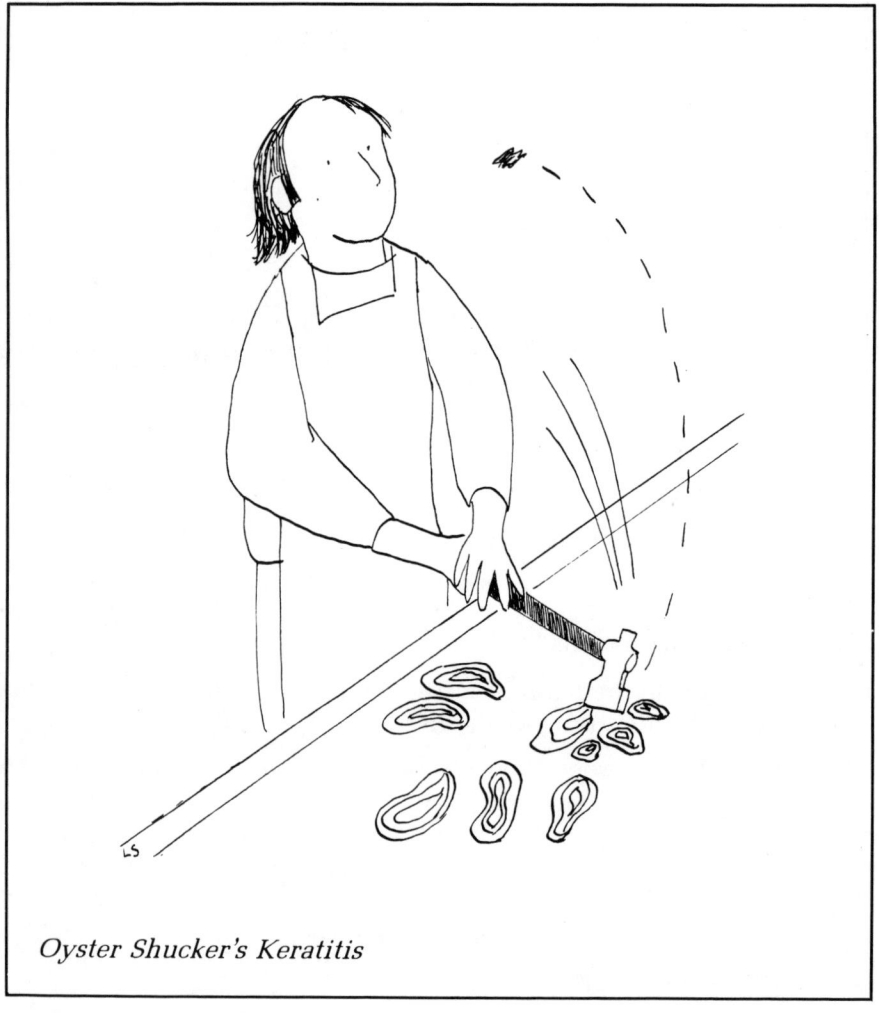

Oyster Shucker's Keratitis

ORGANIST'S CRAMP

see OCCUPATIONAL NEUROSIS

Hunter, D. The Diseases of Occupations. 5th ed. London: The English Univ. Press Ltd., 1975

OYSTER SHUCKERS' ASTHMA

SEASQUIRT ASTHMA

Jap. J. Allergol. 16:349, 1967

OYSTER SHUCKER'S KERATITIS

eye irritation and ulceration from contact with small fragments of oyster shell driven off when the shell is hammered in shucking

Brit. Med. J. 1:50, 1896

OYSTER WORKER'S ASTHMA

SEASQUIRT ASTHMA

Hir. J. Med. Sci. 18:141, 1969

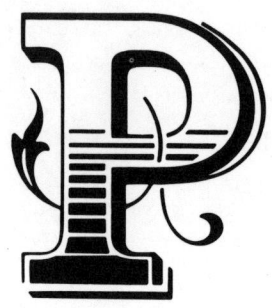

Packing Case Maker's Cramp

see OCCUPATIONAL NEUROSIS

Lancet 2:333, 1886

Pack Palsy

BACKPACK PALSY

Bull. U.S. Army Med. Dept. 2:112, 1944

Paddy Field Foot

IMMERSION FOOT among Vietnam troops in the 1960's

Lancet 1:1043, 1967

Painters' Colic

lead colic occurring in painters handling lead paints

Dana, S. L. Lead Diseases: A Treatise from the French of L. Tanquerel des Planches. Boston: Tappan, 1850

Painter's Cramp

see OCCUPATIONAL NEUROSIS

Brit. Med. J. 1:11, 1886

Painters' Colic

Hunter, D. The Diseases of Occupations. 5th ed. London: The English Univ. Press Ltd., 1975

Paint Gun Injury

accidental injection of paint beneath the skin from contact with an operating pressure paint gun

J. Bone & Joint. Sur. 49A:637, 1967

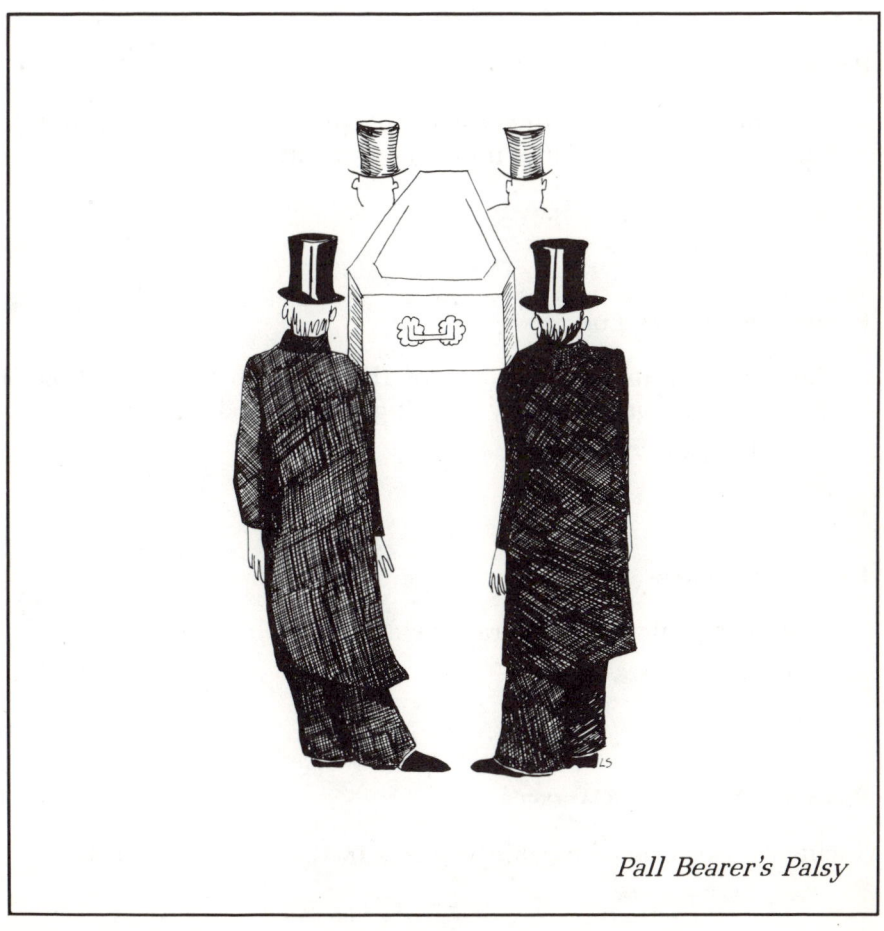

Pall Bearer's Palsy

Pall Bearer's Palsy

altered sensation and reflexes of an upper extremity from pressure caused by carrying a coffin on the shoulder

Brit. Med. J. 2:808, 1966

Pantie-Girdle Syndrome

tingling or swelling of the feet and legs from wearing a constricting pantie-girdle

Brit. Med. J. 2:407, 1972

Paper Folder's Fingers

deviation of the index finger and calluses of the index and middle fingers from folding large numbers of documents

Brit. Med. J. 2:1166, 1954

Paprika Splitter's Lung

allergic inflammatory response of the lungs to the inhalation of capsicum dust generated by splitting paprika pods

Aerzt. Sachver. Ztg. 42:297, 1936

Paraffin Plukes

small skin boils seen in paraffin workers

Brit. Med. J. 2:1528, 1903

Paraffin Workers' Cancer

cutaneous cancer of paraffin workers in the shale oil industry

Brit. Med. J. 2:1108, 1922

Paratrooper's Fracture

fracture of the ankle sustained on landing from a jump

original source not identified

Parsnip Ill

skin irritation of the wrists and forearms of cow parsnip gatherers due to parsnip oil

Brit. J. Derm. 45:301, 1933

Parson's Knee

swelling over the front of the knee cap from the repeated pressure and friction of kneeling

original source not identified

Peach Fever

skin eruption, eye and nose irritation, asthma, fever and malaise seen among peach packers and canners

Brit. Med. J. 1:1076, 1893

Pearl Grinders' Phthisis

bronchitis of pearl button makers due to the inhalation of pearl dust

Brit. Med. J. 1:389, 1892

Pearl Worker's Disease

bronchitis caused by pearl dust inhalation

Thackrah, C. T. The Effects of Arts, Trades and Professions On Health and Longevity. London: Longman, 1832

PEARL WORKER'S OSTEOMYELITIS

Brit. Med. J. 1:910, 1890

Pearl Worker's Osteomyelitis

firm, painful swelling of the bones of the face or extremities developing after exposure to mother-of-pearl dust

JAMA 41:1235, 1903

Peasant's Skin

FARMER'S SKIN

White, R. P. The Dermatogoses or Occupational Affections of the Skin. London: H. K. Lewis, 1928

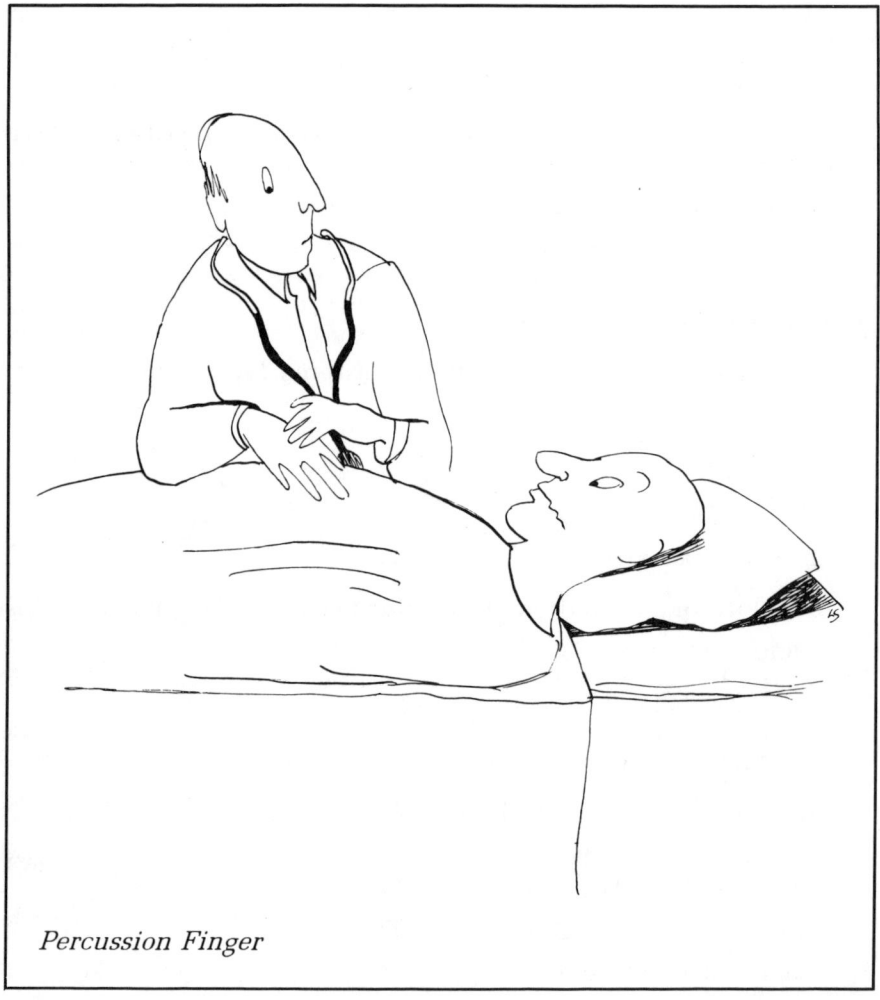

Percussion Finger

Pension Disease

physical, emotional and social degeneration occurring as a result of inactivity in the retirement phase of life

Mech. Illus. 73:10, 1977

Percussion Finger

swelling over the top of the middle finger of physicians who use this finger in bimanual percussion (thumping) of the chest

Brit. Med. J. 2:440, 1949

Permanent Waver's Cramp

see OCCUPATIONAL NEUROSIS

Lancet 1:1195, 1929

Petromortis

carbon monoxide poisoning via exhaust gases of gasoline engines

Lancet 2:317, 1921

Pheasant Hunter's Toe

gout alleged to trauma, fatigue and exposure while hunting

Stedman's Medical Dictionary. 23rd ed. Baltimore: William & Wilkins, 1976

Phosphoritis

reddening and peeling of the skin of workers exposed to phosphorus sesquesulfide in match manufacturing

Bull. de Soc. Franc. de Derm. et Syph. p. 218, Mar. 1929

Phossy

PHOSSY JAW

Brit. Med. J. 1:238, 1892

PHOSSY JAW

degeneration of the jaw bone in match factory workers suffering from chronic phosphorus poisoning (compare LUCIFER MATCH MAKERS' DISEASE)

Brit. Med. J. 1:434, 1863

PHOTOGRAPHER'S DERMATITIS

skin irritation caused by metol contaminated with phenylenediamine

Klin. Wochen. 11:240, 1932

PHOTOGRAPHER'S ECZEMA

PHOTOGRAPHER'S DERMATITIS

JAMA 76:540, 1921

PHOTOGRAPHER'S SKIN DISEASE

PHOTOGRAPHER'S DERMATITIS

Brit. Med. J. 2:648, 1898

PIANIST'S CRAMP

see OCCUPATIONAL NEUROSIS

Lancet 2:333, 1886

PIANOFORTE PLAYER'S CRAMP

see OCCUPATIONAL NEUROSIS

Brit. Med. J. 1:912, 1883

PICKLE JAR TYER'S CRAMP

see OCCUPATIONAL NEUROSIS

Lancet 2:333, 1886

Pig Breeders' Disease

a three phase illness (gastroenteritis, skin eruption and nervous system symptoms) occurring among pig breeders and presumed to be due to a virus

Suppl. to Occup. & Hlth. ILO. Sept. 1938

Pigeon Breeder's Lung

allergic inflammatory response of the lungs to inhaled avian protein

Brit. J. Exp. Path. 13:461, 1932

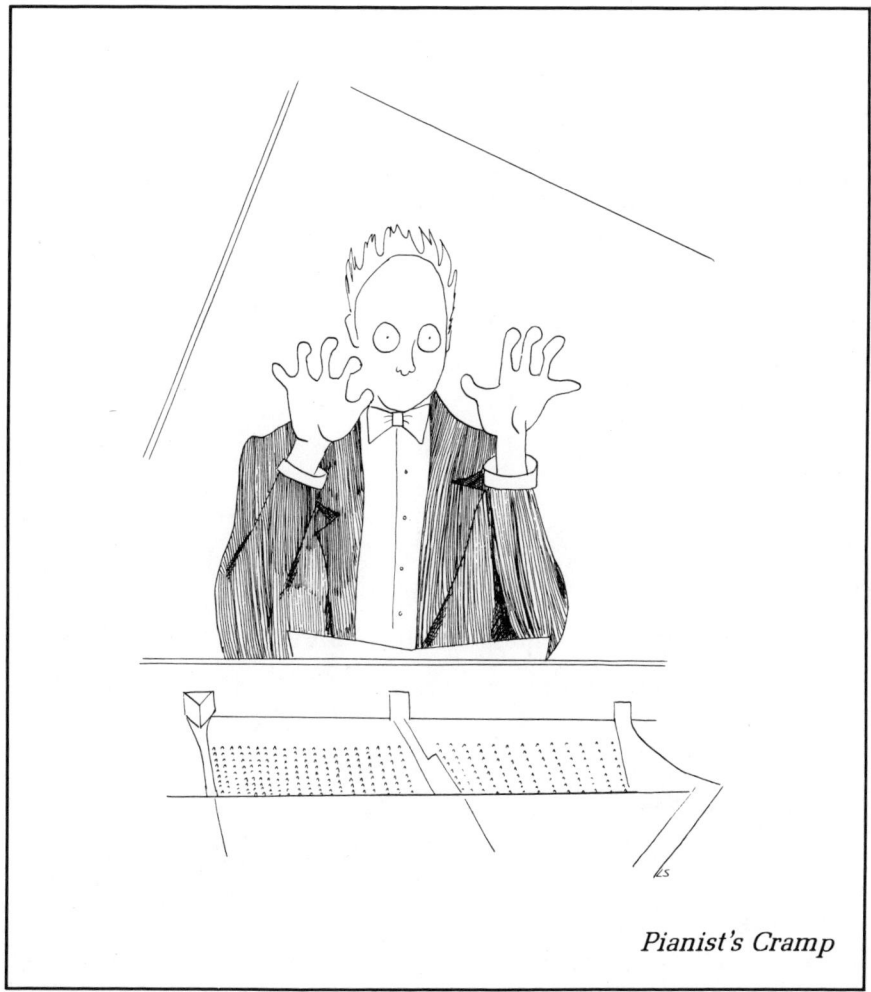

Pianist's Cramp

Pigeon Fancier's Lung

PIGEON BREEDER'S LUNG

Hunter, D. The Diseases of Occupations. 5th ed. London: The English Univ. Press Ltd., 1975

Pig's Feet

swellings over the thumbs of railway carriage cleaners caused by friction from the cleaning brush handle

Brit. Med. J. 1:280, 1927

Pillion Rider's Pelvic Split

damage to the soft tissues between the thighs accompanied by separation of the pelvic bones following motorcycle accidents

Lancet 1:20, 1932

Pilots' Neurosis

AVIATORS' NEUROSIS

JAMA 107:809, 1936

Pilots' Vertigo

spatial disorientation in pilots (compare SATELLITE SICKNESS)

Aerosp. Med. 31:189, 1960

Pineapple Fingers

erosion of the finger tips of pineapple canners caused by contact with the proteolytic enzyme in pineapple juice and the rough spears on the husk

Brit. Med. J. 1:1232, 1955

Pinginits

inflammation of the forearm hair follicles of fishermen from contact with coal tar used on fishing nets

JAMA 104:2326, 1935

Ping Pong Tenosynovitis

inflammation of the tendon sheath of the leg muscle (tibialis anticus) from playing ping pong

Brit. Med. J. 1:1083, 1902

Pitcher's Elbow

pain over either side of the elbow from overexertion

JAMA 153:74, 1953

pain and bone degeneration over the inner side of the elbow

Encyclopedia of Sports Sci. & Med. N.Y.: Macmillan Co., 1971

Pitcher's Glass Arm

painful arm from baseball pitching

JAMA 93:321, 1929

Pitch Worker's Cancer

brownish raised skin lesions following prolonged contact with pitch which sometimes develop into cancer

Arch. Derm. & Syph. 31:721, 1935

Pitch Worker's Papillomata

cancerous changes in the skin due to pitch or tar exposure

Brit. J. Ind. Med. 27:160, 1970

PLANKER'S HAND

loss of hand hair, loosening and discoloration of the fingernails and thickening of the ends of the fingers from "planking" felt hats (kneading the basic felt form of the hat)

Brit. Med. J. 1:379, 1902

PLANKER'S SEGS

callosities over the prominent portions of the palms of the hands from planking felt hat forms

Ann. d' Hyg. 34:133, 1898

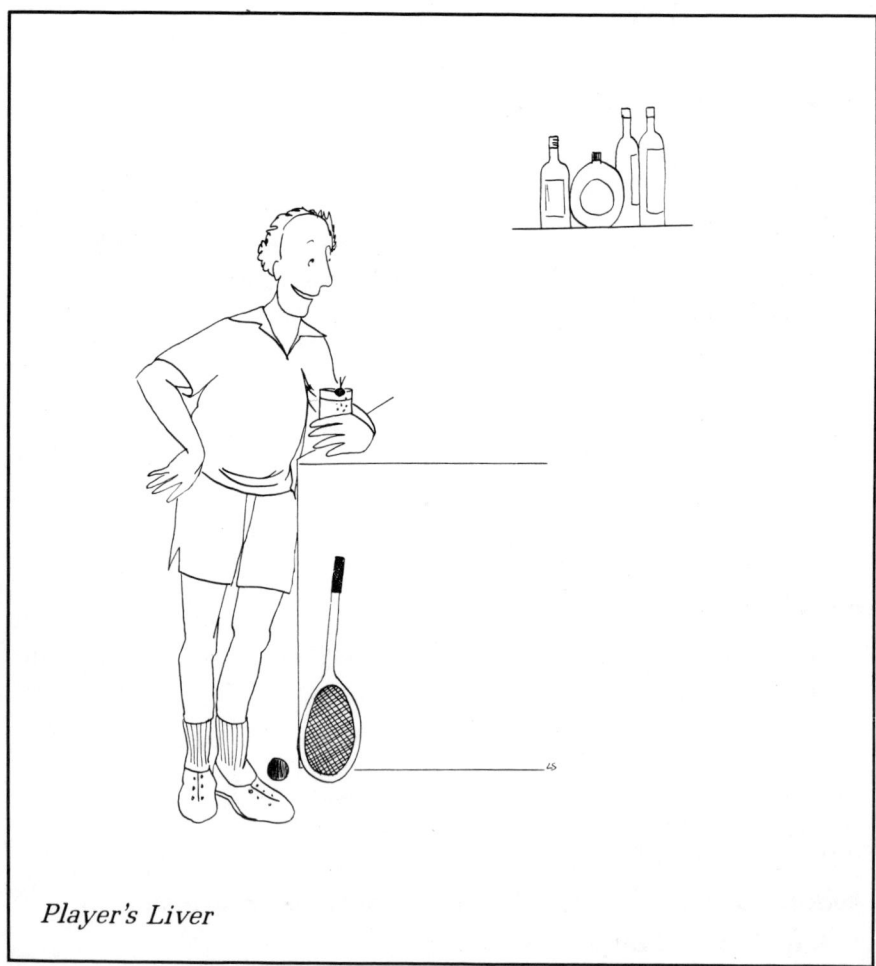

Player's Liver

Plasterer's Bunions

calluses over the knuckle joints of the thumb and index finger from holding the hawk (mortarboard)

Med. Rec. 89:560, 1916

Player's Liver

the hazard of spending more time at the bar talking about squash tennis than on the court playing the game

Encyclopedia of Sport Sci. & Med. N.Y.: Macmillan Co., 1971

Ploughman's Elbow

swelling over the right elbow from operating a farm tractor while leaning on the elbow against the mudguard

Brit. Med. J. 2:1358, 1958

Plumbers' Colic

lead colic among plumbers

Dana, S. L. Lead Diseases: A Treatise from the French of L. Tanquerel des Planches. Boston: Tappan, 1850

Pneumatic Drill Disease

PNEUMATIC HAMMER DISEASE

International Classification of Diseases. 8th rev. USDHEW Pub. Hlth. Serv. Pub. No. 1963, 1968

Pneumatic Hammer Disease

blanching and altered sensation of the fingers and hands of stone cutters who use vibratory tools

Proc. Staff Meet. Mayo Clinic 8:345, 1933

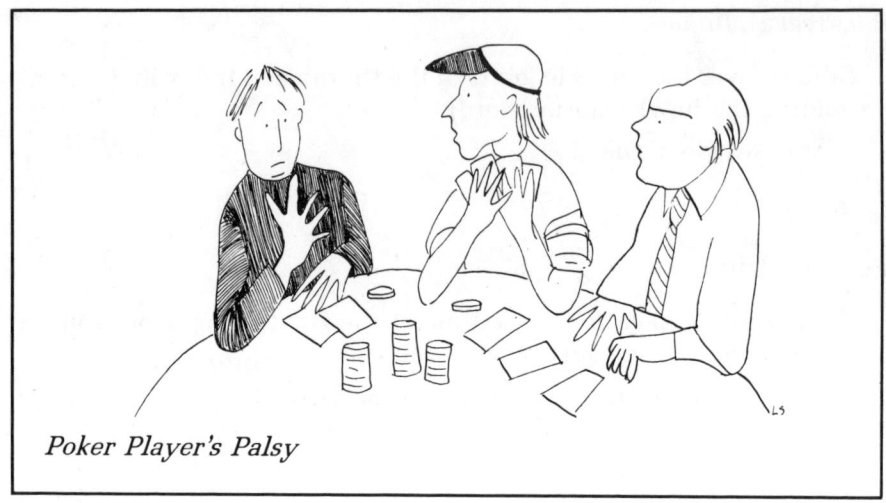
Poker Player's Palsy

POKER PLAYER'S PALSY

numbness and tingling of the ring and little fingers resulting from prolonged pressure of the elbow on the card table

N. Eng. J. Med. 259:620, 1958

POLAR ANEMIA

anemia in natives of temperate climates who are exposed to Arctic or Antarctic conditions

Stedman's Medical Dictionary. 23rd ed. Baltimore: William & Wilkins, 1976

weakness and heart trouble alleged to dietary deficiencies among Antarctic explorers

Brit. Med. J. 1:781, 1914

POLICEMEN'S DISEASE

painful ankle or foot from walking a beat

Billing's Natl. Med. Dict., 1890

POLICEMAN'S HEEL

painful heel

original source not identified

POLISHER'S KERATITIS

small vacuoles in the cornea of the eye associated with pain and light sensitivity following exposure to toluol, xylol, and methyl, ethyl and butyl acetate and other chemical irritants

   Arch. Gewerbepath. ü. Gewerbehyg. 15:37, 1956

POLISHERS' NODULES

hard brown skin nodules seen in emery polishers from pressure and friction

   Derm. Wochenschr. 81:1103, 1925

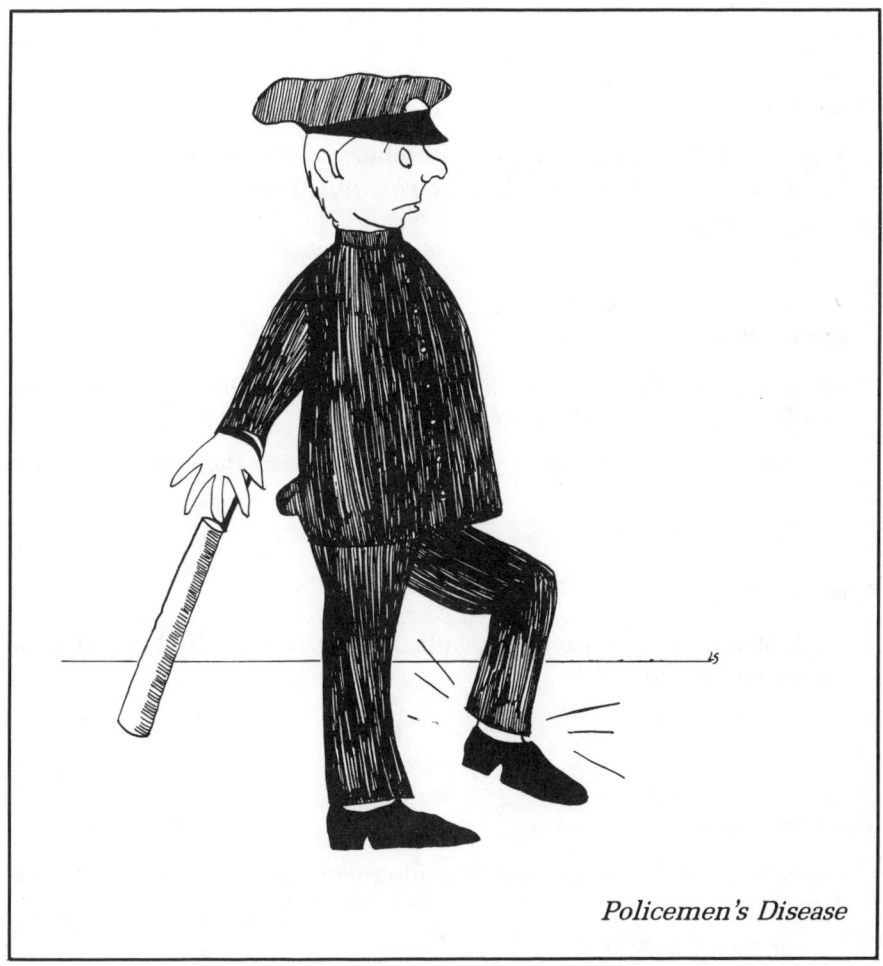

Policemen's Disease

TRADE DISEASES

Polymer Fume Fever

fever, chills, general aching and soreness of the throat, accompanied by weakness, sweating, nausea and vomiting, following the inhalation of a sublimate from heated polytetrafluoroethylene

Lancet 2:1008, 1951

Pope

injury to the anterior thigh muscle (rectus femoris) from a football injury

Lancet 2:790, 1888

Pork Finger

finger redness and pain among butchers, farmers and cooks caused by infection with *Erysipelothrix rhusiopathiae*

Lancet 1:680, 1953

Porter's Bursitis

swelling over the lower neck from carrying boxes balanced high on the back

Hunter, D. The Diseases of Occupations. 5th ed. London: The English Univ. Press Ltd., 1975

Porter's Neck

neck strain or fracture as a result of carrying 200 lb. bags of meal balanced on the head

Brit. Med. J. 2:16, 1968

Potters' Asthma

chronic chest disease (silicosis) among workers in the pottery industry

Brit. Med. J. 2:489, 1876

Potter's Colic

abdominal colic of lead intoxication from the lead glazes used in pottery

> Dana, S. L. Lead Diseases: A Treatise from the French of L. Tanquerel des Planches. Boston: Tappan, 1850

Potters' Consumption

silicotuberculosis occurring in workers employed in the pottery industry

> Brit. Med. J. 2:489, 1876

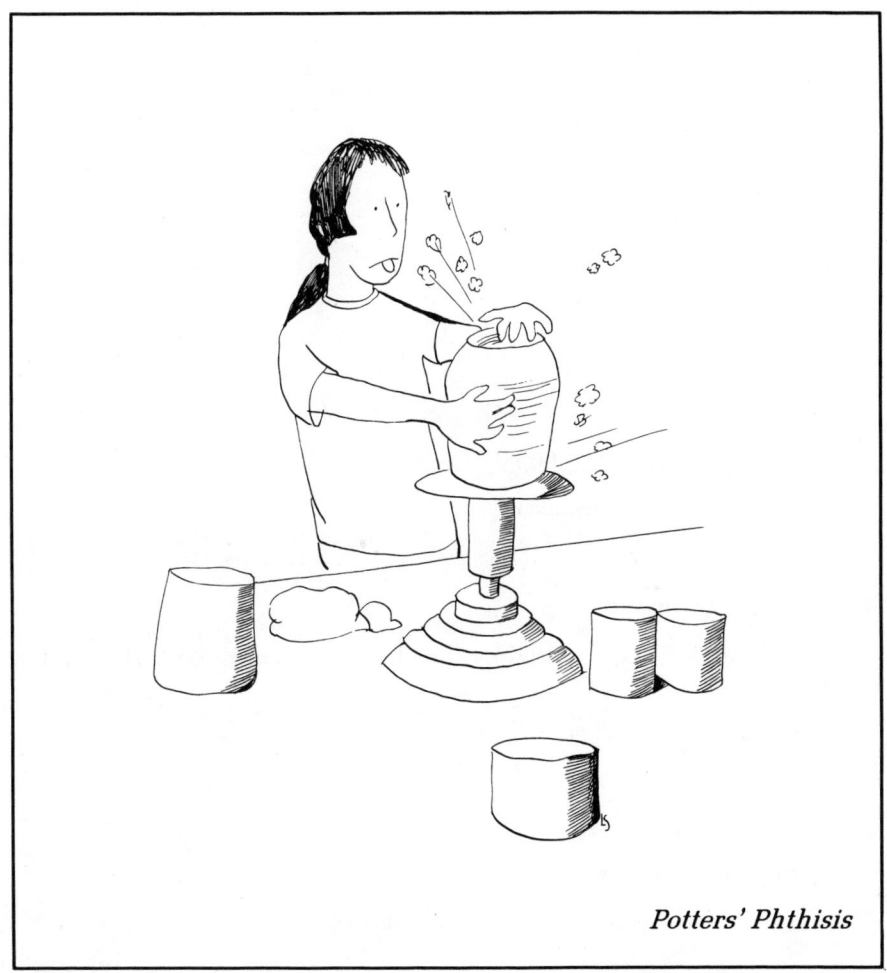

Potters' Phthisis

TRADE DISEASES

POTTERS' DISEASE
>   POTTERS' ASTHMA
>> Lancet 2:234, 1876

POTTERS' ECZEMA
> skin eruption of the hands and forearms of pottery workers from exposure to dust, frit or turpentine
>> Brit. Med. J. 2:491, 1908

POTTERS' LUNG
>   POTTERS' ASTHMA
>> Brit. Med. J. 1:766, 1889

POTTERS' PHTHISIS
>   POTTERS' ASTHMA
>> Lancet 2:1369, 1893

POTTERS' ROT
>   POTTERS' CONSUMPTION
>> original source not identified

POTTERS' SILICOSIS
> fibrotic lung disease caused by the chronic inhalation of silicon dioxide
>> Pub. Hlth. Bull. No. 244, Washington, 1939

POTTERS' TUBERCULOSIS
>   POTTERS' CONSUMPTION
>> International Classification of Diseases. 8th rev. USDHEW Pub. Hlth. Serv. Pub. No. 1963, 1968

Pottery Fireman's Cataract

cataract resulting from prolonged exposure of the eye to infrared radiation from the furnace

>Hunter, D. The Diseases of Occupations. 5th ed. London: The English Univ. Press Ltd., 1975

Pottery Workers' Silicosis

POTTERS' ASTHMA

>Oliver, T. Dangerous Trades. London: J. Murray, 1902

Poucey Chest

byssinosis caused by pouce, the French word for flax dust

>Brit. Med. J. 1:703, 1889

Poultry Keeper's Lung

allergic inflammatory response of the lungs to inhaled poultry dust

>Ger. Med. Mon. 15:245, 1970

Poultryman's Itch

dermatitis caused by contact with the poultry fungus *Trichophyton gallinae*

>International Classification of Diseases. 8th rev. USDHEW Pub. Hlth. Serv. Pub. No. 1963, 1968

Powder Headache

NITROCLYCERINE HEADACHE

>JAMA 32:671, 1899

PREACHERS' VOICE

CHORDITIS TUBEROSA

International Classification of Diseases. 8th rev. USDHEW Pub. Hlth. Serv. Pub. No. 1963, 1968

PRESSURE GUN INJECTION INJURY

accidental injection of foreign material beneath the skin by a pressure gun (compare GREASE GUN INJURY)

J. Bone Joint. Surg. 43A:485, 1961

PRINTER'S ASTHMA

bronchial asthma due to gum acacia and other allergens used in the color printing process

J. Allergy 12:290, 1941

PRINTER'S INK DERMATITIS

skin irritation of the face and neck from contact with para-red used in the ink

JAMA 91:870, 1928

PRINTER'S PALSY

chronic antimony intoxication

Dorland's Medical Dictionary. 25th ed. Phila.: W. B. Saunders, 1974

PRINTERS' PHTHISIS

pulmonary tuberculosis among printers due to poor working conditions and exposure to silica dust

JAMA 75:1438, 1920

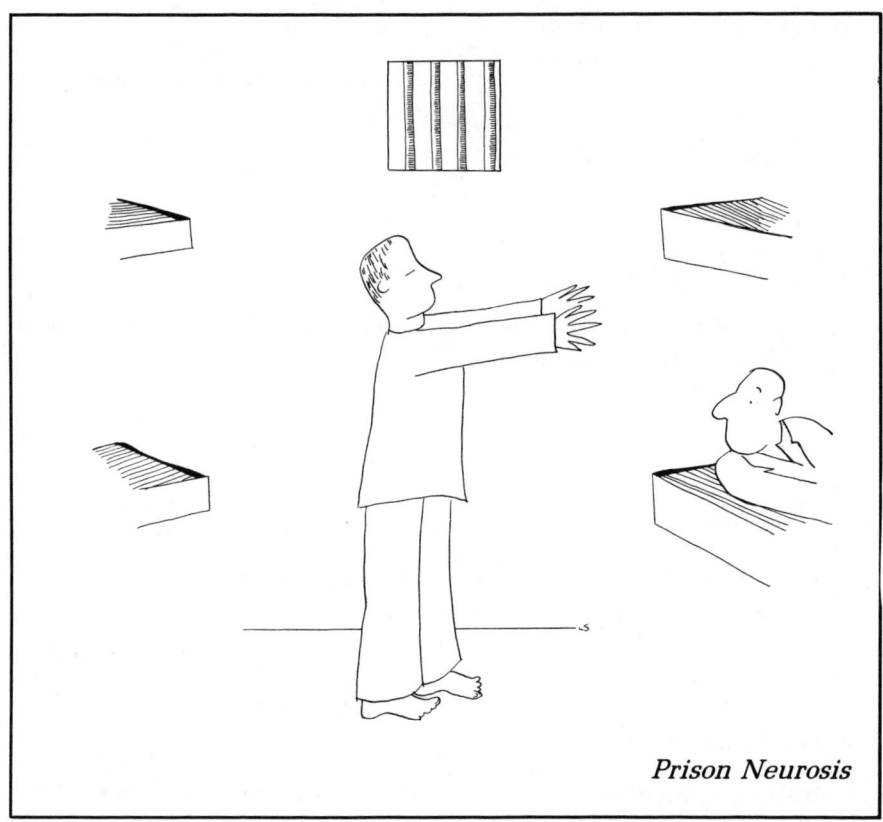
Prison Neurosis

Prison Neurosis

restlessness, irritability, insomnia, gastrointestinal disturbances and weight loss among prisoners

J. Mental & Nerv. Dis. 50:319, 1919

Prizefighter's Ear

deformity of the ear from repeated trauma

Sat. Eve. Post 31:2, 1909

Professional Cramp

see OCCUPATIONAL NEUROSIS

Brit. Med. J. 2:1166, 1888

TRADE DISEASES

PROOFREADER'S PROSTATITIS

inflammation of the prostate gland from reading sexually stimulating material

N. Eng. J. Med. 280:1130, 1969

PROPELLER FRACTURE

fracture of the arm at the elbow caused by a backfire when hand-cranking an airplane engine

Lancet 1:293, 1919

PROSECTOR'S WART

skin tuberculosis contracted by medical pathologists

Arch. Derm. 100:380, 1969

PSYCHOANALYST'S DISEASE

numbness and tingling of the hands with finger weakness from ulnar nerve pressure caused by resting the elbows on an armchair

N. Eng. J. Med. 259:302, 1958

PUDDLERS' CATARACT

cataract among iron smelters from prolonged exposure of the eye to infrared radiation

Brit. J. Ophth. 5:193, 1921

PULLED JOCKEY MUSCLE

tear of the thigh muscle (gracilis) from forcefully pulling the knees in while jump-riding

Encyclopedia of Sport Sci. & Med. N.Y.: Macmillan Co., 1971

Pump Bumps

calluses of the heel at the upper edge of the shoe occurring in box lacrosse players

Encyclopedia of Sport Sci. & Med. N.Y.: Macmillan Co., 1971

Pumpkin Carvers' Palm

knife laceration of the nondominant hand sustained by those who carve jack-o-lanterns

N. Eng. J. Med. 298:348, 1978

Punch Drunk Syndrome

traumatic brain damage of prizefighters

JAMA 91:1103, 1928

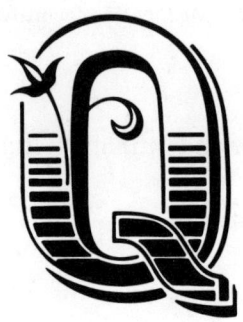

Quick Draw Leg

bullet wound of the leg sustained while practicing a fast draw from a gun-belt holster (compare GUNFIGHTER WOUND)

JAMA 196:1083, 1966

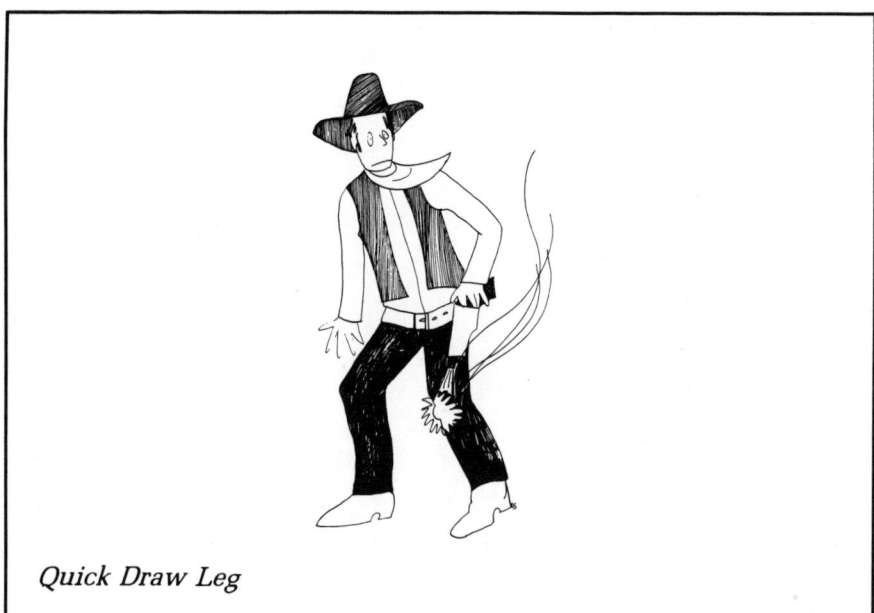

Quick Draw Leg

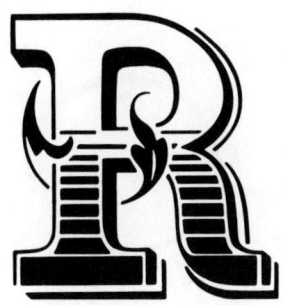

Racers' Humpback

permanent curvature of the upper back from the slouching position used by bicycle racers

Encyclopedia of Sports Sci. & Med. N.Y.: Macmillan Co., 1971

Radiologist's Cancer

skin cancer following damage by exposure to x-rays

Brit. Med. J. 2:272, 1897

Radiowave Sickness

multiple ill-defined symptoms attributed to microwave exposure (compare MICROWAVE NEUROSIS)

Am. J. Epid. 97:223, 1973

Rag Picker's Disease

RAG SORTER'S DISEASE

Ann. N.Y. Acad. Sci. 174:577, 1970

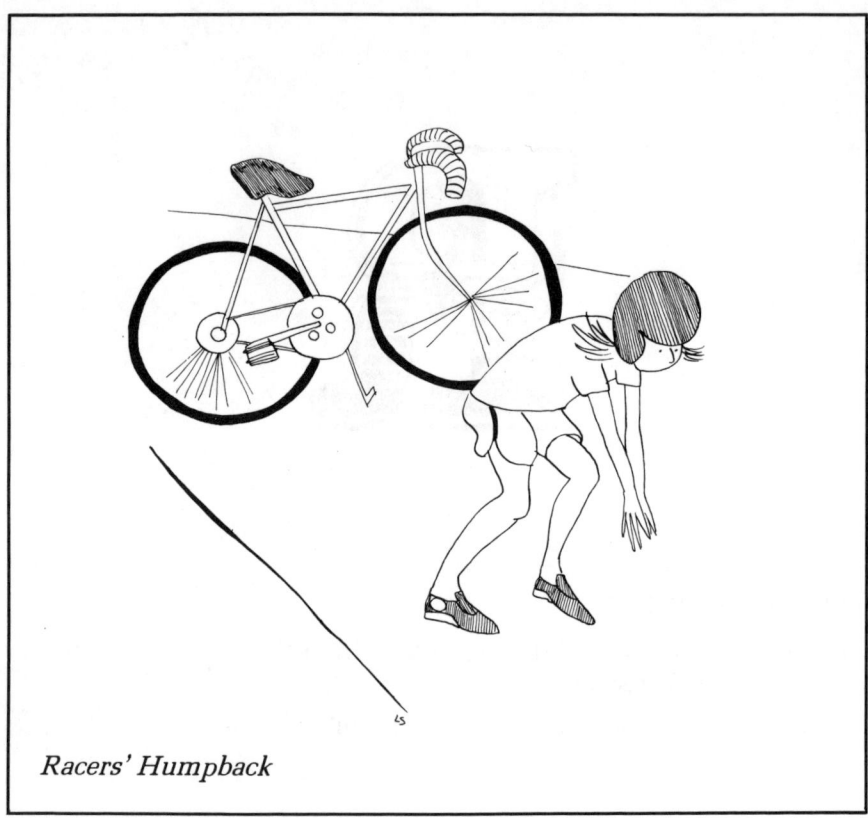

Racers' Humpback

RAG SORTER'S DISEASE

pulmonary anthrax characterized by fever, chills, headache, cough and rapid pulse in the early stages

Lancet 2:640, 1886

RAILROAD NEUROSIS

COMPENSATION NEUROSIS

original source not identified

RAILWAY BRAIN

nervous symptoms following a railway accident

Bost. Med. & Surg. J. 119:133, 1888

Railway Brain Strain

nervous symptoms among railway employees due to excessive overtime work

> N. Eng. Med. Month. 26:36, 1907

Railway Spine

concussion resulting from a railway accident

> N. Eng. Med. Month. 27:185, 1908

traumatic neurosis following a spine injury

> Erichsen, J. E. On Railway and Other Injuries of the Nervous System. London: Walton & Maberly, 1866

Railway Strain

job stress suffered by engineers and signalmen

> Brit. Med. J. 1:740, 1896

Rand Miners' Phthisis

progressive pulmonary disability (silicosis) among the Rand gold field miners of S. Africa

> Brit. Med. J. 2:919, 1905

Reapers' Keratitis

grain fiber irritation of farmers' eyes

> JAMA 81:780, 1918

Red Disease (mal rouge)

flushing and itching of the skin when workers exposed to calcium cyanamide ingest alcohol (compare DEGREASER'S FLUSH)

> Arch. Mal. Profess. 15:282, 1954

Red-out

throbbing head pain, eye discomfort and cerebral confusion or unconsciousness seen in flying personnel subjected to high centrifugal forces

Av. Med. 15:304, 1944

Red Phthisis

deposition of iron dust in the lung resulting in siderosis

Dtsch. Arch. Klin. Med. 2:116, 1867

Reflex Horn Syndrome

tendency for auto drivers waiting behind other cars at a light to blow their horns when the light turns green

N. Eng. J. Med. 294:908, 1976

Reverse Ear

outward bulging of the eardrum and possible rupture which may occur when a diver ascends improperly from a dive

Brit. Med. J. 2:192, 1963

Rice Paddy Dermatitis

skin irritation of rice paddy laborers caused by fertilizers and insecticides

A Barefoot Doctor's Manual USDHEW Pub. No. (NIH) 75-695, 1974

Rice Field Fever

infection by *Leptospira batavia* occurring among rice harvest workers

Dorland's Medical Dictionary. 25th ed. Phila.: W. B. Saunders, 1974

Rice Worker's Coniomycosis

cough and shortness of breath following exposure to rice straw dust

Med. Lavoro 49:368, 1958

Rice Workers' Dermatitis

irritation of the hands and feet of rice workers from contact with the pricking weed *Naia*

Schwartz, L. Occupational Diseases of the Skin. Phila.: Lea & Febiger, 1957

eczema among rice workers due to mosquito bites, poor hygiene and mechanical irritation from rice grain

JAMA 84:1770, 1925

Rider's Bone

bone formation in the muscle of the inner thigh from repeated strains in horseback riding

Oliver, T. Dangerous Trades. London: J. Murray, 1902

Rider's Bursa

swellings of the inner thigh and leg from horseback riding

Brit. Med. J. 2:38, 1893

Rider's Hygroma

RIDER'S BURSA

Brit. Med. J. 2:38, 1893

Rider's Leg

strain of the inner thigh muscles from horseback riding

Milit. Surg. 63:507, 1928

Rider's Sprain

sprain of the inner thigh muscles near the pelvis from strenuous horseback riding

Lancet 2:133, 1882

Rider's Tendon

RIDER'S LEG

Stedman's Medical Dictionary. 23rd ed. Baltimore: William & Wilkins, 1976

Rider's Thigh

RIDER'S SPRAIN

Lancet 2:133, 1882

Rider's Vertigo

motion sickness

Dorland's Medical Dictionary. 25th ed. Phila.: W. B. Saunders, 1974

Rifle Sling Palsy

numbness in the fourth and fifth fingers and partial paralysis of the hand caused by nerve pressure produced by a rifle sling

U.S. Armed Forces M.J. 6:353, 1955

Riveter's Wrist

wrist soreness from the use of vibratory tools (compare JACKHAMMER ARTHROPATHY)

original source not identified

Road Rash

severe scrapes, sores and bruises from skateboard accidents

Changing Times 32:41, 1978

ROENTGENOLOGIST'S CANCER

cancer of the hand from exposure to ionizing radiation

Dorland's Medical Dictionary. 25th ed. Phila.: W. B. Saunders, 1974

ROOT PULLER'S FRACTURE

fracture of a prominence of one of the vertebral bodies in the neck or upper back sustained while using a long handled shovel (compare SHOVELER'S FRACTURE)

Amer. J. Roent. 115:540, 1972

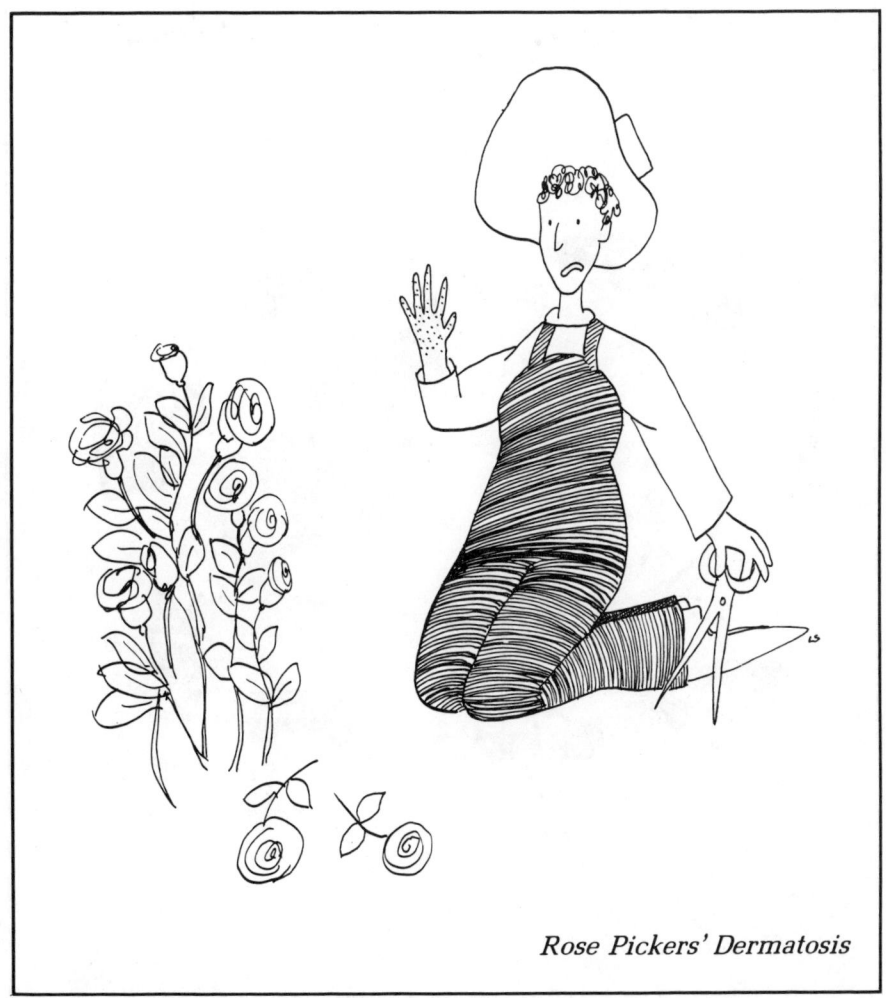

Rose Pickers' Dermatosis

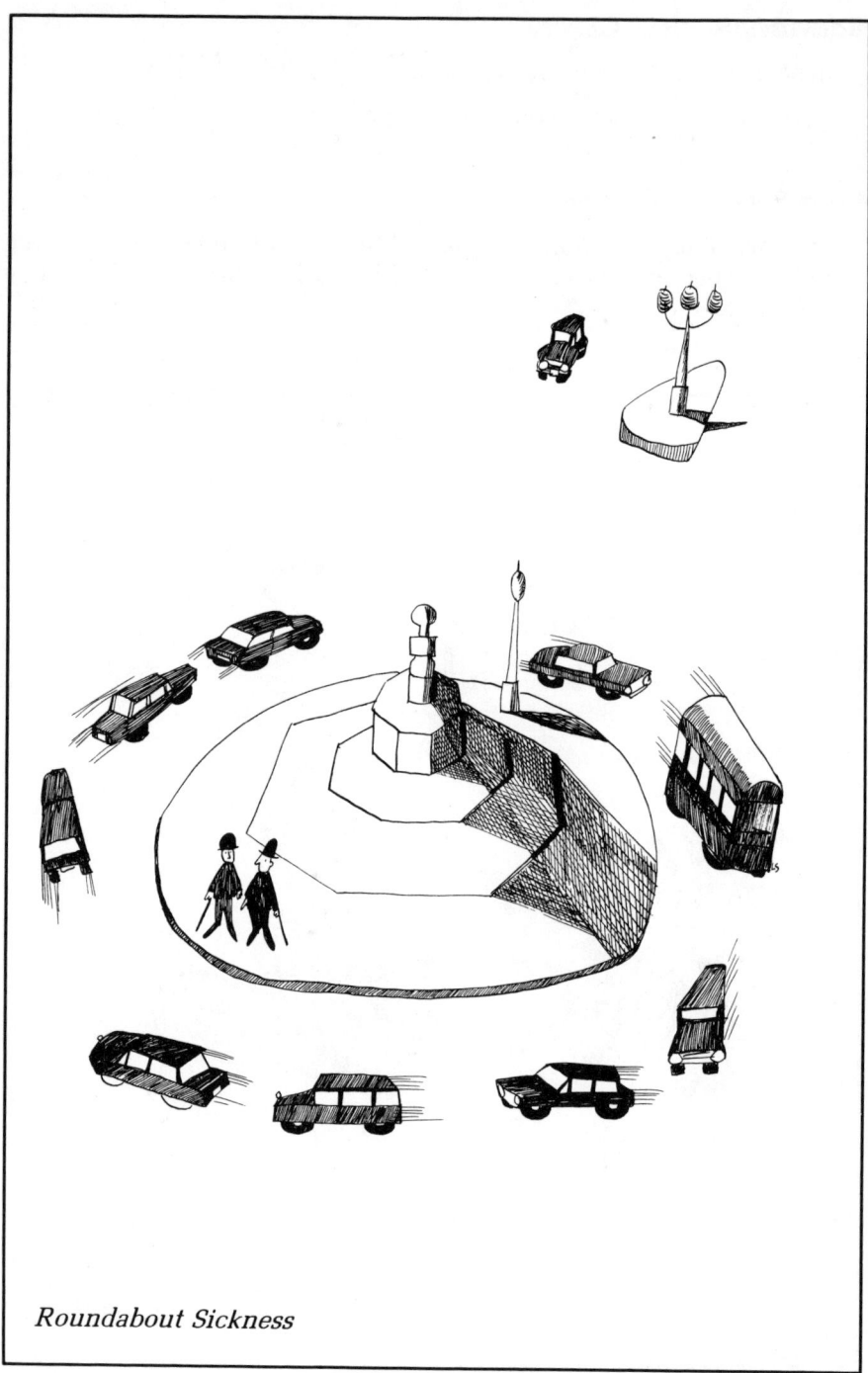

Roundabout Sickness

Rose Pickers' Dermatosis

irritation of gardeners' hands from the pricks of rose thorns

Schwartz, L. Occupational Diseases of the Skin. Phila.: Lea & Febiger, 1957

Rouge Polisher's Lung

deposition of iron dust in the lungs of workers using jewellers' rouge (ferric oxide) to polish silver

original source not identified

Roundabout Sickness

motion sickness

International Classification of Diseases. 8th rev. USDHEW Pub. Hlth. Serv. Pub. No. 1963, 1968

Rucksack Paralysis

motor and sensory changes in the upper extremity from compression of the brachial nerves by the rucksack harness (compare BACKPACK PALSY)

Munch. Med. Wschr. 40:121, 1893

Runner's Cramp

pain across the arch of the foot and the anterior leg from strenuous running

USN Med. Bull. 4:25, 1910

Runner's High

feeling of exhilaration from jogging

McCalls 105:61, 1978

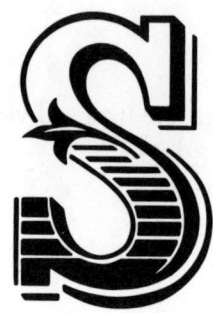

Saddler's Cramp

see OCCUPATIONAL NEUROSIS

Hunter, D. The Diseases of Occupations. 5th ed. London: The English Univ. Press Ltd., 1975

Saddle Sore

irritation of the buttocks from saddle friction

original source not identified

Sailmaker's Cramp

see OCCUPATIONAL NEUROSIS

Hunter, D. The Diseases of Occupations. 5th ed. London: The English Univ. Press Ltd., 1975

Sailor's Cramp

see OCCUPATIONAL NEUROSIS

Hunter, D. The Diseases of Occupations. 5th ed. London: The English Univ. Press Ltd., 1975

Sailor's Skin

premature ageing of the exposed skin due to solar radiation

Unna P. G., The Histopathology of the Diseases of the Skin. Edinburgh, 1896

Sailor's Stomach

peptic ulcer among navy personnel due to social, job and dietary factors

J. Roy. Nav. Med. Serv. 58:12, 1972

Salem Sarcoid

beryllium disease among employees in a fluorescent lamp plant in Salem, Massachusetts

Hunter, D. The Diseases of Occupations. 5th ed. London: The English Univ. Press Ltd., 1975

Salivation Disease

irritation of the mouth with increased saliva formation seen in mercury intoxication

original source not identified

Salt Water Boils

inflammation of the wrists and forearms of deep sea fishermen caused by chaffing from their oilskin sleeves

Brit. Med. J. 2:917, 1938

Salt Water Sores

skin infections on the hands, knees and feet of fishermen following minor trauma

Med. J. Austral. 2:352, 1949

SANDBLASTER'S ASTHMA

fibrotic lung disease caused by the chronic inhalation of silica sand

International Classification of Diseases. 8th rev. USDHEW Pub. Hlth. Serv. Pub. No. 1963, 1968

SANDBLASTER'S LUNG

SANDBLASTER'S ASTHMA

International Classification of Diseases. 8th rev. USDHEW Pub. Hlth. Serv. Pub. No. 1963, 1968

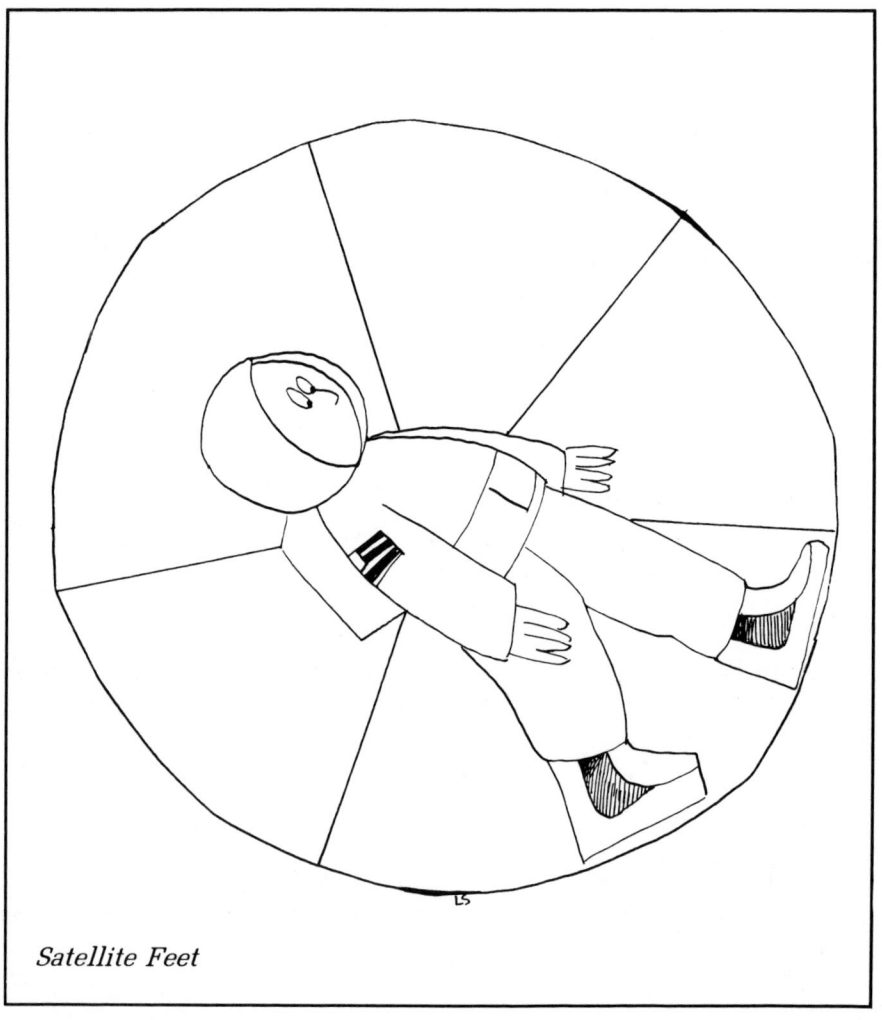

Satellite Feet

SANDBLASTER'S PHTHISIS

SANDBLASTER'S ASTHMA

International Classification of Diseases. 8th rev. USDHEW Pub. Hlth. Serv. Pub. No. 1963, 1968

SANDBLASTER'S SILICOSIS

SANDBLASTER'S ASTHMA

Hare Juah 81: 326, 1971

SANDBLASTER'S TUBERCULOSIS

silicotuberculosis

International Classification of Diseases. 8th rev. USDHEW Pub. Hlth. Serv. Pub. No. 1963, 1968

SATELLITE FEET

anticipated foot complaints in spacemen who may have to adapt to a concave walking surface in a spaceship

Lansberg, M. P. A Primer of Space Medicine. Amsterdam: Elsevier, 1960

SATELLITE SICKNESS

disturbed spatial orientation peculiar to the circumstances of space flight (compare PILOTS' VERTIGO)

Lansberg, M. P. A Primer of Space Medicine. Amsterdam: Elsevier, 1960

SAUNA TAKER'S DISEASE

allergic inflammatory response of the lungs to the inhalation of contaminated moisture in a sauna bath

JAMA 236:2209, 1976

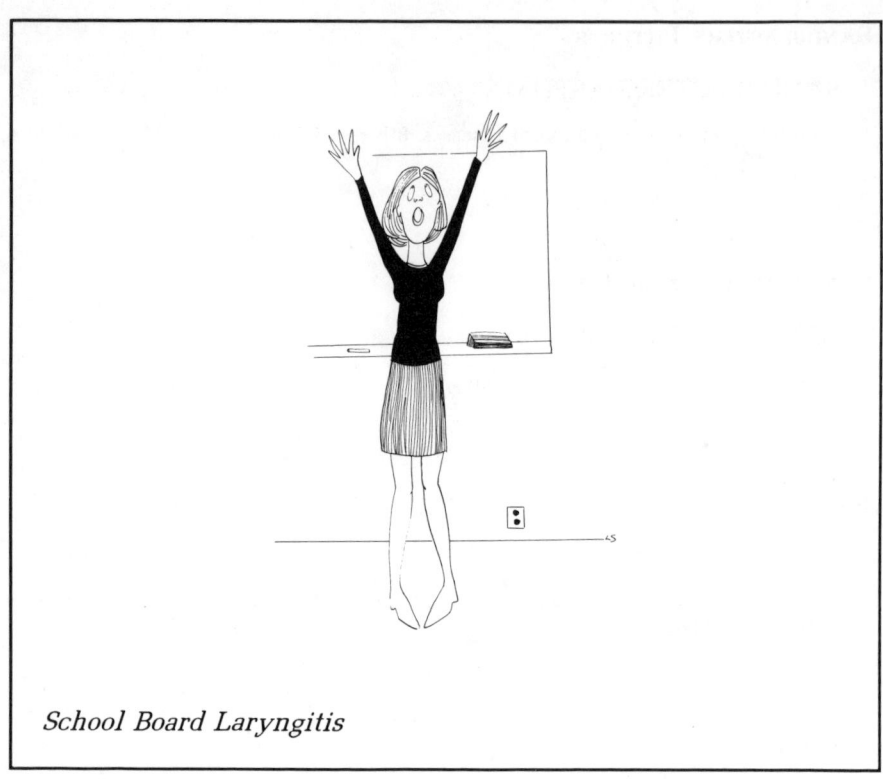

School Board Laryngitis

Sawyer's Cramp

see OCCUPATIONAL NEUROSIS

> Hunter, D. The Diseases of Occupations. 5th ed. London: The English Univ. Press Ltd., 1975

Scandinavian Blubberfinger

SPAEK FINGER

> Canad. M. A. J. 76:455, 1957

Schneeberg Tumor

lung cancer among the Schneeberg miners due to radioactive ores (compare MALA METALLORUM)

> International Classification of Diseases. 8th rev. USDHEW Pub. Hlth. Serv. Pub. No. 1963, 1968

School Board Laryngitis

husky, worn-out voice of the over-worked schoolteacher
Brit. Med. J. 2:750, 1890

School Board Sore Throat

throat irritation among teachers from the inhalation of blackboard eraser dust
Lancet 1:920, 1889

School Desk Dermatitis

irritant dermatitis from a fiberglass reinforced plastic school chair
Arch. Derm. 105:890, 1972

School Phobia

JOB PHOBIA
Am. J. Orthopsychiat. 11:702, 1941

Scissor Grinder's Disease

deposition of iron dust in the lungs
Stedman's Medical Dictionary. 23rd ed. Baltimore: William & Wilkins, 1976

Scissor Sharpener's Cramp

see OCCUPATIONAL NEUROSIS
Hunter, D. The Diseases of Occupations. 5th ed. London: The English Univ. Press Ltd., 1975

Scissors' Palsy

see OCCUPATIONAL NEUROSIS
Brit. Med. J. 1:1316, 1900

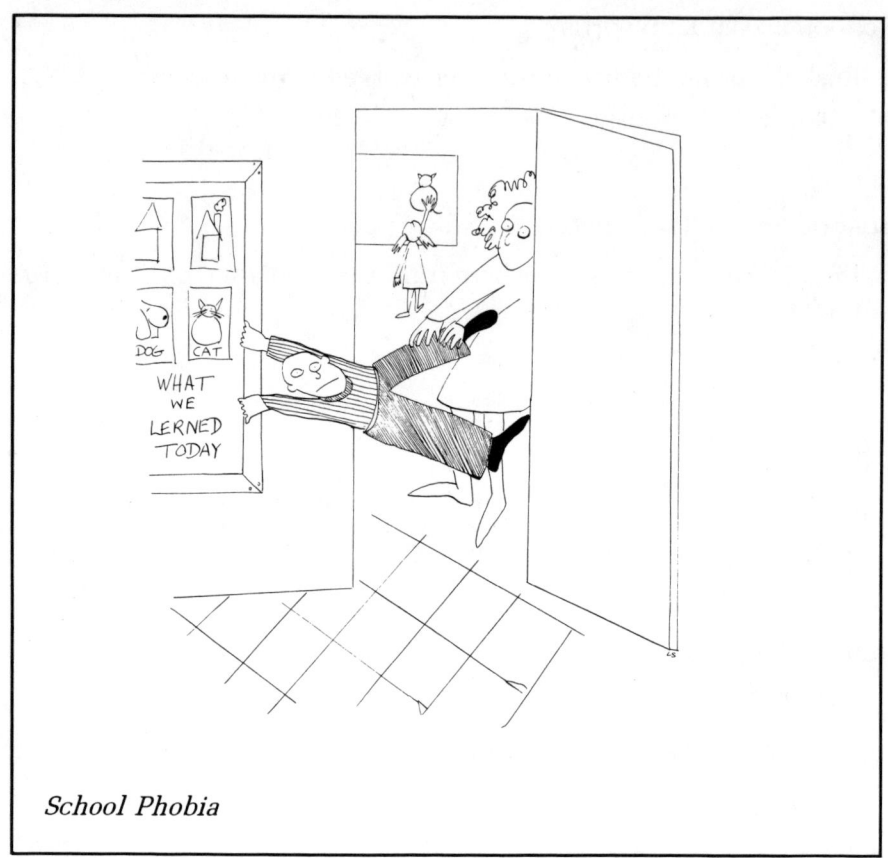

School Phobia

Scribe's Palsy
    WRITER'S CRAMP
        Brit. Med. J. 2:394, 1861

Scrivener's Cramp
    WRITER'S CRAMP
        Brit. Med. J. 1:87, 1878

Scrivener's Palsy
    WRITER'S CRAMP
        Lancet 2:709, 1864

SCRIVENER'S SPASM

WRITER'S CRAMP

Gowers, W. R. A Manual of Diseases of the Nervous System. London, 1893

SCROTAL SOOT CANCER

cancer of the scrotum from soot exposure while cleaning chimneys

Edin. Med. J. 22:135, 1876

SCRUMPOX

eruption of the face (impetigo) occurring in rugby team players from close contact at the scrum (scrimmage) (compare FOOTBALL IMPETIGO)

JAMA 26:1276, 1896

SEABATHER ERUPTION

itchy dermatitis among Florida swimmers confined to the covered parts of the body, believed to be due to a fluke *Schistosome cercaria*

Arch. Derm. & Syph. 60:227, 1949

SEALERS' FINGER

finger infection among seal hunters believed due to erysipeloid (compare FISH HANDLERS' DISEASE)

Acta. Path. Micro. 16:407, 1949

SEAL FINGER

SEALERS' FINGER

Canad. M. A. J. 76:455, 1957

SEAMSTRESS' PALSY

see OCCUPATIONAL NEUROSIS

Brit. Med. J. 2:394, 1861

SEAMSTRESS'S CRAMP

hand cramp from sewing

Brit. Med. J. 1:11, 1886

SEASQUIRT ASTHMA

nasal irritation with sneezing, cough, shortness of breath and wheezy respiration occurring in oyster and pearl farm workers caused by inhaling droplets of seasquirt body fluids

Jap. J. Allergol. 16:668, 1967

SEAT BELT SYNDROME

internal abdominal injuries from an incorrectly adjusted seat belt

Lancet 1:1370, 1967

SEA WATER BOILS

SALT WATER BOILS

Brit. Med. J. 1:1144, 1966

SEMPSTRESS' CRAMP

see OCCUPATIONAL NEUROSIS

Lancet 2:709, 1864

SEWAGE WORKER'S SYNDROME

attacks of chills, fever and malaise presumably from a toxin in sewage sludge

Lancet 2:478, 1976

Sewer Disease

fibrotic lung disease (silicosis) occurring in workers digging sewers in sandstone

> Hunter, D. The Diseases of Occupations. 5th ed. London: The English Univ. Press Ltd., 1975

Sewer Fume Poisoning

hydrogen sulfide intoxication in sewer workers

> J. Amer. Coll. Emerg. Phys. 4:141, 1975

Sewer's Cramp

see OCCUPATIONAL NEUROSIS

> Ann. Surg. 63:155, 1916

Sewing Spasm

hand cramp from sewing

> Stedman's Medical Dictionary. 23rd ed. Baltimore: William & Wilkins, 1976

Shearer's Knuckles

thickening of the skin over the knuckles of the left hand caused by pressures against the hand during the sheep shearing process

> Aust. N.Z. J. Surg. 42:192, 1972

Sheffield Grinders' Disease

silicosis among the grinders of razors, forks, knives, saws and other edge tools in Sheffield, England

> Brit. Med. J. 1:491, 1857

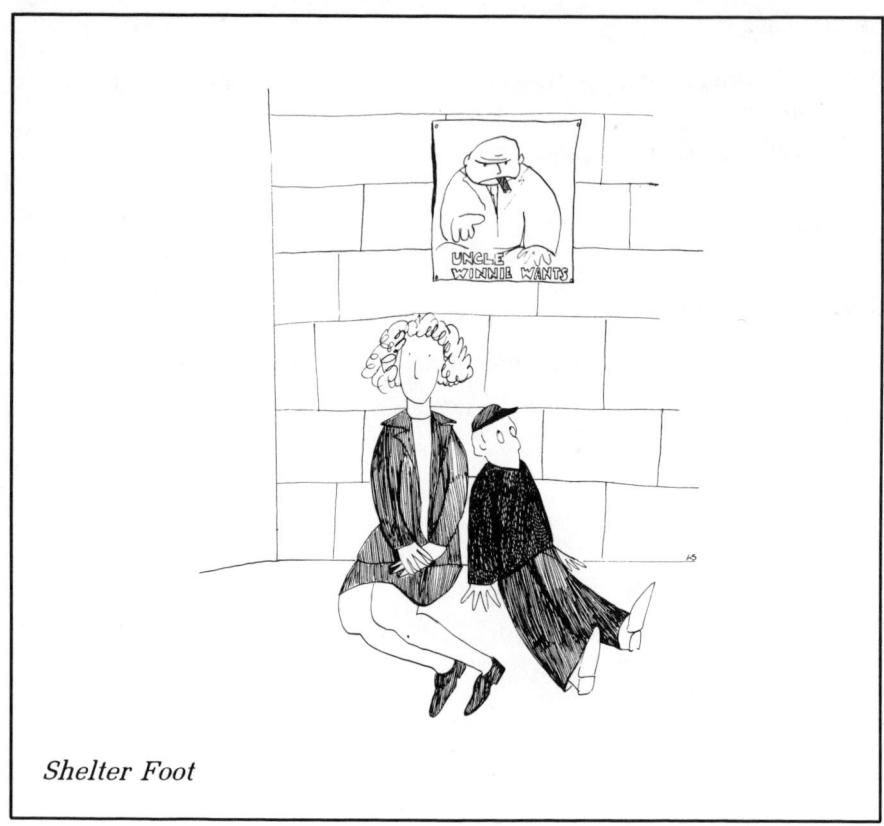

Shelter Foot

SHELL SHOCK

> neurosis due to the tensions of war
>
> Lancet 2:63, 1915

SHELTER FOOT

> swelling of the feet of those spending a night in a sitting position in an air raid shelter, caused by venous stagnation
>
> Lancet 2:659, 1941

SHELTER LEG

> swelling of the leg from sitting overnight in an air raid shelter
>
> Brit. Med. J. 3:109, 1973

Shin Splints

soreness and swelling of the leg muscles from strain or an actual tear in the tibialis posticus muscle

> Thorndike, A. Athletic Injuries; Prevention, Diagnosis & Treatment. Phila.: Lea & Febiger, 1938

Ship Fever

typhus fever occurring as a result of unsanitary conditions on shipboard

> original source not identified

Ship Sickness

incapacitating disability afflicting emigrants, allegedly due to unsanitary conditions aboard ship

> Bost. Med. & Surg. J. 36:103, 1847

Shipyard Conjunctivitis

epidemic eye infection, occasionally involving the cornea, among shipyard personnel, characterized by eyelid swelling, tearing, and discharge

> Arch. Ophth. 28:581, 1942

Shipyard Disease

SHIPYARD CONJUNCTIVITIS

> International Classification of Diseases. 8th rev. USDHEW Pub. Hlth. Serv. Pub. No. 1963, 1968

Shipyard Eye

SHIPYARD CONJUNCTIVITIS

> Indust. Med. 12:184, 1943

Shipyard Keratoconjunctivitis

SHIPYARD CONJUNCTIVITIS

International Classification of Diseases. 8th rev. USDHEW Pub. Hlth. Serv. Pub. No. 1963, 1968

Shoddy Disease

SHODDY FEVER

Brit. Med. J. 1:644, 1889

Shoddy Fever

headache, sickness, dryness of the mouth, shortness of breath and productive cough from the dust produced by reprocessing wool rags

Thackrah, C. T. The Effects of Arts, Trades and Professions on Health and Longevity. London: Longman, 1832

Shoemaker's Breast

darkening of the skin associated with irritation of the hair cells on the front of the chest caused by pressure from holding the shoe and soiling of the skin by pitch

J. Ind. Hyg. 6:67, 1924

Shoemaker's Chest

hollow deformity at the base of the breast bone caused by pressure of the last against the chest

Thackrah, C. T. The Effects of Arts, Trades and Professions On Health and Longevity. London: Longman, 1832

Shoemaker's Cramp

see OCCUPATIONAL NEUROSIS

Lancet 2:709, 1864

Shoemakers' Polyneuropathy

neuritis of the extremities among artisan employees in Italian shoe factories from an unknown cause

Boll. Soc. Med. Chir. di Pavia 1:131, 1957

Shoemaker's Spasm

see OCCUPATIONAL NEUROSIS

Oliver, T. Dangerous Trades. London: J. Murray, 1902

Shoemaker's Ulcer

gastric ulcer and other stomach diseases believed due to pressure of the boots held against the abdomen

Brit. Med. J. 2:832, 1886

Shoeworkers' Neuropathy

SHOEMAKERS' POLYNEUROPATHY

Elect. Clin. Neurophys. 16:493, 1976

Shooters' Deafness

noise-induced hearing loss from gun-fire

original source not identified

Shooting Gallery Lead Poisoning

intoxication from lead dust exposure in shooting galleries

Indust. Med. 16:421, 1947

Shoveler's Disease

SHOVELER'S FRACTURE

Arch. Orthop. Unfallchir. 37:223, 1936

Shoveler's Fracture

fracture of the prominence (spinous process) of a vertebra in the neck (7–C) due to excessive muscular strain while using a shovel (compare ROOT PULLER'S FRACTURE)

Lancet 1:174, 1945

Shovel Sickness

SHOVELER'S FRACTURE

Deutsch. Med. Wchnschr. 61:1271, 1935

Shuttle Maker's Disease

irritation of the eyes and nose, sneezing, headache, dizziness, faintness, shortness of breath, and other symptoms caused by W. African boxwood dust exposure

JAMA 58:38, 1912

Side-swipe Fracture

left elbow fracture sustained by auto drivers involved in accidents when their left elbow protrudes through the car window (compare TRAFFIC FRACTURE)

Georgia Med. Assoc. J. 42:211, 1953

Sightseers' Headache

headaches among frequenters of museums, picture galleries and exhibitions, from a multitude of causes

Lancet 1:1043, 1888

Silk Handler's Disease

skin irritation from an antimildew solution containing cresol used on raw silk prior to weaving

Acta. Dermat. Venereol. 15:25, 1934

Silk-weavers' Nails

comb or rake-like shape of the fingernails of Japanese art silk-weavers deliberately done to assist in working with the threads

Arch. Derm. 71:525, 1955

Silk Winders' Dermatosis

hand eruption of silk handlers presumed to be caused by the decomposition products of dead silkworm pupae

White, R. P. The Dermatogoses or Occupational Affections of the Skin. London: H. K. Lewis, 1928

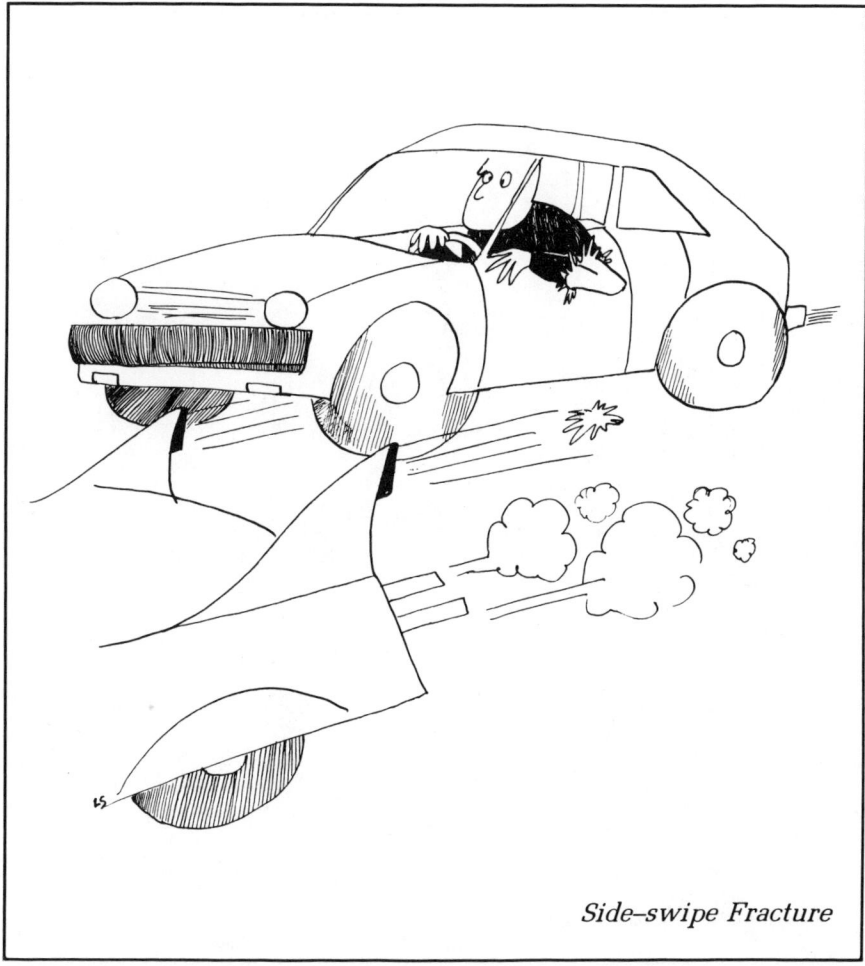

Side-swipe Fracture

Silo Disease

asphyxiation from exposure to carbon dioxide in silos

Ind. Med. & Surg. 25:402, 1956

Silo Filler's Disease

nitrous fume intoxication from fresh silage characterized by cough, shortness of breath and weakness, followed after an interval by a second more severe phase of fever, chills, severe shortness of breath and cyanosis

Univ. Minn. M. Bull. 27:203, 1956

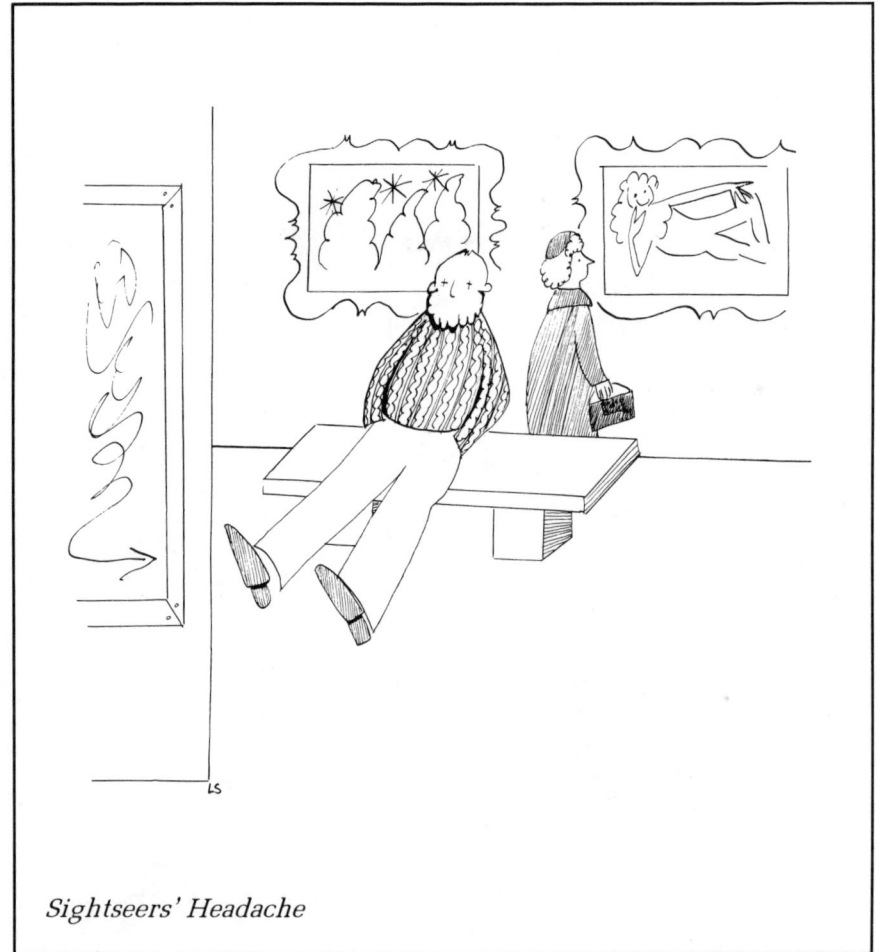

Sightseers' Headache

Silo Filler's Lung

SILO FILLER'S DISEASE

JAMA 63:1570, 1914

Silo Worker's Asthma

SILO FILLER'S DISEASE

Hunter, D. The Diseases of Occupations. 5th ed. London: The English Univ. Press Ltd., 1975

Silver Polishers' Lung

deposition of iron dust in the lungs of workers using jewellers' rouge (ferric oxide) to polish silver

original source not identified

Singer's Knots

vocal cord nodules from overuse of the voice

Singer, K. Diseases of the Musical Profession. (tr. by W. Lakond, Greensberg, N.Y., 1932)

Singer's Nodes

SINGER'S KNOTS

JAMA 33:1090, 1899

Singer's Nodules

SINGER'S KNOTS

Lancet 2:363, 1894

Skateboarder's Elbow

fracture of the elbow from a skateboard accident

Changing Times 32:41, 1978

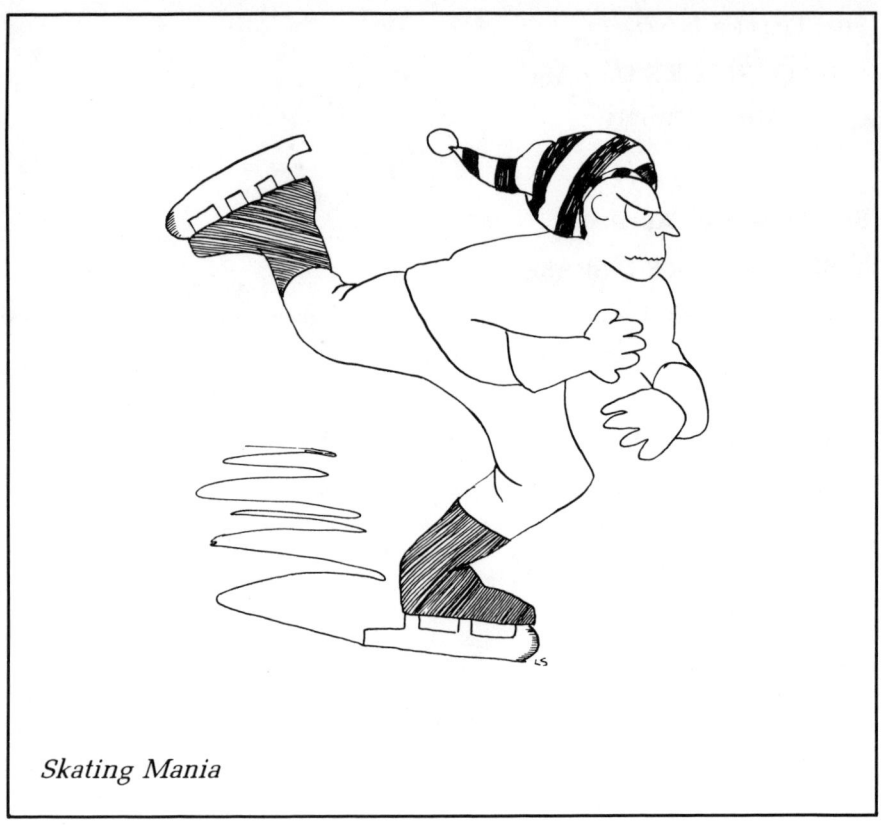

Skating Mania

Skating Mania

restlessness, insomnia and depression from prolonged ice skating
Lancet 2:1175, 1885

Ski-boot Neuropathy

numbness and tingling of the soles of the feet from pressure of the boot top against the leg nerves
N. Eng. J. Med. 288:420, 1973

Slag Cough

chronic bronchitis among iron workers
original source not identified

SLATE DRESSER'S LUNG

schistosis, the deposition of slate dust in the lungs

original source not identified

SLATE MINER'S LUNG

SLATE DRESSER'S LUNG

International Classification of Diseases. 8th rev. USDHEW Pub. Hlth. Serv. Pub. No. 1963, 1968

SLATE MINER'S PHTHISIS

SLATE DRESSER'S LUNG

International Classification of Diseases. 8th rev. USDHEW Pub. Hlth. Serv. Pub. No. 1963, 1968

SLATE WORKER'S LUNG

SLATE DRESSER'S LUNG

Hunter, D. The Diseases of Occupations. 5th ed. London: The English Univ. Press Ltd., 1975

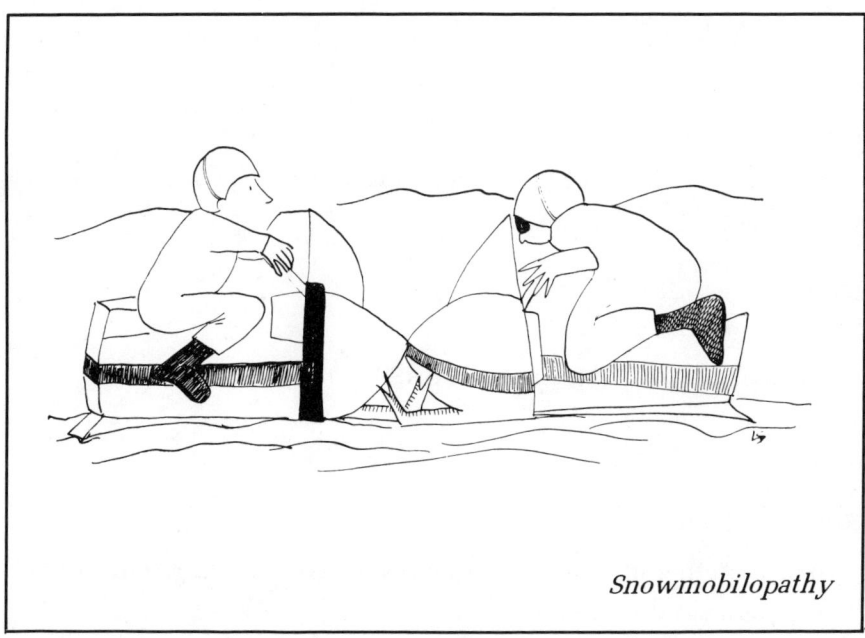

Snowmobilopathy

TRADE DISEASES

Sling Palsy

RIFLE SLING PALSY

Milit. Med. 131: 161, 1966

Slug Happiness

PUNCH DRUNK SYNDROME

Brit. Med. J. 2:793, 1950

Smallpox Handler's Lung

headache, chills, aching, malaise and pneumonitis from the inhalation of smallpox virus

Lancet 2:312, 1944

Smarts, The

photosensitivity of the skin of pitch workers with severe smarting of the exposed parts of the body (compare TAR SMARTS)

Brit. Med. J. 2:370, 1948

Smelter's Ague

METAL FUME FEVER in smelter workers

original source not identified

Smelter's Fever

SMELTER'S AGUE (compare BRASS FOUNDERS' AGUE)

JAMA 87:2107, 1926

Smelters' Itch

skin irritation of smelter workers believed due to arsenical salts

original source not identified

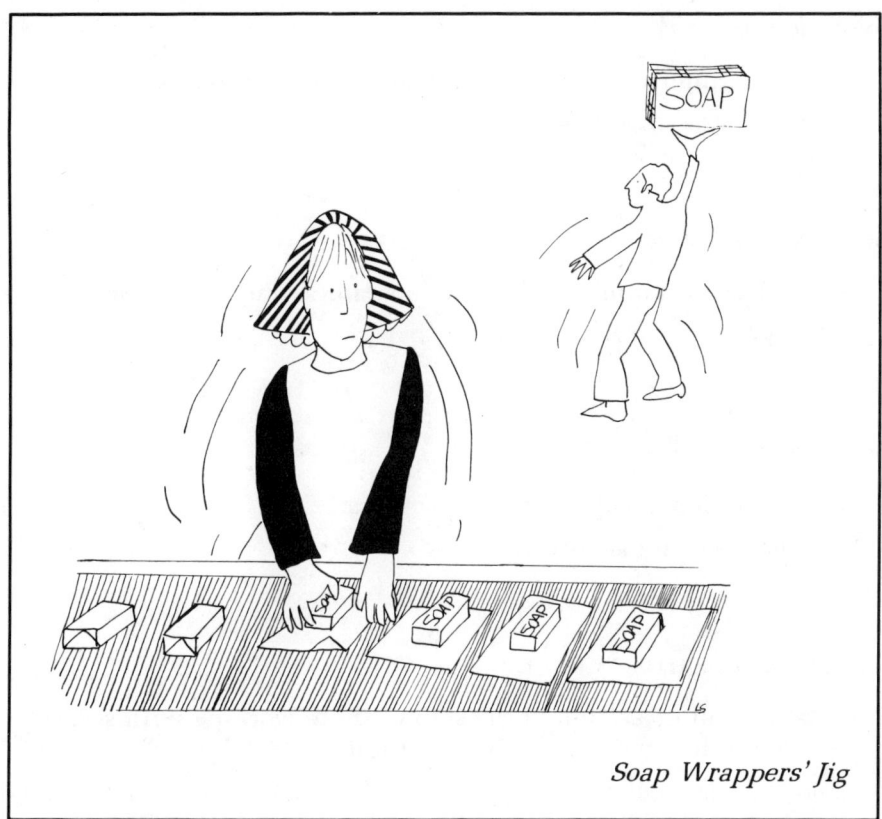

Soap Wrappers' Jig

Smelters' Shakes

SMELTERS' AGUE

original source not identified

Smith's Cramp

see OCCUPATIONAL NEUROSIS

Brit. Med. J. 2:165, 1890

Snow Blindness

light sensitivity, tearing, small corneal ulcers and retinal damage from reflected ultraviolet rays

Ophth. Record 9: 117, 1900

Snowmobilopathy

any of the injuries possible from snowmobile accidents

N. Eng. J. Med. 286:845, 1972

Soap Wrappers' Jig

unusual work motions peculiar to operators who wrap soap

Brit. J. Ind. Med. 11:279, 1954

Soda Ulcer

skin ulceration affecting caustic workers

original source not identified

Solders' Dermatitis

irritation and ulceration of the skin of those working with soft solder, caused by zinc salts in Baker's solution

Brit. Med. J. 2:38, 1946

Soldiers' Feet

pain, swelling and redness of the feet due to fatigue

Brit. Med. J. 2:871, 1879

Soldiers' Heart

shortness of breath, dizziness, fatigue and chest pain in soldiers on active duty

Lancet 2:1279, 1910

a variety of morbid states resulting from the physical and emotional stresses of military life

Lancet 1:985, 1917

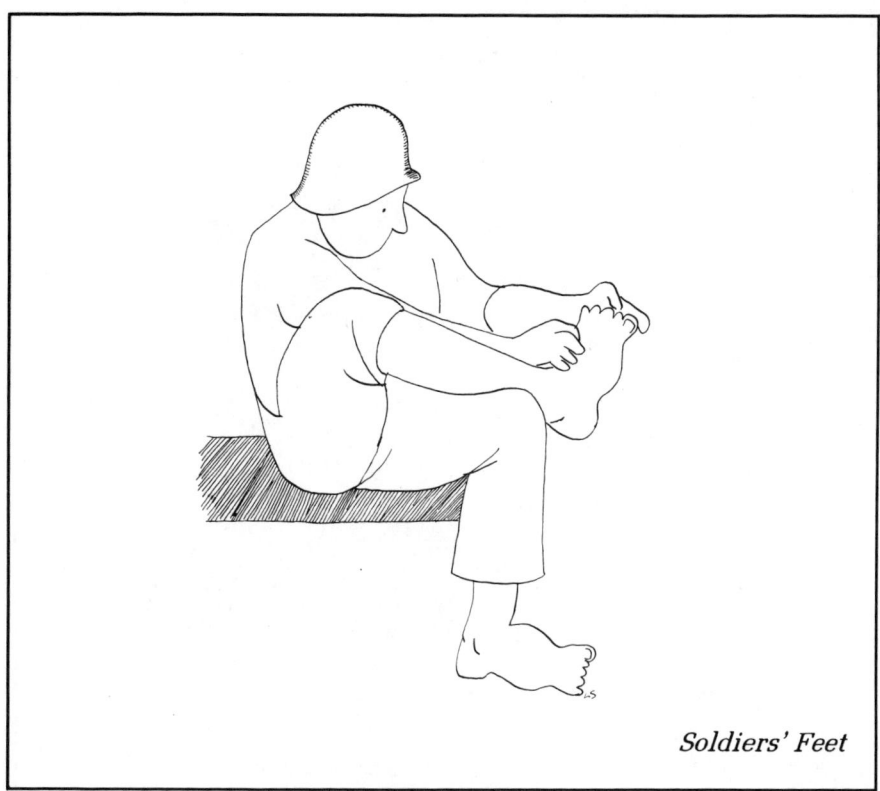

Soldiers' Feet

Soldier's Spot

a white spot seen on the external surface of the heart at postmortem alleged to friction and pressure from carrying a full soldier's pack

Lancet 1:368, 1864

Sonic Boom Stress

psychologic and physiologic effects produced by the sonic booms of supersonic aircraft

JAMA 211:1288, 1970

Soot Lung

deposition of soot in the lungs of workers in a lampblack factory

Med. Welt. 20:253, 1951

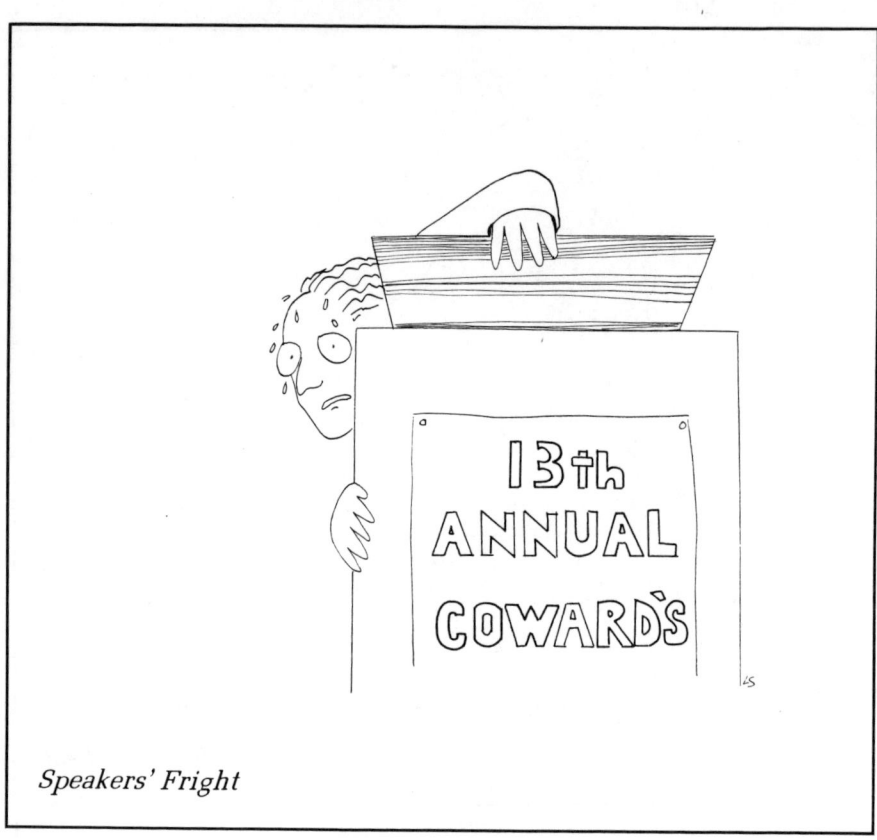

Speakers' Fright

Space Ebullism

vaporization of body fluids in outer space decompression

Lansberg, M. P. A Primer of Space Medicine. Amsterdam: Elsevier, 1960

Spaek Finger

finger infection among Norwegian seal hunters due to *Erysipelothrix rhusiopathiae*

Acta. Path. Micro. Scand. 26:407, 1949

Speakers' Fright

anxiety and tension related to making a public speech

Brit. Med. J. 2:1055, 1958

SPEAKER'S THROAT
CHORDITIS TUBEROSA
International Classification of Diseases. 8th rev. USDHEW Pub. Hlth. Serv. Pub. No. 1963, 1968

SPECK FINGER
SPAEK FINGER
Canad. M.A.J. 76:455, 1957

SPEED FEVER

the exhilarating sensation of speed and power engendered by certain automobiles

Lansberg, M. P. A Primer of Space Medicine. Amsterdam: Elsevier, 1960

SPEKKFINGER
SPAEK FINGER
Acta. Chir. Scand. Supp. 177, 1953

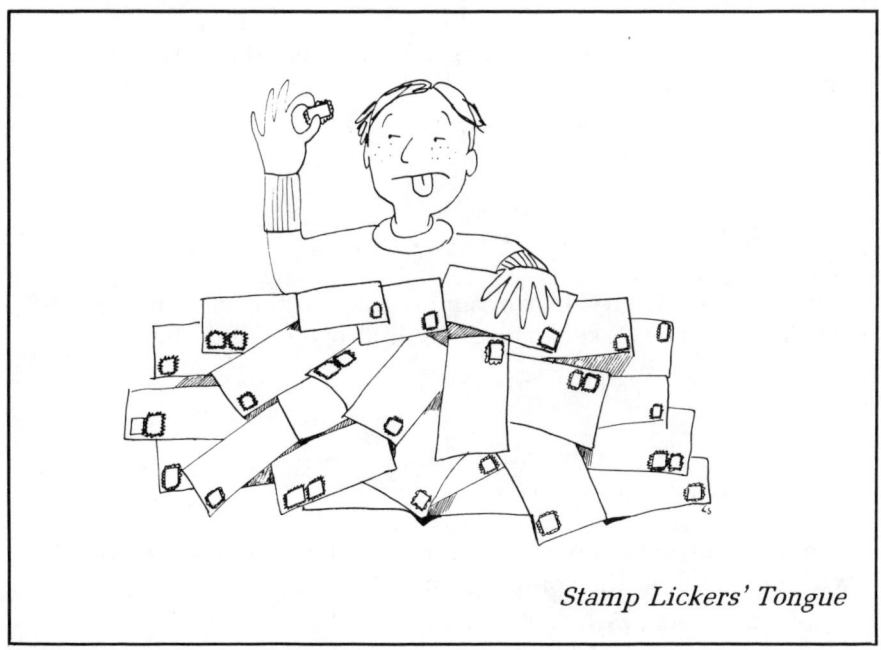

Stamp Lickers' Tongue

Spelter Fever

METAL FUME FEVER due to the inhalation of zinc fumes generated in metal smelting

original source not identified

Spelter Shakes

METAL FUME FEVER symptoms in coppersmiths

Thackrah, C. T. The Effects of Arts, Trades and Professions On Health and Longevity. London: Longman, 1832

Spinners' Cancer

MULE SPINNERS' CANCER

Lancet 2:1336, 1927

Spinners' Eczema

hand irritation of flax spinners who cleanse the yarn with contaminated water

Brit. J. Derm. 1:140, 1889

Spinners' Eye

pain, light sensitivity, tearing and redness of the eyes among artificial-silk factory workers caused by hydrogen sulfide fumes

Klin. Monatsbl. Augenh. 123:440, 1953

Spinners' Folliculitis

skin irritation of the lower extremities of flax workers due to contact with oils used on the spinning mills

Brit. J. Derm. 2:15, 1890

Spinners' Phthisis

BYSSINOSIS (compare COTTON SPINNERS' PHTHISIS)

N. Eng. M. Surg. J., 1831

Splitters' Knee

swelling over the inner side of the knee of slate splitters caused by pressure from the slate press

Suppl. to Occup. & Hlth. ILO Sept., 1938

Sponge Divers' Disease

BENDS

International Classification of Diseases. 8th rev. USDHEW Pub. Hlth. Serv. Pub. No. 1963, 1968

dermatitis caused by contact with the sea anemone

Hunter, D. The Diseases of Occupations. 5th ed. London: The English Univ. Press Ltd., 1975

Sponge Fisher's Disease

redness, blistering and gangrenous skin lesions caused by the poisonous secretions of the sponge parasite *Sagarsia rosea*

Grèce Med. 13:14, 1905

Sports Anemia

transient anemia caused by the increased demands made upon the body during training periods

Med. Sport (Roma) 26:120, 1973

Sports Pubic Osteoarthropathy

atrophic changes of the pelvic arch (pubis) as a result of constant strain of this area in broad jumpers and football players

Encyclopedia of Sports Sci. & Med. N.Y.: Macmillan Co., 1971

Spring Finger

pain and swelling of the fingers with impaired flexion caused by the use of a compressed air hammer

> Monatsschr. J. Unfallh. 52:106, 1949

Sprinter's Fracture

fracture of the anterior spine of the pelvic bone, the ilium, due to an intense muscular pull at the start of a sprint

> Dorland's Medical Dictionary. 25th ed. Phila.: W. B. Saunders, 1974

Stage Fright

anxiety related to making a public stage appearance

> original source not identified

Staggers

dizziness, ringing in the ears and nausea associated with DECOMPRESSION SICKNESS

> original source not identified

Stamp Lickers' Tongue

ulcers of the tongue and mouth seen among workers applying gum stamps, due to irritation from the adhesive materials

> Oliver, T. Dangerous Trades. London: J. Murray, 1902

Stapled Finger Syndrome

crushing and puncturing injuries caused by staples ejected from an electric stapling machine

> N. Eng. J. Med. 296:1005, 1977

Steamer Leg

swelling of the leg from venous stasis alleged to sitting with the leg flexed over the rail of a deck chair

Brit. Med. J. 3:109, 1973

Steam Fitter's Asthma

fibrotic lung disease caused by the inhalation of asbestos dust

Dorland's Medical Dictionary. 25th ed. Phila.: W. B. Saunders, 1974

Steel Grinder's Disease

deposition of iron dust in the lungs

Stedman's Medical Dictionary. 23rd ed. Baltimore: William & Wilkins, 1976

Steel Grinder's Phthisis

STEEL GRINDER'S DISEASE

original source not identified

Stitch

pain in the side believed due to a strain of the abdominal ligaments resulting from any jolting activity such as cross-country running, camel riding, motor-cycling, etc.

Brit. Med. J. 1:207, 1945

Stock Car Kidney

elevated blood pressure, albumin in the urine and kidney scarring alleged to repeated abdominal trauma in stock car racing

Lancet 1:125, 1972

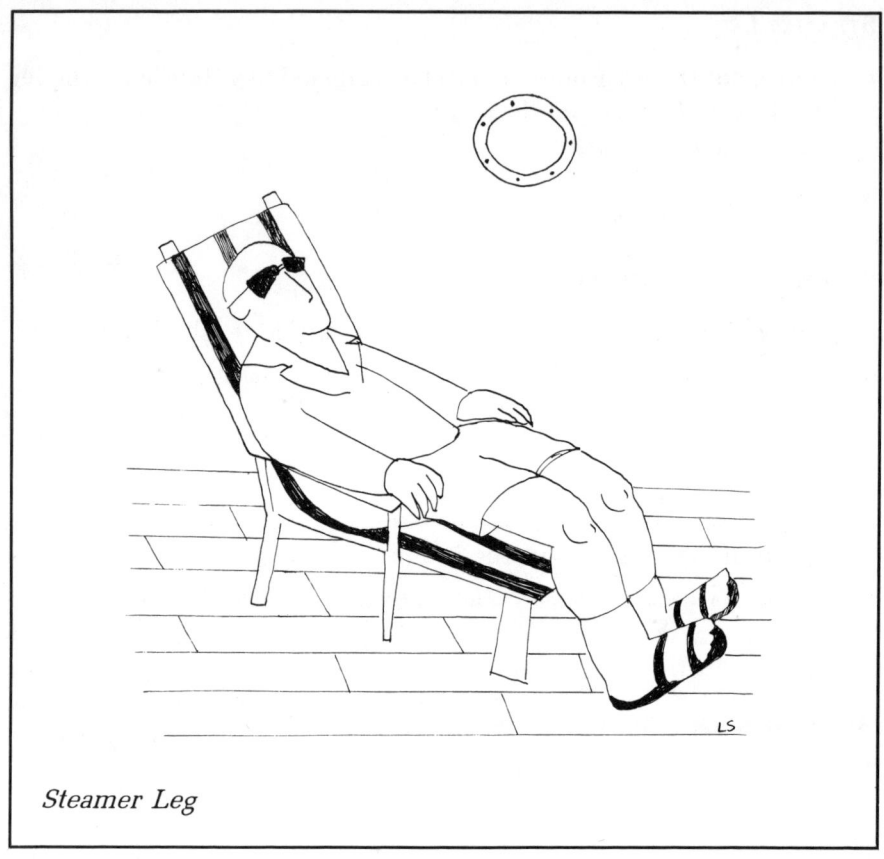
Steamer Leg

STOKERS' CRAMPS

    heat cramps seen in boiler stokers

        Brit. Med. J. 1:65, 1929

STONE CARRIER'S PARALYSIS

    RUCKSACK PARALYSIS

        Munsch. Med. Wschr. 40:121, 1893

STONE CUTTER'S ASTHMA

    fibrotic lung disease caused by the inhalation of silica dust

        Anat. corporis humani. Utrecht 2:13, 1672

Stone Cutter's Consumption

loss of appetite, weakness, shortness of breath, blood spitting and emaciation

Brit. Med. J. 1:80, 1868

Stone Cutter's Lung

silicosis

International Classification of Diseases. 8th rev. USDHEW Pub. Hlth. Serv. Pub. No. 1963, 1968

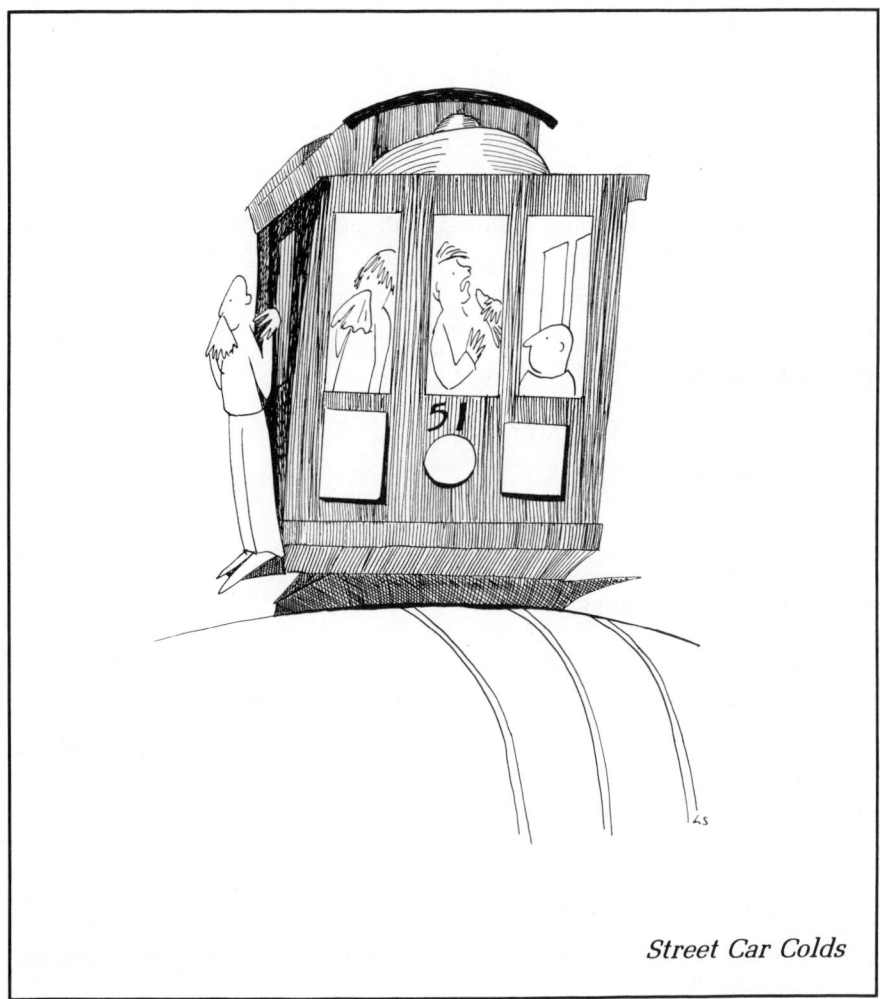

Street Car Colds

TRADE DISEASES

Stone Cutter's Phthisis

cough, asthmatic breathing, hoarseness, fever and emaciation

N. Eng. J. Med. 1:357, 1831

Stone Hewer's Phthisis

silicosis

Hunter, D. The Diseases of Occupations. 5th ed. London: The English Univ. Press Ltd., 1975

Stone Mason's Asthma

silicosis

International Classification of Diseases. 8th rev. USDHEW Pub. Hlth. Serv. Pub. No. 1963, 1968

Stone Mason's Cramp

see OCCUPATIONAL NEUROSIS

Brit. Med. J. 1:188, 1894

Stone Mason's Disease

silicosis

International Classification of Diseases. 8th rev. USDHEW Pub. Hlth. Serv. Pub. No. 1963, 1968

Stone Mason's Lung

silicosis

International Classification of Diseases. 8th rev. USDHEW Pub. Hlth. Serv. Pub. No. 1963, 1968

Stone Mason's Phthisis

silicosis

International Classification of Diseases. 8th rev. USDHEW Pub. Hlth. Serv. Pub. No. 1963, 1968

Stone Mason's Tuberculosis

silicotuberculosis

International Classification of Diseases. 8th rev. USDHEW Pub. Hlth. Serv. Pub. No. 1963, 1968

Strawberry Picker's Foot Drop

numbness, tingling and paralysis of the foot due to pressure on the popliteal nerve from squatting with the knee flexed and the leg pressed against the ground

Brit. Med. J. 2:520, 1977

Strawberry Picker's Peroneal Palsy

leg symptoms from compression of the peroneal nerve by crouching

Duodecim (Helsinki) 92:242, 1976

Straw Plaiter's Cramp

see OCCUPATIONAL NEUROSIS

Brit. Med. J. 1:110, 1896

Street Car Colds

upper respiratory infections associated with bronchitis and pneumonia from the crowded conditions in street cars

Lancet 1:320, 1903

Stress Dyspepsia

abdominal pain, vomiting and weight loss associated with long work hours

Lancet 2:449, 1944

Strikers' Arthritis

wrist and elbow soreness among forgemen from jarring of the extremity

Oliver, T. Dangerous Trades. London: J. Murray, 1902

Stucco Boils

skin irritation of exposed body surfaces among gypsum wallboard workers due to occlusion of the hair follicles by gypsum dust

JAMA 91:1738, 1928

Student's Elbow

elbow pain produced by pressure against the desk

International Classification of Diseases. 8th rev. USDHEW Pub. Hlth. Serv. Pub. No. 1963, 1968

Stud Gun Injury

any penetrating injury by the metallic studs fired from an explosive-charged tool

N. Eng. J. Med. 267:1020, 1962

Sugar Beet Pollinosis

irritation of the eyes and nose and bronchial asthma in sugar beet pollinators caused by sensitivity to the pollen

Jap. J. Allergol. 21:235, 1972

SUGAR BOILS
> infections in small skin wounds among workers in the sugar refining industry
>> Brit. Med. J. 2:77, 1936

SUGAR CANE CUTTERS' CRAMPS
> heat cramps among field workers
>> Hunter, D. The Diseases of Occupations. 5th ed. London: The English Univ. Press Ltd., 1975

SUGAR CANE LUNG
> BAGASSOSIS
>> original source not identified

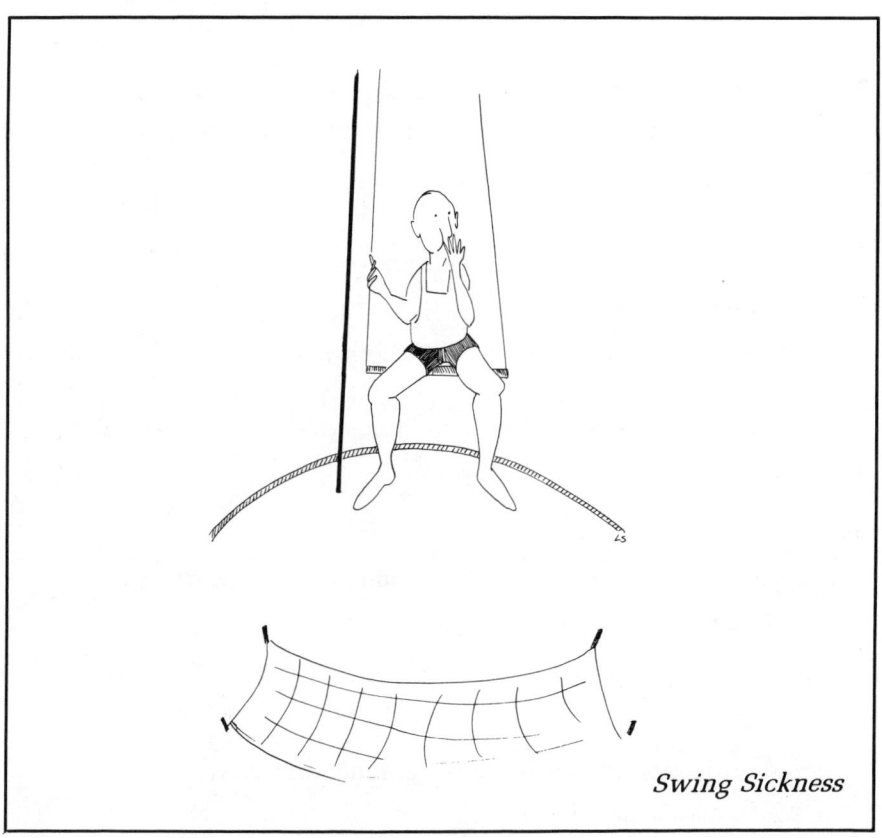

Swing Sickness

SUGAR MAKER'S LYMPHADENITIS

bacterial infection of the skin spreading to the lymph nodes
original source not identified

SUGAR WORKER'S ITCH

secondary infection of minor skin breaks
White, R. P. The Dermatogoses or Occupational Affections of the Skin. London: H. K. Lewis, 1928

SUGAR WORKER'S NEURITIS

BEET SUGAR WORKER'S NEURITIS
J. Ind. Hyg. 16:118, 1934

SUPERSONIC SICKNESS

ill-defined symptoms alleged to noise and vibration among jet test pilots
JAMA 135:933, 1947

SUPERSONIC SYNDROME

multiple injuries incurred by jet pilots who must bail out at high speeds
Stedman's Medical Dictionary. 23rd ed. Baltimore: William & Wilkins, 1976

SURFERS' EAR

overgrowth of the ear canal bone noted in cold water surfers
AMA Arch. Otolaryngol. 103:58, 1977

SURFERS' FOOT

fungus infection of the feet seen among surfers
Med. J. Austral. 18:420, 1939

Surfers' Knobs

SURFERS' KNOTS

International Classification of Diseases. 8th rev. USDHEW Pub. Hlth. Serv. Pub. No. 1963, 1968

Surfers' Knots

soft tissue swellings of the foot and leg caused by surfboard trauma

JAMA 192:223, 1965

Surfers' Nodules

SURFERS' KNOTS—"the prestige of the surfer is proportional to the size of his nodule"

original source not identified

Surfing Leash Injury

injuries sustained by the impact of an uncontrolled surfboard leashed to the swimmer

N. Eng. J. Med. 295:287, 1976

Sweat Band Dermatitis

forehead irritation caused by thioprene latex used as a sizing agent in sweat band cloth

Acta. Derm. Venereol. 27:287, 1947

skin irritation from chrome-tanned leathers used in sweat bands

JAMA 169:1747, 1959

Swell Foot

swelling, redness and pain of the foot from marching, jumping or dancing

Stedman's Medical Dictionary. 23rd ed. Baltimore: William & Wilkins, 1976

Swimmer's Conjunctivitis

SWIMMING POOL CONJUNCTIVITIS

International Classification of Diseases. 8th rev. USDHEW Pub. Hlth. Serv. Pub. No. 1963, 1968

Swimmer's Cramp

see OCCUPATIONAL NEUROSIS

JAMA 59:53, 1912

Swimmer's Dermatitis

SWIMMER'S ITCH

Dorland's Medical Dictionary. 25th ed. Phila.: W. B. Saunders, 1974

Swimmer's Ear

an infection of the external ear canal

original source not identified

Swimmers' Itch

skin eruption seen in swimmers caused by the snail parasite *Schistosoma cercariae*

Geograph. Rev. 42:212, 1952

Swimmer's Nose

redness and peeling of the nose due to sun and water exposure

Cent. Afr. J. Med. 17:232, 1971

Swimmers' Osteoma

SURFERS' EAR

World Wide Abst. 6(1):7, 1963

Swimming Pool Conjunctivitis

redness, swelling and tearing of the eyes caused by an infection which is spread via swimming pools

JAMA 86:966, 1926

Swimming Pool Granuloma

non-ulcerating, firm swelling among swimmers caused by *Mycobacterium balnei*

Arch. Derm. 88:158, 1963

Swimming Pool Rash

skin eruption among swimmers using pools which have not been adequately disinfected

Brit. Med. J. 2:344, 1976

Swimming Tank Conjunctivitis

SWIMMING POOL CONJUNCTIVITIS

Deut. Med. Wochen. 39:63, 1913

Swineherds' Disease

infectious disease (leptospirosis) occurring among those who attend, slaughter, or process swine, characterized by fever, headache, dizziness, nausea and generalized aching

J. Path. Bact. 34:545, 1931

Swing Sickness

motion sickness

J. Av. Med. 17:86, 1946

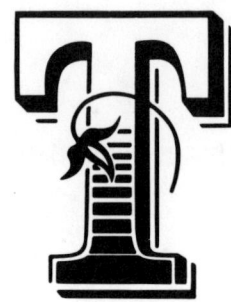

Tabacosis

deposition of tobacco dust in the lungs
>Versamml. Naturforsch. u. Aertzle. p. 271, 1865

tobacco poisoning
>Dorland's Medical Dictionary. 25th ed. Phila.: W. B. Saunders, 1974

Tacklers' Exostosis

overgrowth of bone of the arm seen in football players as a result of repeated local trauma
>J. Sports Med. 3:238, 1975

Tailor's Ankle

swelling over the ankle from sitting on the floor with the legs crossed
>Dorland's Medical Dictionary. 25th ed. Phila.: W. B. Saunders, 1974

Tailor's Bunion

inflammation and swelling of the fifth toe from pressure caused by sitting in the legs-crossed position

Stedman's Medical Dictionary. 23rd ed. Baltimore: William & Wilkins, 1976

Tailor's Callosities

hand calluses from the use of scissors

Hunter, D. The Diseases of Occupations. 5th ed. London: The English Univ. Press Ltd., 1975

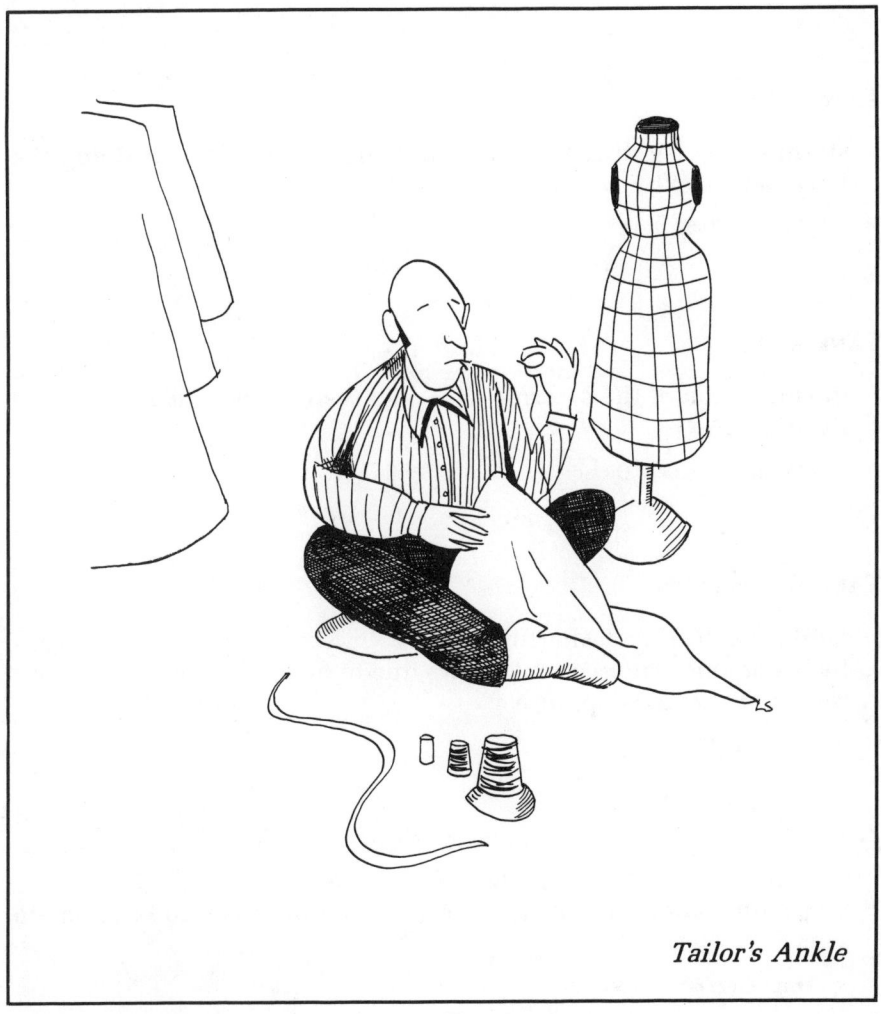

Tailor's Ankle

TRADE DISEASES

Tailor's Cramp

see OCCUPATIONAL NEUROSIS

Lancet 2:333, 1886

Tailors' Phthisis

tuberculosis among tailors during the sweat shop era

Hunter, D. The Diseases of Occupations. 5th ed. London: The English Univ. Press Ltd., 1975

Tango Foot

strain of the leg muscle (tibialis anticus) among dancers doing the tango and maxixe

JAMA 62:1507, 1914

Tank Ear

inflammation of the external ear canal seen in swimmers (compare BEACH EAR)

Dorland's Medical Dictionary. 25th ed. Phila.: W. B. Saunders, 1974

Tank Exhaustion

headache, dizziness, shortness of breath, vomiting and mental confusion among armored tank crews due to heat, poor ventilation and carbon monoxide exposure

Lancet 1:1156, 1920

Tanners' Ulcer

finger ulceration in tannery workers from exposure to bichromate salts

Ann. Surg. 63:155, 1916

Taravana Diving Syndrome

unconsciousness or paralysis after a strenuous series of deep water dives made by the pearl divers of the South Pacific Tuamotu Archipelago

Nat. Acad. Sci. Pub. No. 1341, 1965

Tar Smarts

dermatitis and photosensitivity of the exposed parts of the body among those employed in the distillation of coal (compare SMARTS)

Lancet 1:1153, 1965

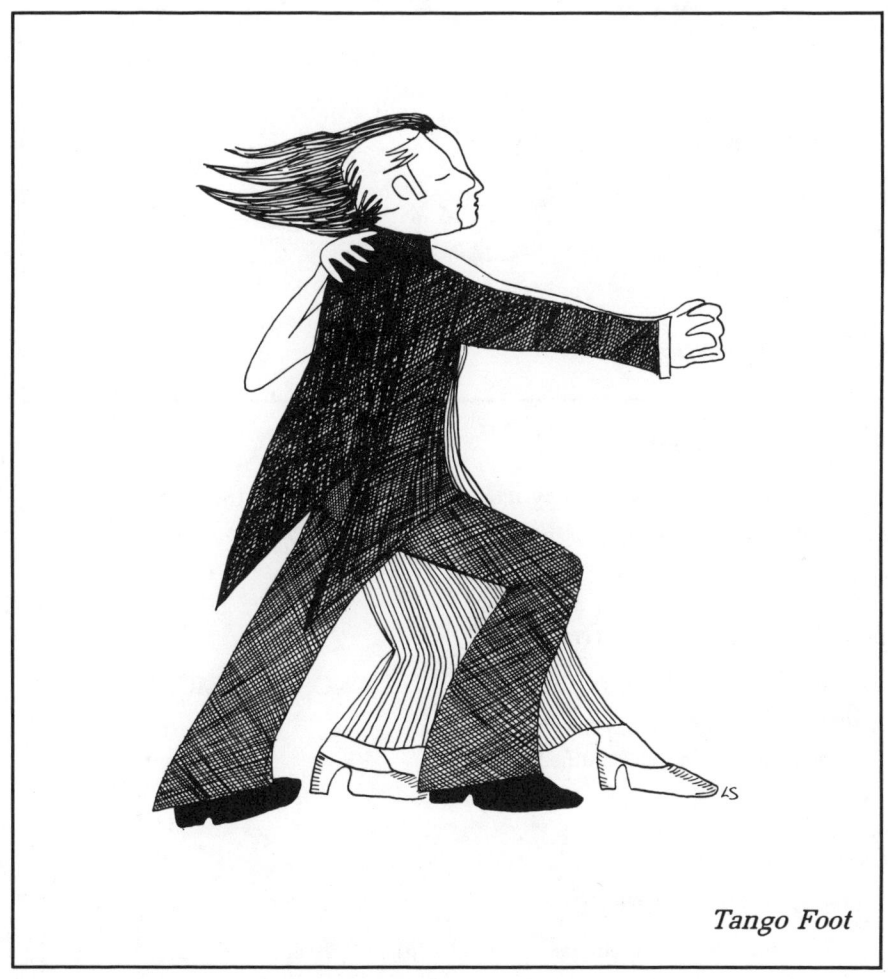

Tango Foot

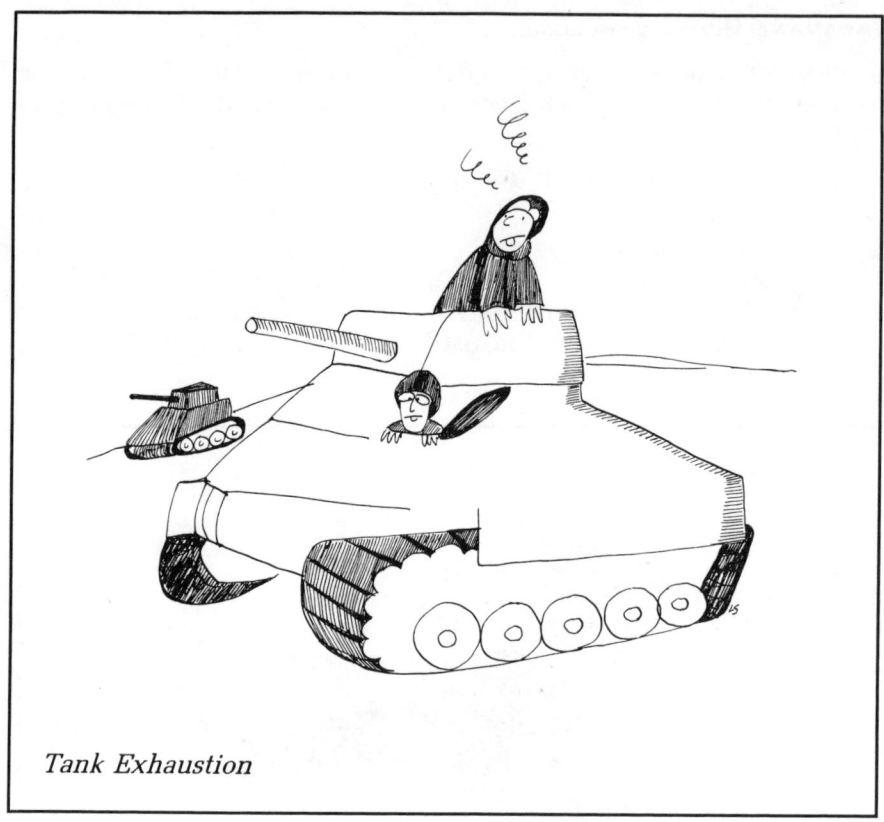

Tank Exhaustion

Tar Workers' Cancer

skin cancer observed in workers manufacturing tar paper

J. Cut. Dis. 28:644, 1910

Tar Workers' Dermatitis

any of the tar lesions such as T. MELANOSIS, T. MOLLUSCA, T. SMARTS, T. ITCH, T. CANCER

original source not identified

Teacher's Node

CHORDITIS TUBEROSA

Dorland's Medical Dictionary. 25th ed. Phila.: W. B. Saunders, 1974

TEACHER'S NODULE
CHORDITIS TUBEROSA
Dorland's Medical Dictionary. 25th ed. Phila.: W. B. Saunders, 1974

TEA FACTORY COUGH
weight loss, fatigue and cough among tea factory workers
Castellani, A., A J Chambers. Manual of Tropical Medicine. London: Bailliere, 1919

TEA MAKER'S ASTHMA
allergic inflammatory response of the lungs to inhaled tea fluff
Brit. J. Ind. Med. 27:181, 1970

TEA TASTERS' COUGH
cough, weight loss and debility among tea tasters who hold tea leaves in their hands and snuff the tea leaf dust
U.S. Nav. Med. Bull. 14:669, 1920

TEA TASTER'S DISEASE
TEA FACTORY COUGH
Arlidge, J. T. The Hygiene, Diseases And Mortality of Occupations. London: Percival, 1892

TELEGRAPH CLERK'S CRAMP
see OCCUPATIONAL NEUROSIS
Brit. Med. J. 1:515, 1875

TELEGRAPHERS' CRAMPS
see OCCUPATIONAL NEUROSIS
International Classification of Diseases. 8th rev. USDHEW Pub. Hlth. Serv. Pub. No. 1963, 1968

TELEGRAPHIC COMPLAINT

see OCCUPATIONAL NEUROSIS

Brit. Med. J. 1:515, 1875

TELEGRAPHIC MALADY

see OCCUPATIONAL NEUROSIS

Lancet 1:585, 1875

TELEGRAPHIST'S CRAMP

see OCCUPATIONAL NEUROSIS

Brit. Med. J. 2:880, 1882

TELEGRAPHIST'S PARALYSIS

see OCCUPATIONAL NEUROSIS

Lancet 2:1034, 1934

TELEGRAPHIST'S SPASM

see OCCUPATIONAL NEUROSIS

Oliver, T. Dangerous Trades. London: J. Murray, 1902

TELEGRAPH WRITER'S CRAMP

see OCCUPATIONAL NEUROSIS

Brit. Med. J. 1:515, 1875

TELEPHONE EAR

headache, dizziness, insomnia and other symptoms alleged to overuse of the telephone

Lancet 2:1369, 1892

Telephone Paralysis

partial vocal paralysis alleged to excessive use of the telephone

JAMA 35:844, 1900

Telephoner's Impetigo

staphylococcal infection of the ear from overuse of the telephone

Arch. Derm. 112:1178, 1976

Telephone Tinnitus

ringing in the ear, nervousness, dizziness and ear pain from prolonged use of the telephone

Brit. Med. J. 2:672, 1889

Television Angina

attacks of angina pectoris provoked by violence or excitement in television stories

JAMA 169:2064, 1959

Television Epilepsy

precipitation of a seizure via the photic stimulation of television flicker

Lancet 2:926, 1970

Television Glaucoma

eye disease precipitated by watching television due to an unstable intraocular tension and the accommodation effort required in a dark room

Brit. Med. J. 2:98, 1953

TELEVISION LEGS

loss of normal flexibility in the legs and lower back of youngsters who spend long hours slumped in front of TV sets

JAMA 166:2066, 1958

TELEVISION NECK

limited neck motion accompanied by pain among persons who watch TV for prolonged periods of time

JAMA 149:1332, 1952

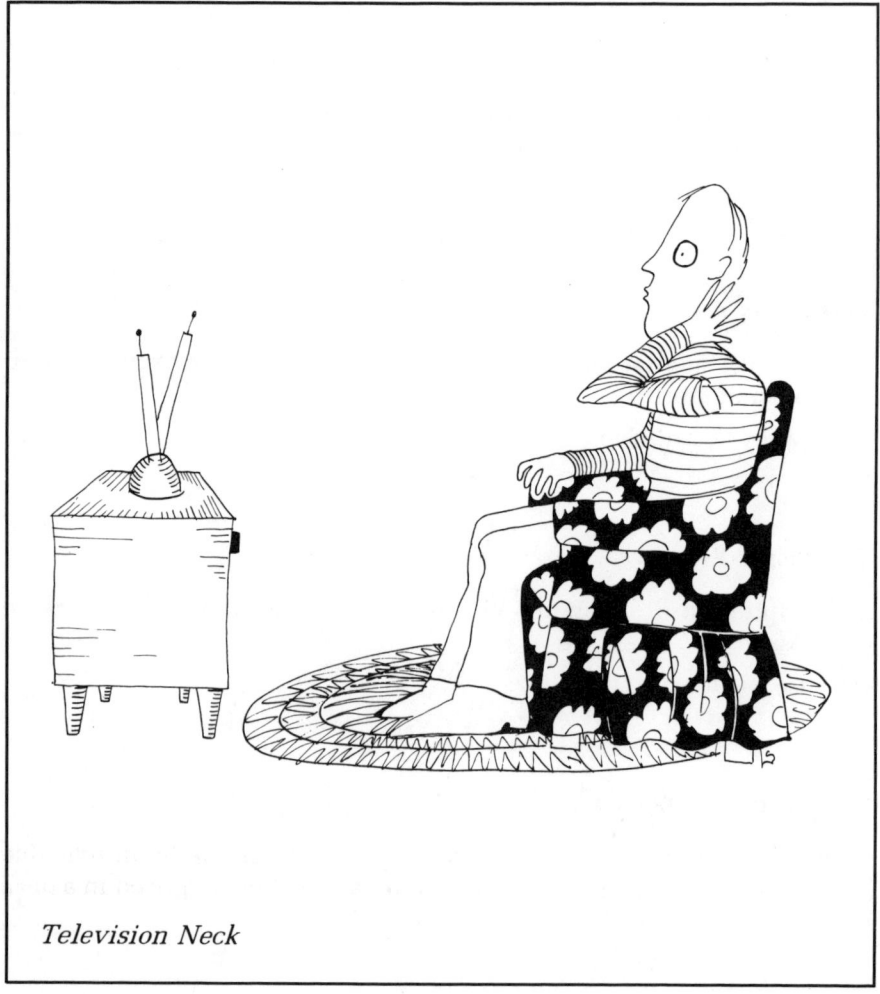

Television Neck

TENNIS BLISTERS
>blister formation on the hands or feet of tennis players
>>Brit. Med. J. 2:173, 1931

TENNIS ELBOW
>pain over the lateral side of the elbow
>>Deut. Med. Wochen. N 44:713, 1900
>
>numbness and weakness of the hand from radial nerve strain
>>JAMA 57:1698, 1911

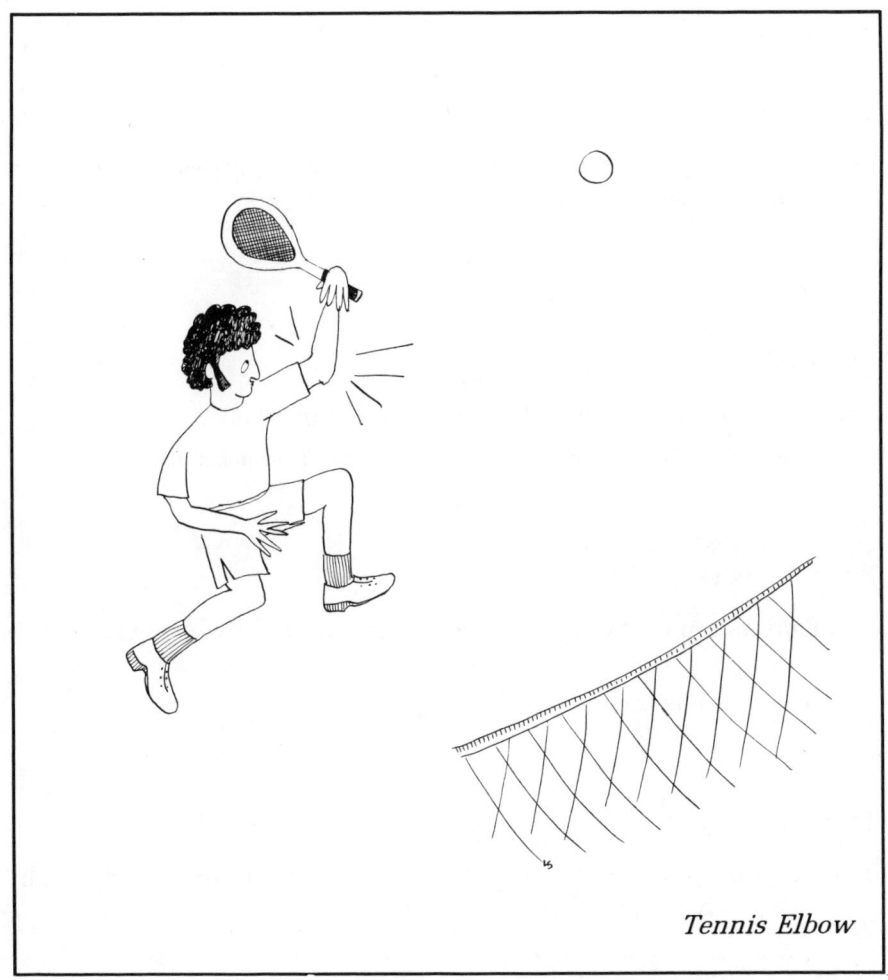

Tennis Elbow

TRADE DISEASES

Tennis Leg

pain in the calf of the leg from a tear of the gastrocnemius muscle while playing tennis

Brit. Med. J. 1:611, 1931

Tennis Thumb

inflammation and calcification of the long flexor tendon of the thumb

Lancet 1:1151, 1951

Tennis Toe

pain and bleeding beneath the nail from excess pressure of the box toe of a sneaker

Arch. Derm. 107:918, 1973

Tennis Wrist

inflammation of the wrist tendons in tennis players

Dorland's Medical Dictionary. 25th ed. Phila.: W. B. Saunders, 1974

Ten-pin Finger

inflammation of the middle finger joints caused by excessive bowling

Brit. Med. J. 1:542, 1963

Testitis

anxiety over proficiency flight check-rides occurring among flight crews (compare CHECKITIS)

Av. Sp. Environ. Med. 46:1407, 1975

THRESHER'S DISEASE

fever, cough, sweating, headaches and weakness presumed to be due to a fungus in the dust given off by grain threshing machines

Schweiz. Med. Wschr. 76:988, 1946

THRESHERS' ITCH

skin eruption among grain handlers caused by the grain mite *Pyemotes ventricosus*

JAMA 91:1129, 1928

THRESHER'S LUNG

allergic inflammatory response of the lungs to the inhalation of moldy grain dust

Acta. Med. Scand. 125:191, 1946

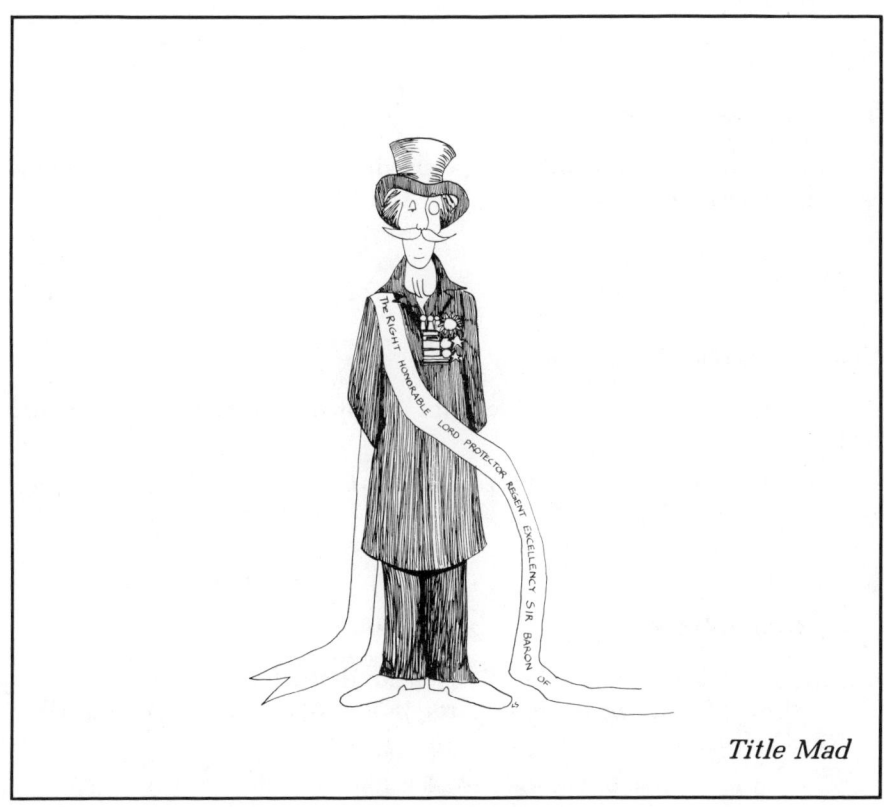

Title Mad

TRADE DISEASES

Threshing Disease

THRESHER'S LUNG

Schweiz. Med. Wchnschr. 76:988, 1946

Threshing Fever

THRESHER'S LUNG

JAMA 110:1696, 1938

Tight Girdle Syndrome

vigorous neck pulses, gastrointestinal symptoms and shortness of breath caused by wearing a tight girdle

N. Eng. J. Med. 288:584, 1973

Tileburners' Anemia

hookworm infection in tile burners due to unsanitary work conditions (compare BRICKBURNERS' ANEMIA)

Brit. Med. J. 2:640, 1883

Timber Porter's Shoulder

swelling over the collar bone from pressure and friction of carrying timbers

Hunter, D. The Diseases of Occupations. 5th ed. London: The English Univ. Press Ltd., 1975

Time Zone Syndrome

fatigue, tenseness and irritability from disturbance of the circadian rhythm of the body (compare JET LAG and TRAVEL DYSRHYTHMIA)

Stedman's Medical Dictionary. 23rd ed. Baltimore: William & Wilkins, 1976

Tin Miner's Lung

stannosis, deposition of tin dust in the lungs, usually not associated with pulmonary impairment

> original source not identified

Tin Plate Millman's Cataract

cataract resulting from prolonged exposure of the eye to infrared radiation from the hot metal

> Brit. J. Ophth. 5:194, 1921

Tin Plate Worker's Cataract

TIN PLATE MILLMAN'S CATARACT

> Hunter, D. The Diseases of Occupations. 5th ed. London: The English Univ. Press Ltd., 1975

Tin Smelters' Pneumoconiosis

deposition of tin oxide dust in the lungs

> Brit. Med. J. 1:598, 1955

Tinsmith's Cramp

see OCCUPATIONAL NEUROSIS

> Hunter, D. The Diseases of Occupations. 5th ed. London: The English Univ. Press Ltd., 1975

Title Mad

ambitious folly with a mania for having a title: president, emperor, king, count, duke, etc.

> Lancet 1:787, 1867

TNT Jaundice

toxic jaundice caused by trinitrotoluene intoxication, seen among ordnance employees

Lancet 2:552, 1941

Tobacco Croppers' Sickness

weakness, nausea and vomiting among tobacco croppers who pick the leaves, presumably due to a non-nicotine agent in tobacco sap

Fla. Med. Assoc. J. 57:13, 1970

Tobacosis

asthma and fever in tobacco workers from the inhalation of tobacco dust (compare TABACOSIS)

Dtsch. Arch. Klin. Med. 2:116, 1866

Toilet Seat Dermatitis

skin irritation of the buttocks and thighs from a red stain used on a toilet seat

Arch. Derm. & Syph. 27:976, 1933

Toilet Seat Neuropathy

foot paralysis from compression of the peroneal nerve between a heavy thigh and the toilet seat

N. Eng. J. Med. 280:1484, 1969

Tonoko Lung

silicosis, believed caused by tonoko, which is used in processing furniture and contains 50% quartz

Tohoku J. Exp. Med. 114:295, 1974

Tourist Hepatitis

viral hepatitis contracted by the traveler from contaminated drinking water

Brit. Med. J. 1:189, 1977

Tourists' Disease

gastroenteritis, affecting tourists, due to an enteropathogen: staphylococcus, salmonella, etc.

JAMA 147:358, 1951

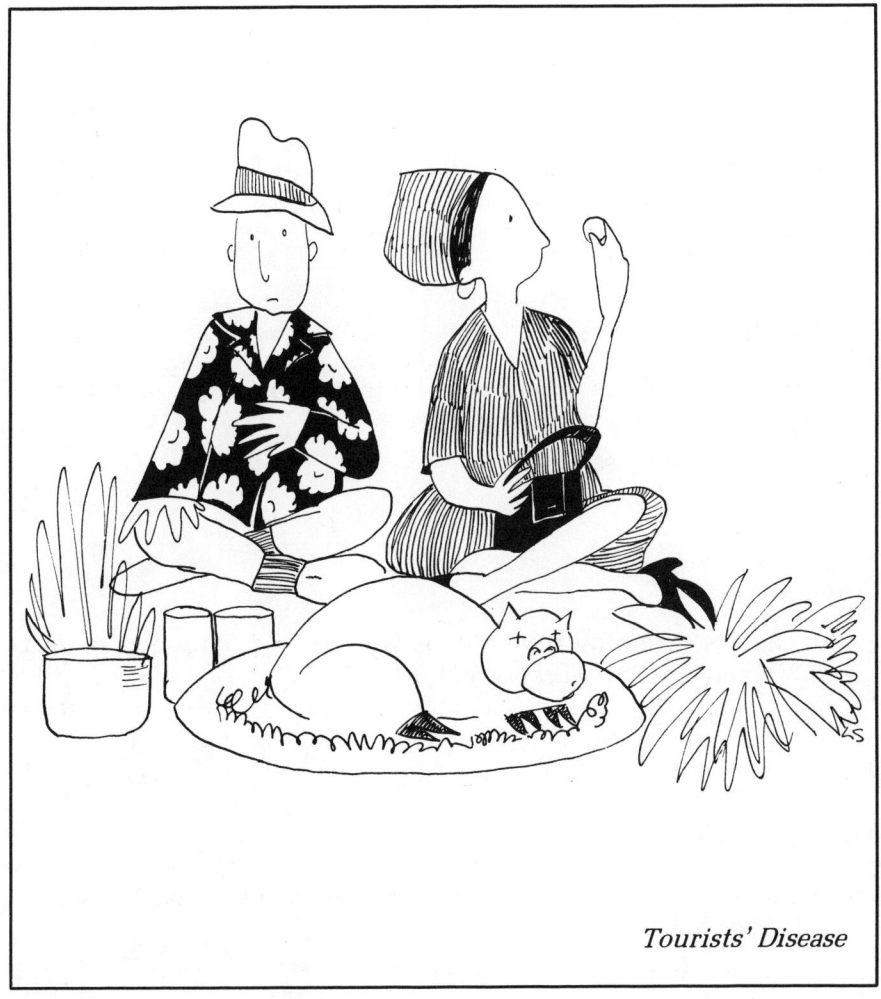

Tourists' Disease

TRADE DISEASES

Tourniquet Paralysis

altered sensation or muscle paralysis due to prolonged application of a tight tourniquet

Milit. Med. 131:161, 1966

Town-dweller's Lung

silicosis in city dwellers due to the inhalation of siliceous dust

Brit. Med. J. 1:476, 1938

Toxigenic Turista

TRAVELER'S DIARRHEA

N. Eng. J. Med. 292:969, 1975

Tractor Sickness

dizziness and nausea experienced by tractor operators, presumably from carbon monoxide intoxication

Practitioner 139:90, 1937

Trade Cancers

skin cancers occurring among trade workers; e.g., chimney sweeps, paraffin and coal tar workers and others

Brit. J. Derm. 21:190, 1909

Trade Dermatitis

skin diseases of the trades; e.g., miners, housewives, chocolate workers, rubber workers, etc.

Lancet 2:732, 1908

Trade Holes

ulcerative skin lesions in tannery workers due to contact with chrome and alkaline solutions

Brit. J. Ind. Med. 12:73, 1955

Traffic Fracture

elbow fracture of a driver whose protruding elbow is struck by a passing vehicle (compare SIDE-SWIPE FRACTURE)

J. Indiana M. 26:509, 1933

Train Sickness

motion sickness

International Classification of Diseases. 8th rev. USDHEW Pub. Hlth. Serv. Pub. No. 1963, 1968

Transkei Dust Disease

silicosis among Transkei South African women who grind corn indoors using quartzite grinding stones

Lancet 1:289, 1968

Trap Drummer's Neurosis

see OCCUPATIONAL NEUROSIS

Med. News 82:257, 1903

Travel Dysrhythmia

malaise and disturbance of sleep, temperature and endocrine rhythms within the body due to rapid travel across time zones (compare TIME ZONE SYNDROME, JET LAG)

original source not identified

Traveler's Ankle

ankle swelling from decreased circulation related to sitting on a bus or airplane for prolonged periods

Brit. Med. J. 3:109, 1973

Traveler's Back

back pain beginning in the buttocks and progressing to the lower spine, caused by sitting in a restricted space without moving for long periods as in a car, bus or plane

Brit. Med. J. 4:551, 1973

Traveler's Diarrhea

self-limiting illness characterized by abdominal cramps, nausea, malaise, diarrhea, vomiting and chills or fever due to a gastrointestinal pathogen

JAMA 180:107, 1962

Travelers' Edema

swelling of the ankles and legs of travelers who sit or stand for long periods of time

Brit. Med. J. 1:322, 1946

Traveler's Psychosis

mental disturbance related to travel, ranging from tension, apprehension and insecurity to acute hallucinations and delusions, resulting from a sense of isolation, alcohol or drug withdrawal, disturbances of biologic rhythms, etc.

Brit. Med. J. 2:133, 1968

Travel Fever

an urge to roam

Lansberg, M. P. A Primer of Space Medicine. Amsterdam: Elsevier, 1960

Travel Sickness

motion sickness

> International Classification of Diseases. 8th rev. USDHEW Pub. Hlth. Serv. Pub. No. 1963, 1968

Treadler's Cramp

see OCCUPATIONAL NEUROSIS

> Lancet 1:434, 1891

Trench Back

back injury caused by falling earth or sandbags during WWI

> Brit. Med. J. 2:215, 1915

Trench Bite

TRENCH FROSTBITE

> Brit. Med. J. 1:515, 1915

Trench Diarrhea

diarrhea due to poor sanitation in the trenches in WWI

> Dorland's Medical Dictionary. 25th ed. Phila.: W. B. Saunders, 1974

Trench Enteritis

TRENCH DIARRHEA

> Lancet 1:689, 1916

Trench Fever

a *Rickettsial* infection of the troops in WWI, transmitted by the body louse, characterized by fever and aching of the shins

> Bost. Med. & Surg. J. 177:596, 1917

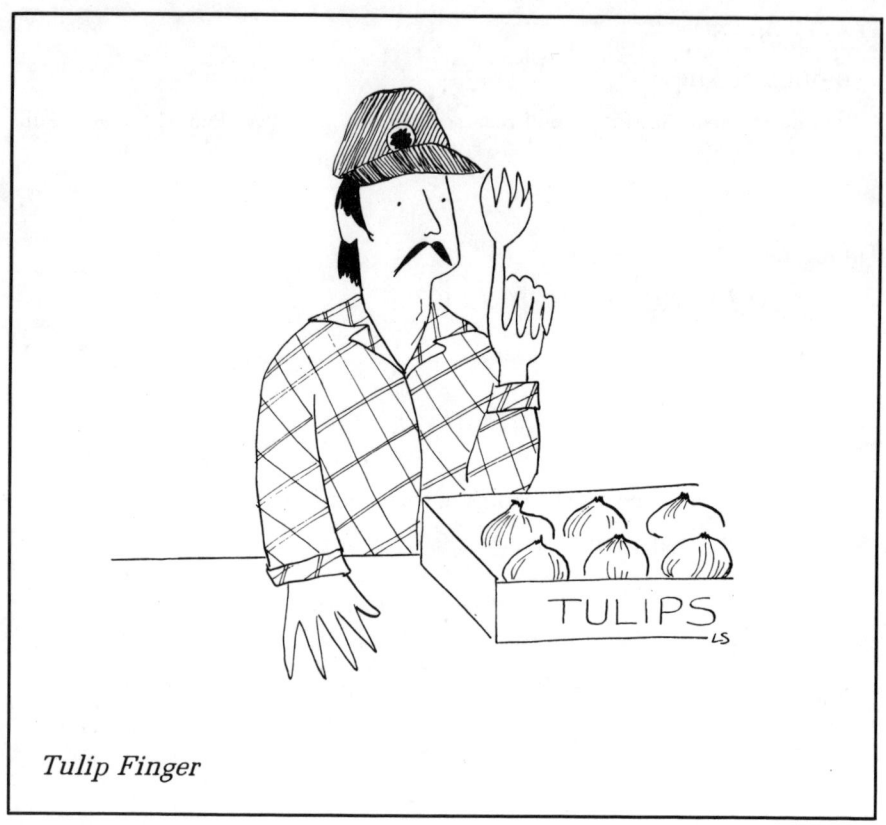

Tulip Finger

Trench Foot

IMMERSION FOOT

Bost. Med. & Surg. J. 176:301, 1917

Trench Frostbite

frostbite among WWI troops

Brit. Med. J. 1:352, 1915

Trench Hand

contracture of the hand following severe frostbite among WWI troops

Dorland's Medical Dictionary. 25th ed. Phila.: W. B. Saunders, 1974

Trench Hemeralopia

disturbance of night vision among WWI troops (the term was used incorrectly since nyctalopia is implied)

Lancet 2:853, 1917

Trench Leg

TRENCH SHIN

Stedman's Medical Dictionary. 23rd ed. Baltimore: William & Wilkins, 1976

Trench Lung

attacks of rapid breathing among the soldiers in trenches during WWI

Dorland's Medical Dictionary. 25th ed. Phila.: W. B. Saunders, 1974

Trench Mouth

ulcerations of the mouth and gums of WWI troops due to a spirochetal infection

Lancet 2:46, 1940

Trench Nephritis

acute kidney infection among WWI troops probably related to unsanitary conditions

Lancet 1:391, 1916

Trench Rheumatism

inflammation of the muscles and tendons with stiffness and deformity of the back and legs occurring in WWI soldiers as a result of exposure in cold, damp trenches

Lancet 1:991, 1917

TRENCH SHIN

tendon inflammation related to the wearing of tight puttees by WWI soldiers

Brit. Med. J. 2:939, 1915

TRIGGER FINGER

a sudden check to voluntary extension or flexion of a finger which can be overcome by pressure, at which time an audible snap may be heard

Brit. Med. J. 2:28, 1885

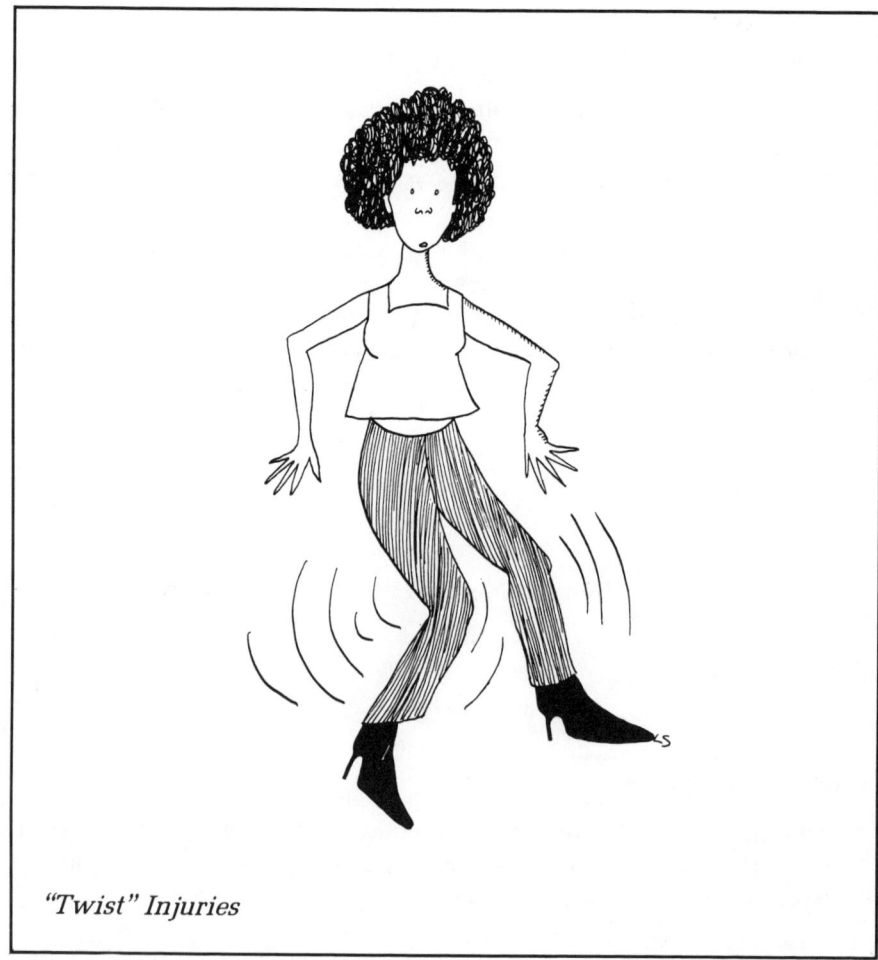

"Twist" Injuries

Tropical Immersion Foot

redness, swelling and tenderness of the feet and ankles after prolonged exposure to water at tropical temperatures as seen among Vietnamese combat forces

Lancet 2:1185, 1973

Tropical Service Ecthyma

DESERT SORES or chronic ulcerative skin lesions occurring among British and African troops from local trauma and lack of personal hygiene

Brit. Med. J. 2:96, 1942

Trumpeter's Parotitis

swelling and pain of the salivary gland from air entry into the duct while playing wind instruments

Mschr. Ohrenheilk 98:101, 1964

Trumpet Player's Cramp

see OCCUPATIONAL NEUROSIS

Hunter, D. The Diseases of Occupations. 5th ed. London: The English Unv. Press Ltd., 1975

Tulip Finger

tingling of the fingertips beneath the nails with occasional separation of the nails and a rash on the fingers affecting workers in the bulb fields

Brit. Med. J. 2:255, 1935

Tunnel Anemia

TUNNEL WORKERS' ANEMIA

Trop. Dis. 36: 537, 1898

TUNNEL DISEASE

DECOMPRESSION SICKNESS

Dorland's Medical Dictionary. 25th ed. Phila.: W. B. Saunders, 1974

TUNNEL WORKERS' ANEMIA

Stedman's Medical Dictionary. 23rd ed. Baltimore: William & Wilkins, 1976

TUNNEL WORKERS' ANEMIA

hook worm infection of tunnel workers due to unsanitary conditions

Hunter, D. The Diseases of Occupations. 5th ed. London: The English Univ. Press Ltd., 1975

TURF TOE

sprain of the great toe of football players using stiff shoes on a hard surface

Med. Sci. Sports 8:81, 1976

TURISTA

TRAVELER'S DIARRHEA

Original sorce not identified

TV-MEDICITIS

tendency of television viewers to "catch" a disease portrayed in a television script (compare VIDEO VOODOO)

JAMA 187:307, 1964

TWISTER'S CRAMP

OCCUPATIONAL NEUROSIS of loom workers

J. Ind. Hyg. 2:191, 1921

"Twist" Injuries

knee and wrist injuries resulting from performing the dance known as the "twist"

Brit. Med. J. 1:803, 1962

Typesetter's Cramp

see OCCUPATIONAL NEUROSIS

Brit. Med. J. 1:11, 1886

Typewriter's Cramp

see OCCUPATIONAL NEUROSIS

Lancet 1:49, 1898

Typist's Cramp

see OCCUPATIONAL NEUROSIS

International Classification of Diseases. 8th rev. USDHEW Pub. Hlth. Serv. Pub. No. 1963, 1968

Typist's Neuritis

see OCCUPATIONAL NEUROSIS

Lancet 2:1052, 1908

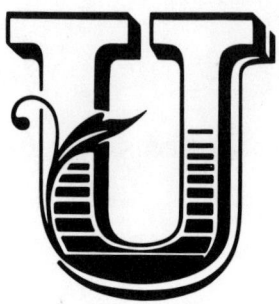

ULTRASONIC SICKNESS

headache, dizziness, nausea, and fatigue with or without hearing loss believed associated with exposure to ultra-audible sound

Amer. Ind. Hyg. Assoc. Quart. 9:57, 1947

UNIFORM RASH

skin irritation of the neck, chest, arms and abdomen of nurses from wearing new uniforms, the causative agent not being identified

Brit. Med. J. 1:423, 1973

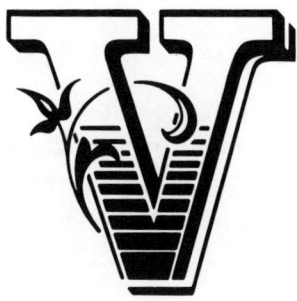

Vaccinator's Thumb

accidental innoculation of the thumb while expelling smallpox vaccine from a small tube

Lancet 1:1422, 1966

Vagabonds' Disease

discoloration of the skin of scavengers caused by long-continued exposure, dirty habits and irritation from vermin

Tr. Clin. Soc. London 9:44, 1876

Vagabonds' Pigmentation

VAGABONDS' DISEASE

Dorland's Medical Dictionary. 25th ed. Phila.: W. B. Saunders, 1974

Vagrants' Disease

VAGABONDS' DISEASE

Stedman's Medical Dictionary. 23rd ed. Baltimore: William & Wilkins, 1976

VANADIUM LUNG

cough, shortness of breath and asthmatic breathing among vanadium workers

Arch. Gewerbepath. u. Gewerbehyg. 13:73, 1954

VANILLISM

itchy skin eruption from handling raw vanilla or vanilla pods caused by the mite *Tyrophagus siro*

Arch. Mal. Profess. 7:120, 1946

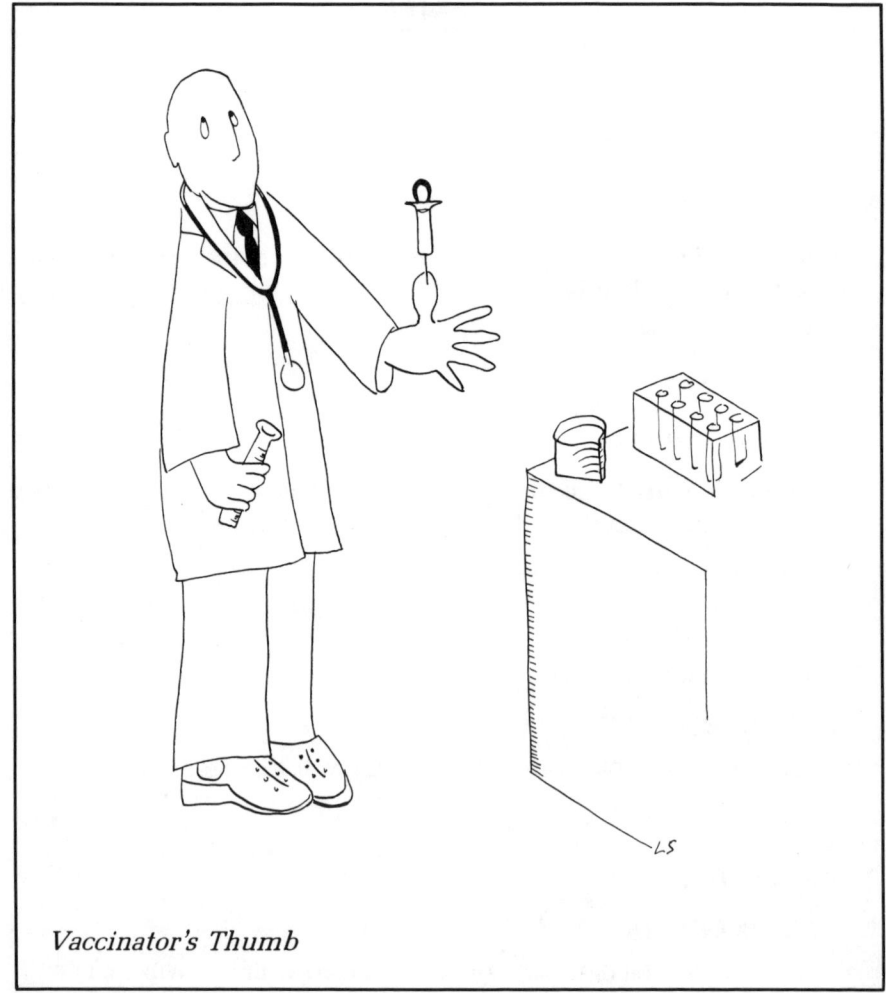

Vaccinator's Thumb

VASODILATOR DISEASE

arterial constrictive phenomena, such as angina pectoris, as a withdrawal effect following exposure to vasodilators as can occur in explosive workers

JAMA 182:101, 1962

VELDT SORE

bacterial skin lesions seen in South African troops

Lancet 1:1108, 1902

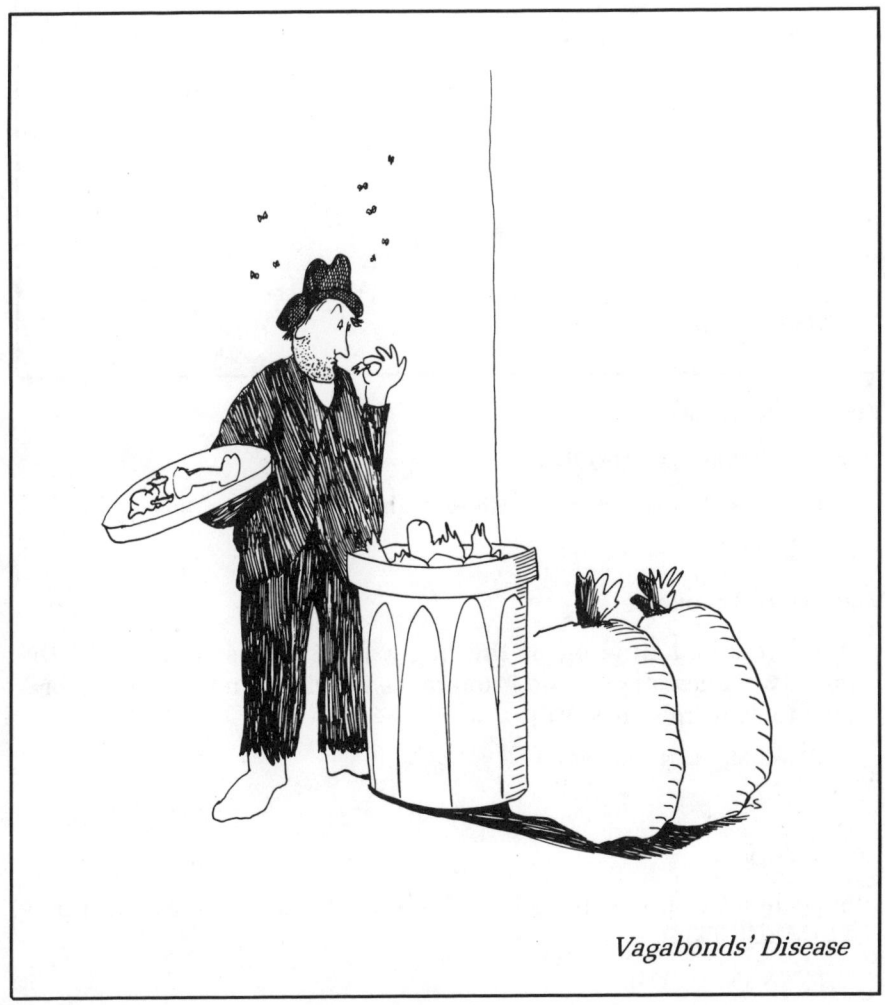

Vagabonds' Disease

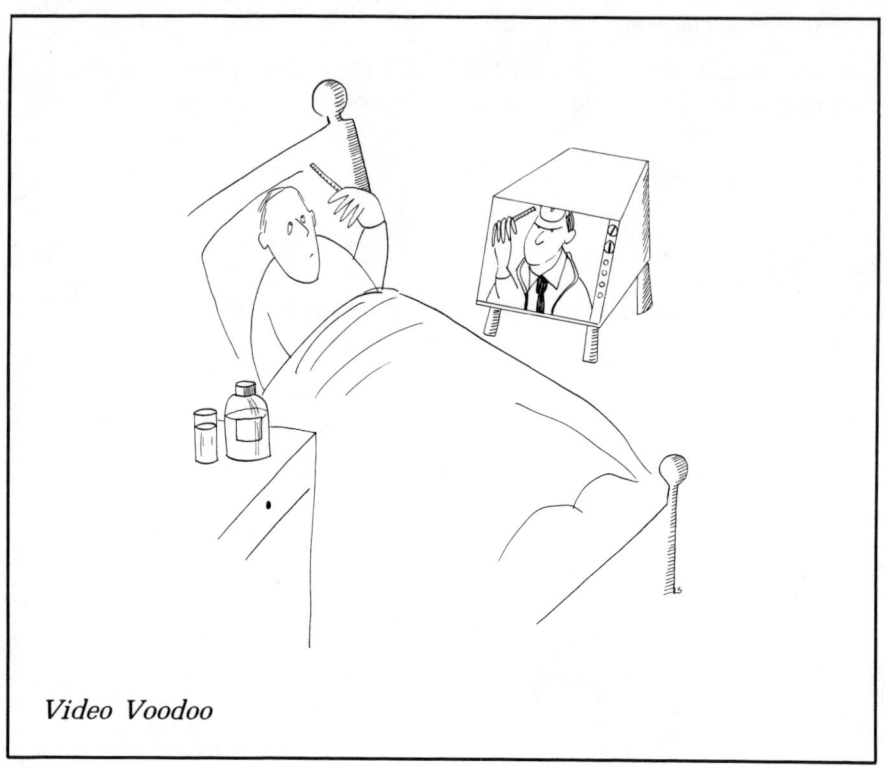
Video Voodoo

VIBRATION DISEASE

VIBRATION SYNDROME

Dorland's Medical Dictionary. 25th ed. Phila.: W. B. Saunders, 1974

VIBRATION SYNDROME

numbness and tingling of the fingers, burning sensations in the hand, weakness of grip and intolerance to cold from the use of vibratory tools (compare VWF)

Canad. M.A.J. 54: 472, 1946

VIDEO VOODOO

hypochondriasis resulting from viewing TV doctor-sagas (compare TV-MEDICITIS)

JAMA 187:296, 1964

Vineyard Sprayer's Lung

pulmonary reaction to copper sulfate in Bordeaux mixture, after years of exposure, characterized by weakness, loss of appetite and weight and shortness of breath

Thorax 24:415, 1969

Violin Cellist's Cramp

see OCCUPATIONAL NEUROSIS

Lancet 2:333, 1886

Violinist's Calluses

fingertip thickenings caused by finger pressure on the strings

Singer, K. Diseases of the Musical Profession. (tr. by W. Lakond, Greensberg, N.Y., 1932)

Violinist's Cramp

see OCCUPATIONAL NEUROSIS

Brit. Med. J. 1:11, 1886

Vocational Cancer

cancer occurring as an occupational disease

Lancet 1:911, 1924

Vocational Phobia

anxiety, depression and other symptoms related to a concern about job performance

Compre. Psychiat. 13:251, 1972

Volkswagon Dermatitis

allergic contact dermatitis caused by rubber bumper guards

Arch. Derm. 103: 85, 1971

VWF (Vibration Induced Whitefinger)

blanching of the fingers with loss of sensation, pain and occasionally degenerative joint changes caused by the use of vibratory tools (compare VIBRATION SYNDROME)

Vibration Syndrome Interim report by the Industrial Injuries Advisory Council Cmnd. 4430 HM Stationery Office, 1970

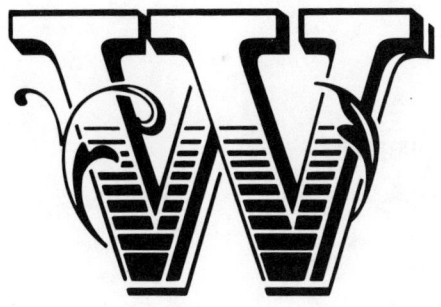

WAITER'S CRAMP

see OCCUPATIONAL NEUROSIS

Hunter, D. The Diseases of Occupations. 5th ed. London: The English Univ. Press Ltd., 1975

WAITER'S SHOULDER

shoulder bursitis from carrying trays in a shoulder-high position

N. Eng. J. Med. 288:799, 1973

WAR DEAFNESS

hearing deficiency produced by the noise from projectile explosions

Lancet 2:852, 1917

WAR EDEMA

tissue swelling as a result of poor nutrition and debilitating diseases during war-time

Brit. Med. J. 2:560, 1917

WAREHOUSEMAN'S ITCH

dermatitis caused by handling irritating substances
Stedman's Medical Dictionary. 23rd ed. Baltimore: William & Wilkins, 1976

WAR FROSTBITE

TRENCH FROSTBITE
Brit. Med. J. 1:352, 1915

WAR HEART

SOLDIERS' HEART
Lancet 1:985, 1917

WAR HYSTERIA

hysteria due to the tensions of war
Lancet 2:79, 1919

WAR MALARIA

benign tertian malaria occurring among British troops in Egypt
Brit. Med. J. 1:162, 1945

WAR NEPHRITIS

acute kidney infection among soldiers during WWI
Lancet 2:119, 1917

WAR NEUROSIS

mental and functional disorders due to the tensions of war
Lancet 2:168, 1918

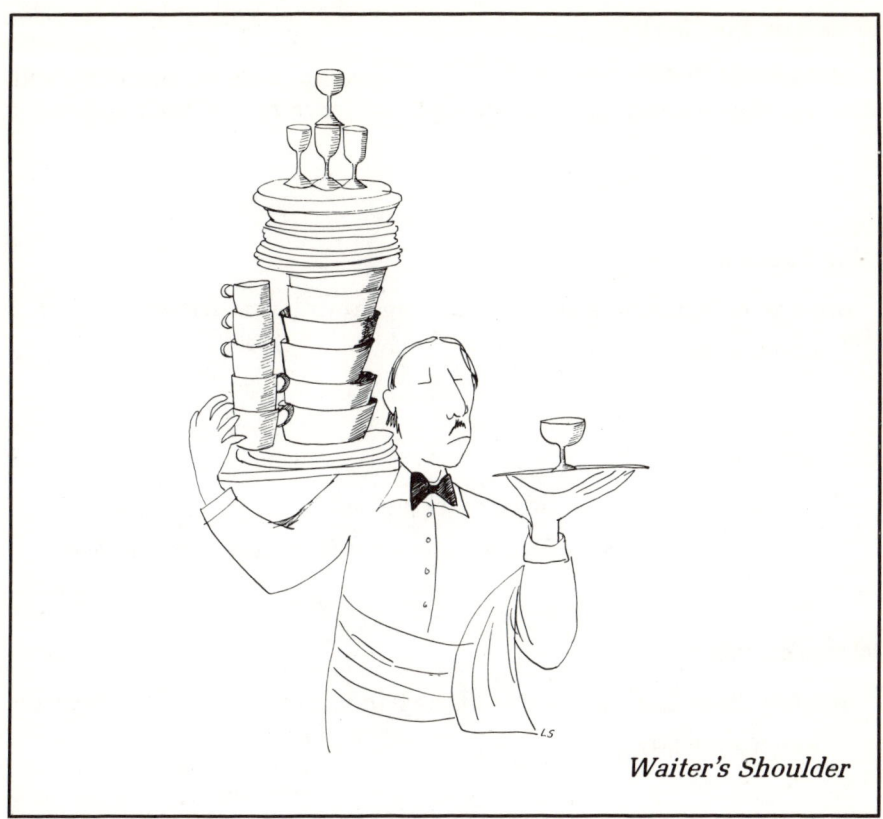
Waiter's Shoulder

War Psychosis

WAR NEUROSIS

Brit. Med. J. 2:64, 1915

War Sailor Syndrome

anxiety and progressive incapacity for work among WWII survivors in the Norwegian merchant marine

T. Norske Laegeforen. 96:868, 1976

War Shock

WAR NEUROSIS

Lancet 2:928, 1917

WAR-TIME POT BELLY

abdominal distension associated with complaints of vomiting and colitis due to voluntary or subconscious depression of the diaphragm

Lancet 1:772, 1917

WAR TREMORS

organic or neurotic tremors resulting from battle trauma

JAMA 70:866, 1918

WASHERMAN'S MARK

skin irritation from laundry marking ink

Stedman's Medical Dictionary. 23rd ed. Baltimore: William & Wilkins, 1976

WASHERMEN'S ITCH

redness, fissuring and peeling of the hands and wrists of laundrymen

Lancet 2:820, 1843

WASHERWOMAN'S DERMATITIS

hand and wrist eczema from cleansers used in doing laundry

White, R.P. The Dermatogoses or Occupational Affections of the Skin. London: H.K. Lewis, 1928

WASHERWOMAN'S FINGER

wrinkling of the skin from prolonged exposure to water

original source not identified

WASHERWOMAN'S HAND

WASHERWOMAN'S FINGER

original source not identified

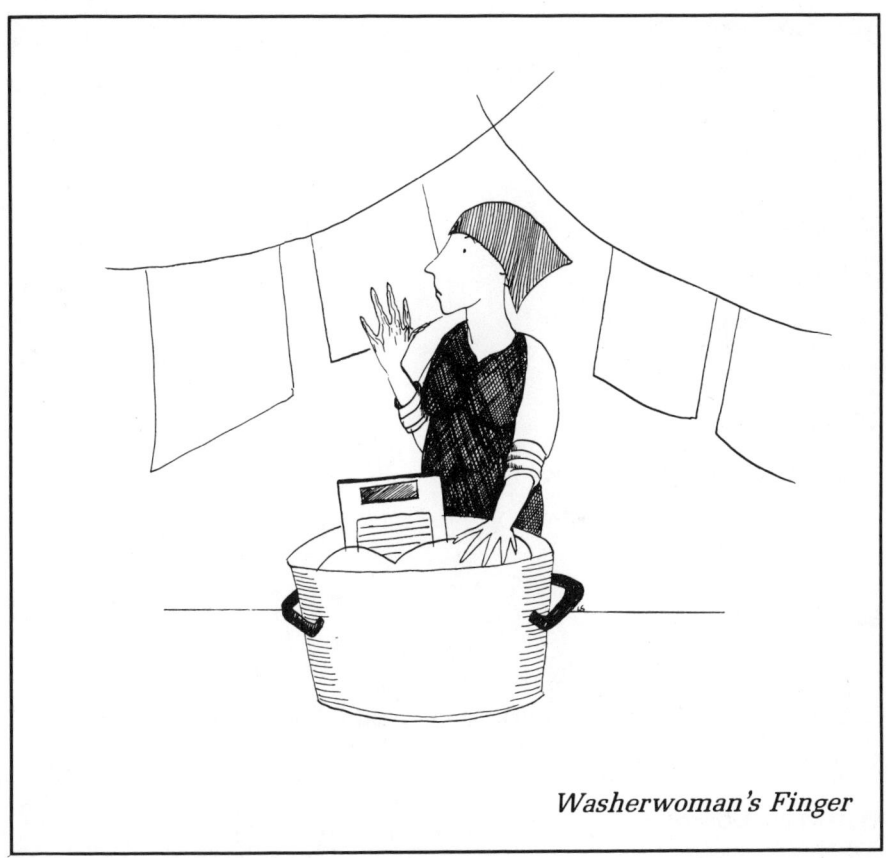

Washerwoman's Finger

WASHERWOMAN'S ITCH
   hand eczema from doing laundry
      Hoblyn's Medical Dictionary, 1844

WASHERWOMAN'S SCALL
   WASHERWOMAN'S ITCH
      Hoblyn's Medical Dictionary, 1844

WASHERWOMEN'S ECZEMA
   WASHERWOMAN'S DERMATITIS
      Brit. Med. J. 2:492, 1908

WATCHMAKER'S CRAMP

see OCCUPATIONAL NEUROSIS

Lancet 2:333, 1886

WAXY FINGERS

DEAD FINGERS

Brit. Med. J. 1:37, 1910

WEAVERS' ASTHMA

BYSSINOSIS in cotton weavers

Acta. Allergol. 22:39, 1967

WEAVER'S BOTTOM

hip bursitis from sitting at the loom

ILO Encyclopedia of Occupational Health and Safety. N.Y.: McGraw Hill, 1972

WEAVERS' COUGH

shortness of breath and cough among cotton weavers ascribed to loom mildew

Brit. Med. J. 1:455, 1927

WEAVER'S CRAMP

see OCCUPATIONAL NEUROSIS

Brain 4:257, 1881

WEAVER'S DEAFNESS

hearing loss caused by loom noise

Hunter, D. The Diseases of Occupations. 5th ed. London: The English Univ. Press Ltd., 1975

WEAVERS' TONSILS

chronic tonsillitis among weavers from "sucking weft"; i.e., threading loom shuttles by sucking the cotton weft through the shuttle eye

Brit. Med. J. 2:770, 1902

WEIGHT LIFTER'S BLACKOUT

loss of consciousness while lifting weights caused by reduced cardiac output and cerebral blood flow occurring during the lift (Valsalva effect)

Lancet 2:1234, 1973

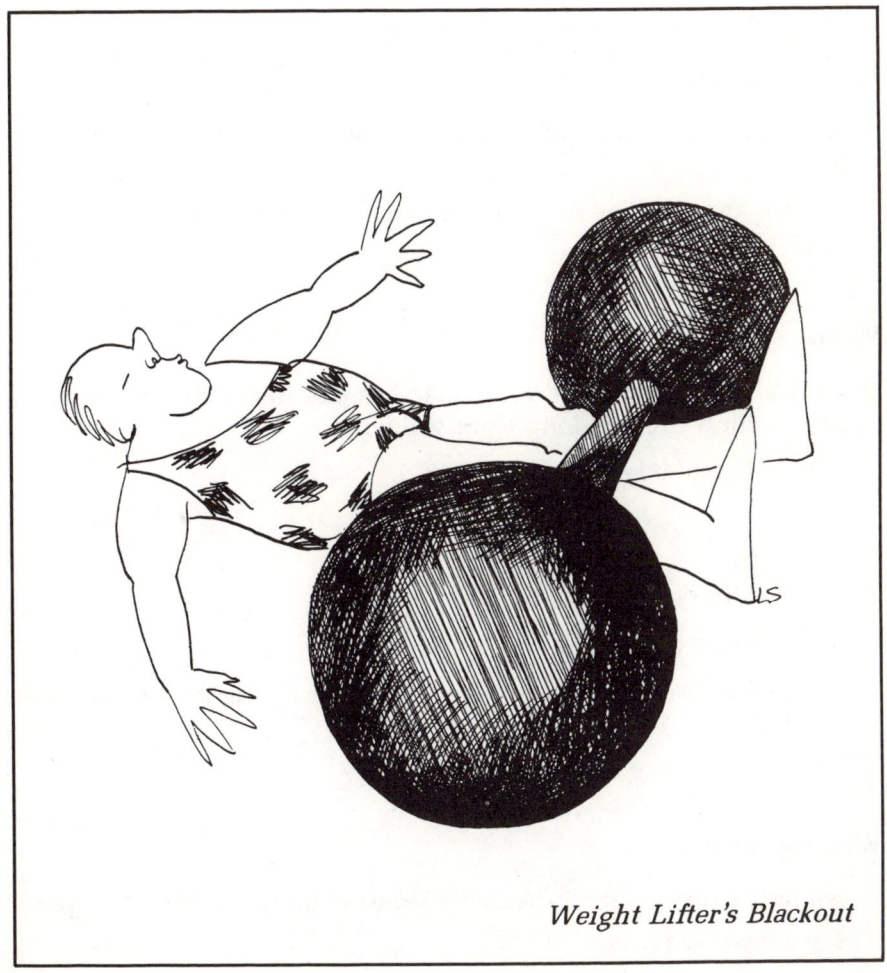

Weight Lifter's Blackout

WELDER'S AGUE

METAL FUME FEVER incurred while welding

Hunter, D. The Diseases of Occupations. 5th ed. London: The English Univ. Press Ltd., 1975

WELDER'S BRONCHITIS

bronchial irritation from the welding fumes

Lakartidningen. 71:479, 1974

WELDER'S CONJUNCTIVITIS

irritation of the eye caused by the ultraviolet radiation from a welding arc

A Report on Electrical Accidents and their Causes. HMSO, 1958

WELDERS' DISEASE

x-ray changes (increased hilar shadows and linear striations) noted on the chest films of long term welders

Arch. Belges Med. Soc. Hyg. 8:507, 1950

WELDERS' EYE FLASH

WELDERS' FLASH

Hunter, D. The Diseases of Occupations. 5th ed. London: The English Univ. Press Ltd., 1975

WELDERS' FLASH

eye irritation or burn in welders exposed to ultraviolet radiation

Brit. Med. J. 2:393, 1949

WELDERS' LUNG

deposition of iron oxide in the lungs (siderosis)

Zbl. Arbeitsmed. 23:286, 1973

WELDERS' SIDEROSIS

WELDERS' LUNG

Lancet 1:789, 1948

WET WINDERS' ACROASPHYXIA

bluish discoloration of the skin and occasionally necrosis of the finger tips of workers exposed to potash alum and other chemicals in wet bobbin winding

Lancet 1:404, 1916

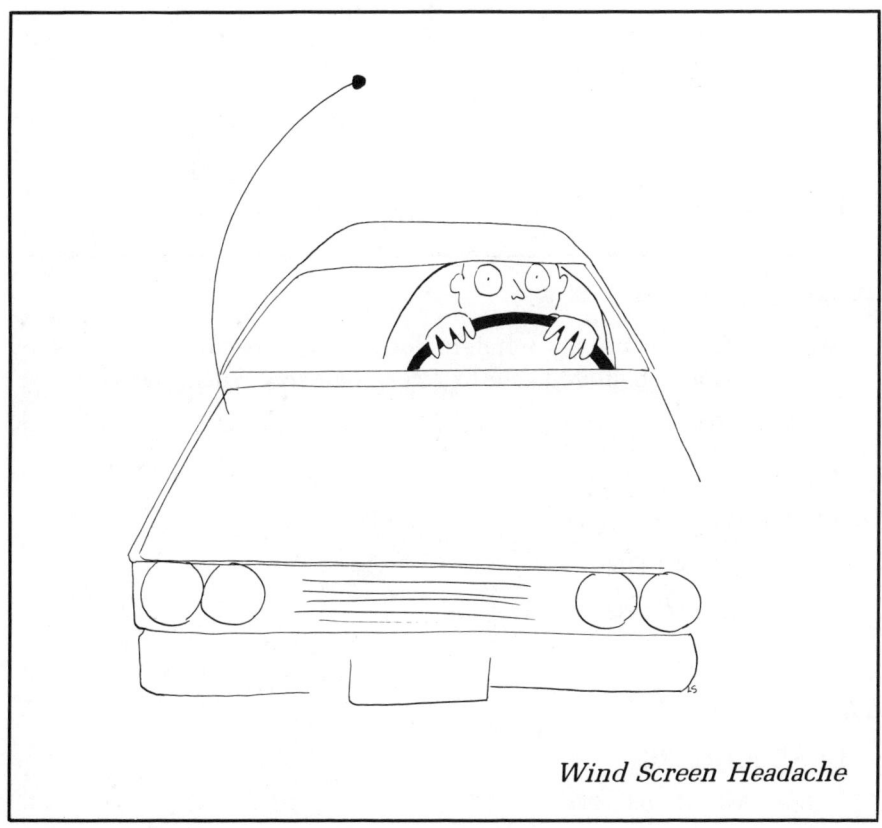

Wind Screen Headache

TRADE DISEASES

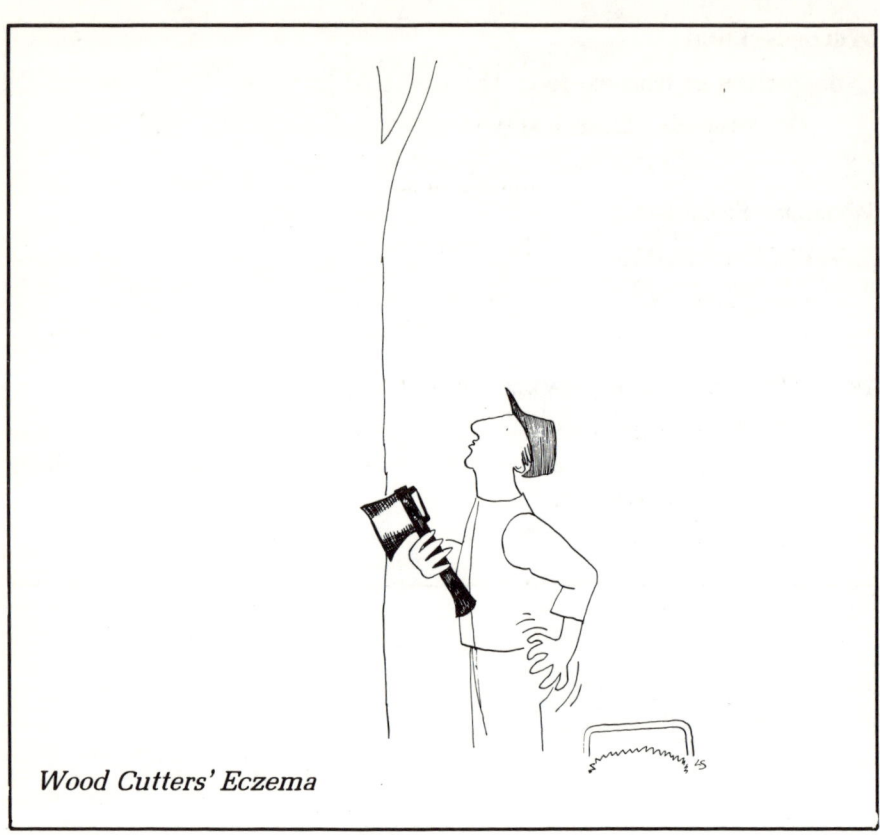

Wood Cutters' Eczema

WHALE FINGER

finger infection among whalers following superficial injuries by wire ropes and believed due to *Erysipelothrix rhusiopathiae*

Lancet 1:680, 1953

WHEAT MILLERS' ASTHMA

THRESHER'S LUNG

JAMA 110:1696, 1938

WHITE FINGER

DEAD FINGERS

Brit. Med. J. 2:1013, 1930

WHITE HAND

VWF

Arch. Gewerbepath. ü Gewerbehyg. 12:102, 1943

WHITE-OUT SYNDROME

psychosis of arctic explorers due to sensory deprivation (compare ARCTIC TEMPER)

Stedman's Medical Dictionary. 23rd ed. Baltimore: William & Wilkins, 1976

WINDOW CLEANER'S FINGER

deformity of the index finger from constant use of the digit to clean the window at the junction of the frame

Brit. Med. J. 2:757, 1954

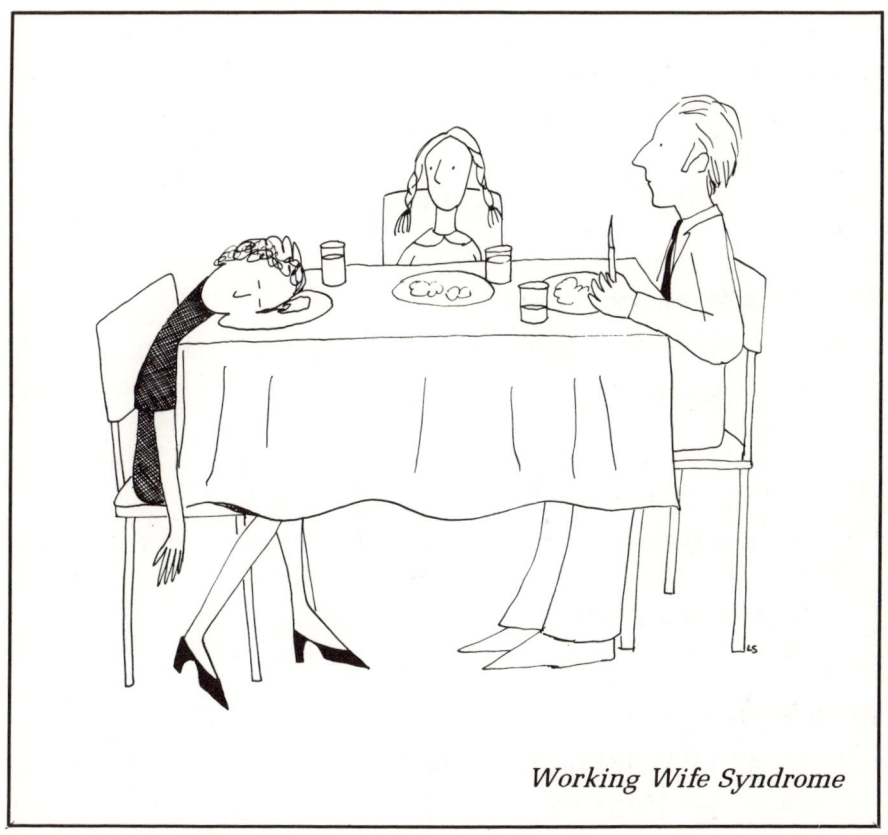

Working Wife Syndrome

TRADE DISEASES

Wind Screen Headache

headache and eyestrain alleged to the sloping windshield of the modern automobile

Brit. Med. J. 2:1123, 1936

Wood Cutters' Disease

contact sensitivity to lichens, among lumbermen

Brit. J. Derm. 77:285, 1965

Wood Cutters' Eczema

red scaling eruption of the skin of wood choppers, cause not known

Arch. Derm. & Syph. 23:1107, 1931

Wood Cutters' Encephalitis

central nervous system infection of woodsmen acquired through tick bites

Dorland's Medical Dictionary. 25th ed. Phila.: W. B. Saunders, 1974

Wood Pulp Worker's Disease

allergic inflammatory response of the lungs to *Alternaria*

Ann. Int. Med. 77:907, 1972

Wood Worker's Dermatitis

irritation of the hands, arms, face and neck from contact with wood dust

East. Afric. Med. J. 21:60, 1944

Wood Worker's Lung

WOOD PULP WORKER'S DISEASE

Ann. Int. Med. 77:907, 1972

WOOL SORTER'S DISEASE

pulmonary anthrax infection following the inhalation of *B. anthracis* from the fleece of infected animals

Lancet 2:920, 1879

WOOL SORTER'S PNEUMONIA

WOOL SORTER'S DISEASE

Dorland's Medical Dictionary. 25th ed. Phila.: W. B. Saunders, 1974

WOOL STAPLERS' DISEASE

pulmonary anthrax among sorters of alpaca, mohair, camels' hair and wool

Brit. Med. J. 1:319, 1878

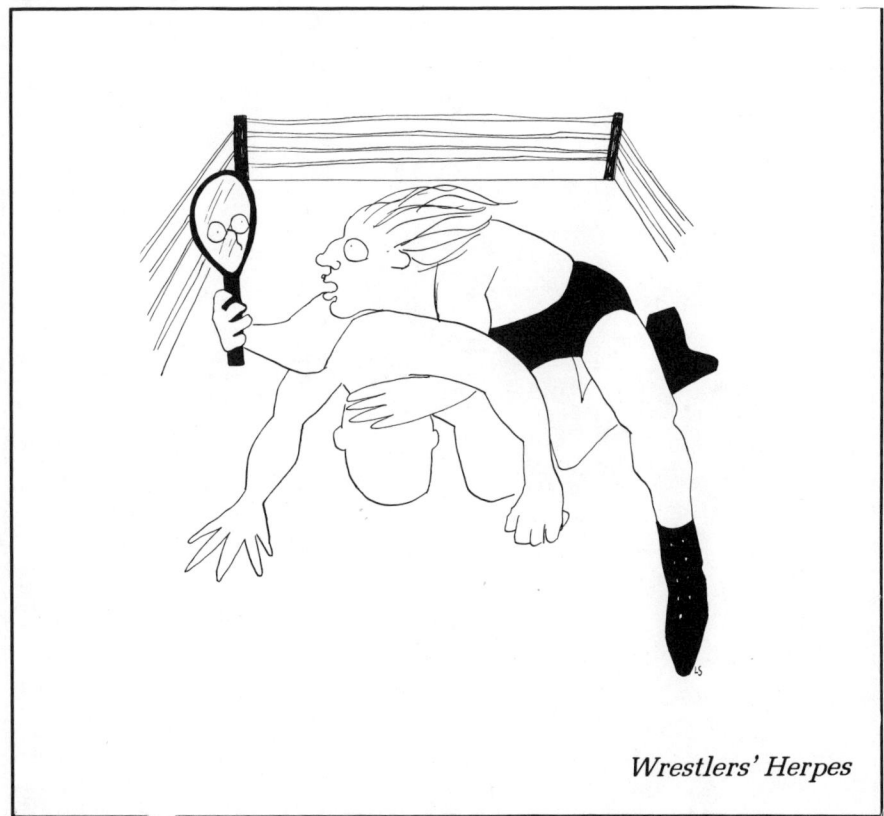

Wrestlers' Herpes

TRADE DISEASES

WOOL TWISTER'S CRAMP

see OCCUPATIONAL NEUROSIS

Hunter, D. The Diseases of Occupations. 5th ed. London: The English Univ. Press Ltd., 1975

WORKER'S CRAMP

see OCCUPATIONAL NEUROSIS

Lancet 2:427, 1914

WORKING WIFE SYNDROME

fatigue, irritability, insomnia, headaches, indigestion and diminished libido from the extra strain of holding two jobs

Lancet 1:312, 1966

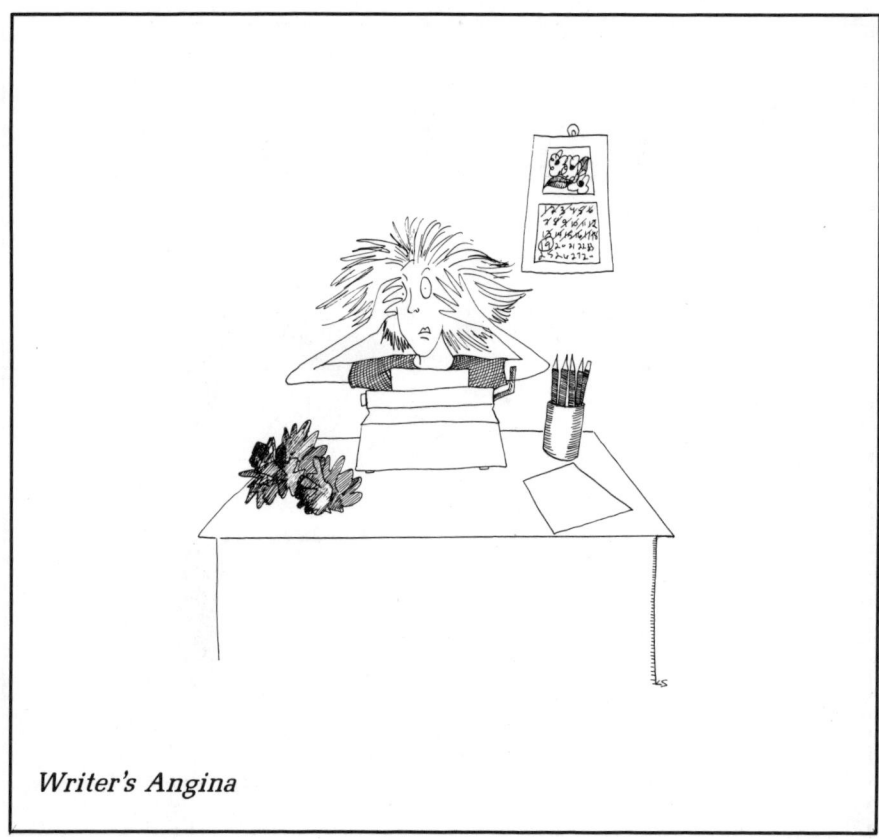

Writer's Angina

WRESTLER'S EAR

deformity of the ear from repeated trauma

original source not identified

WRESTLERS' HERPES

herpes infection among wrestlers wherein the virus gains access through small skin abrasions (compare HERPES GLADIATORUM)

N. Eng. J. Med. 270:979, 1964

WRESTLER'S TRACHOMA

viral eye infection transmitted by close contact while wrestling

Am. J. Ophth. 5:545, 1922

WRINGER INJURY

bruising, laceration and more serious injuries to a hand or arm caught in a washing machine wringer

Am. J. Pub. Hlth. 5:812, 1964

WRITER'S ANGINA

symptoms of coronary insufficiency induced by "writing against time"; i.e., mental anxiety, poor posture and muscle cramping

Lancet 1:157, 1899

WRITER'S CRAMP

see OCCUPATIONAL NEUROSIS

Gowers, W. R. A Manual of Diseases of the Nervous System. London, 1893

WRITER'S NEURALGIA

WRITER'S CRAMP

original source not identified

WRITER'S PARALYSIS
> WRITER'S CRAMP
>> Lancet 2:709, 1864

WRITERS' SYNDROME
> weakness, redundancy, indistinctness, triteness, endlessness and rejection slips noted among physicians whose poorly written manuscripts are not accepted for publication
>> JAMA 181:1124, 1962

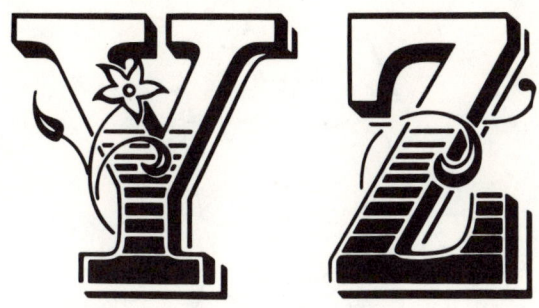

Yoga Foot Drop

paralysis of the foot due to compression of the peroneal nerve from practicing the Yoga kneeling pose; i.e., sitting on the heels

JAMA 217:827, 1971

Zinc Ague

METAL FUME FEVER caused by the inhalation of zinc oxide fumes from any of several sources such as welding, ship-breaking, zinc smelting, galvanizing, metallizing, etc.

JAMA 61:771, 1913

Zinc Chills

ZINC AGUE

Am. J. Med. Sci. 153:376, 1917

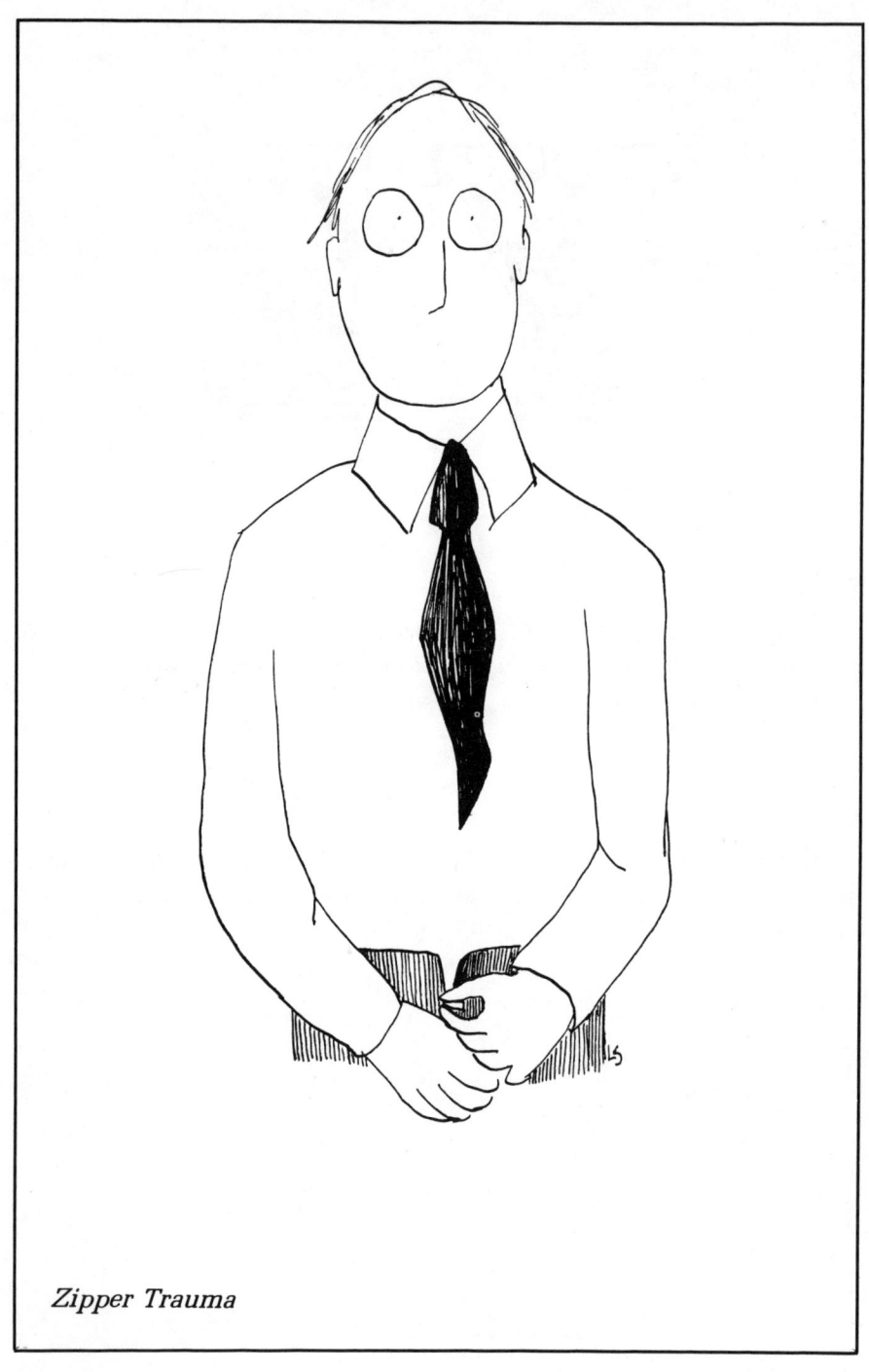

Zipper Trauma

Zinc Colic

chronic zinc intoxication with intermittent abdominal pain

Dorland's Medical Dictionary. 25th ed. Phila.: W. B. Saunders, 1974

Zinc Disease

ZINC AGUE

Brit. Med. J. 2:439, 1947

Zinc Pox

acneiform lesions in the armpits and groins of zinc oxide workers due to mechanical blocking of the skin follicles

Schwartz, L. Occupational Diseases of the Skin. Phila.: Lea & Febiger, 1957

Zinc Shakes

ZINC AGUE

Indust. Med. 12:885, 1943

Zip Fastener Injury

ZIP INJURY

Brit. Med. J. 2:51, 1970

Zip Injury

injury to the penis from entrapment in a zipper

Brit. Med. J. 2:773, 1977

Zipper Trauma

ZIP INJURY

JAMA 107:809, 1936

APPENDIX

Major Body Parts

Ankle
 beat ankle
 dancers' ankle
 deck ankles
 ding string injury
 footballers' ankle
 jockey's ankle
 jogger's petechiae
 policemen's disease
 tailor's ankle
 traveler's edema

Anus and Perineum
 cyclists' neurosis
 jeep disease
 knights' disease
 pillion rider's split
 saddle sore
 weaver's bottom

Arm
 backfire fracture
 backpack palsy
 baseball arm
 cane cutters' tenosynovitis
 chauffeur's fracture
 dhobie itch
 golf arm
 grenade thrower's fracture
 jake paralysis
 knapsack paralysis
 lawn tennis arm
 locksmith's cancer
 lover's palsy
 midwife's disease
 pall bearer's palsy
 parsnip ill
 pearl worker's osteomyelitis
 pinginits
 propeller fracture
 rucksack paralysis
 stone carrier's paralysis
 tackler's exotosis

Back
 bicyclists' hump
 Billingsgate hump
 cyclists' spine
 fish porter's bursitis
 golf back
 hula hoop syndrome
 humpers' lump
 miners' back
 motor headache
 motor driver's spine
 porter's bursitis
 racers' hump back
 railway spine
 trench back
 trench rheumatism

Bladder
 aniline cancer
 dye workers' cancer

Blood
 arctic anemia
 brick burners' anemia
 brick maker's anemia
 miner's anemia
 money rouleaux
 sports anemia
 tile burners' anemia
 tunnel workers' anemia
 war malaria

Breast
 guitar nipple

jogger's nipples
shoemaker's breast

CHEST
cellist's chest
cobblers' chest
shoemaker's breast
shoemaker's chest
maltster's itch
uniform rash

CRAMPS
artificial flower maker's
ballet dancer's
bather's
bathing
bowler's
bricklayer's
button maker's chorea
cabinet makers'
cane cutters'
cellarman's
cellist's
cigarette roller's
cigar maker's
clarinet player's
coachman's
compositor's
comptometer's
cornet player's
cotton twister's
craft palsy
dancers'
diamond cutter's
draper's
drummer's
drummer's neurosis
embroiderer's
engraver's
fencer's
firemen's
flautist's
florist's

flute player's
forge hammer workers'
foundryworker's
furnaceman's
glass blowers'
glass workers'
goldbeater's
haircutter's
hair dresser's
hammer cramp
hammerman's
hammer swinger's
handicraft spasm
harpist's
ironer's
iron workers'
knife sharpener's
knitter's
letter sorter's
linotypist's
locksmith's
machinist's tremor
mason's
metalcasters'
metalworker's
microscope worker's
milker's
milker's spasm
milkmaid's
miners'
money counter's
musician's
musician's neurosis
nailmaker's
nailsmith's
newspaper folder's
orchestra conductor's
organist's
packing case maker's
painter's
permanent waver's
pianist's
pianoforte player's

pickle jar tyer's
printer's
saddler's
sail maker's
sailor's
sawyer's
scissor sharpener's
scissors' palsy
scribe's palsy
scrivener's
scrivener's palsy
scrivener's spasm
seamstress' palsy
seamstress's
sempstress' palsy
sewer's cramp
sewing spasm
shoemaker's
shoemaker's spasm
smith's
stokers'
stone mason's
straw plaiter's
sugar cane cutters'
swimmer's
tailor's
telegraph clerk's
telegraphers'
telegraphic complaint
telegraphic malady
telegraphist's
telegraphist's paralysis
telegraphist's spasm
telegraph writer's
tinsmith's
treadler's
trumpet player's
twister's
typesetter's
typewriter's
typist's
violin-cellist's
violinist's

waiter's
watchmaker's
weaver's
wool twister's
writer's
writer's neuralgia
writer's paralysis

EAR
aviation deafness
aviation otitis
aviator's ear
aviators' vertigo
beach ear
blacksmith's deafness
blacksmith's disease
blast ear
boilermaker's deafness
boilermaker's ear
boxer's ear
chiclero's ulcer
descent sickness
diver's ear
divers' vertigo
ear phone dermatitis
gun fire deafness
jet engine sickness
listening-in dermatitis
pilots' vertigo
prize fighter's ear
rider's vertigo
shooters' deafness
staggers
surfers' ear
swimmer's ear
swimmers' osteoma
tank ear
telephone ear
telephone tinnitus
war deafness
weaver's deafness
wrestler's ear

ELBOW
  baseball pitcher's elbow
  beat elbow
  bricklayer's elbow
  coal miners' elbow
  football goalkeeper's elbow
  golfer's elbow
  gymnast's elbow
  javelin thrower's elbow
  judoman's elbow
  lawn tennis elbow
  little leaguers' elbow
  miner's bursitis
  miner's elbow
  pitcher's elbow
  pitcher's glass arm
  ploughman's elbow
  side swipe fracture
  skateboarder's
  strikers' arthritis
  student's elbow
  tennis elbow
  traffic fracture

EYES
  airman's ptosis
  angel eyes
  arc burn
  arc eye
  arc flash
  artificial silk keratitis
  blacksmith's cataract
  blast blindness
  blue halos
  bottle finisher's cataract
  bottle maker's cataract
  bottle worker's cataract
  brassy eye
  camp eyes
  cataracta electrica
  chain maker's cataract
  cinema eye
  cinema fatigue
  concussion blindness
  cornpickers' pupil
  eclipse blindness
  eclipse burns
  electric arc welder's flash
  electrical opthalmia
  electric flash cataract
  electricians' moons
  electric light blindness
  electric opthalmia
  endoscopist's eye
  eye flash
  firemen's cataract
  firemen's eye
  fireworks blindness
  flash blindness
  flight blindness
  furnaceman's cataract
  furnace workers' cataract
  gas eye
  glass blower's cataract
  glass blower's disease
  glass workers' cataract
  gold smelter's cataract
  harvester's keratitis
  hedgers' cataract
  helicopter flicker disease
  hop eye
  hoppers' eye
  hop picker's opthalmia
  iron puddler's cataract
  Klieg eye
  metal workers' cataract
  miners' nystagmus
  motor conjunctivitis
  motorcyclist's ptosis
  opthalmia militaris
  oyster shucker's keratitis
  polisher's keratitis
  pottery fireman's cataract
  pottery fireman's eye
  puddlers' cataract
  reapers' keratitis

red out
shipyard conjunctivitis
shipyard disease
shipyard eye
shipyard keratoconjunctivitis
spinners' eye
swimmer's conjunctivitis
swimming pool conjunctivitis
swiming tank conjunctivitis
television glaucoma
tin plate millman's cataract
tin plate worker's cataract
trench hemeralopia
welder's conjunctivitis
welder's eye flash
welders' flash
wrestler's trachoma

Face
colliers' stripes
diver's squeeze
football impetigo
hop dermatitis
pearl worker's osteomyelitis
phossy jaw
printer's ink dermatitis
scrumpox

Finger
air hammer disease
anatomic wart
asbestos corns
barbers' disease
barbers' interdigital hair sinus
baseball finger
beer drinker's finger
bird's eyes
blubber finger
bolster finger
bone button makers' disease
bongo drum disease
bulb fingers
chicken neck wringer's finger

confectioners' paronychia
dactylitis discus
dead finger
dissection tuberculoma
draft tendon syndrome
dressmaker's fingers
fishbone furunculosis
fish filleters' wart
fish handler's disease
fish tank granuloma
frisbee finger
furniture polisher's eczema
glass blowers' cramp
granite cutter's ring
grease gun finger
hopper's gout
lasters' disease
milkers' felon
milker's nodules
milkers' panaritium
milkers' vaccinia
milkers' warts
paper folder's finger
pineapple finger
pneumatic hammer disease
poker player's palsy
pork finger
prosector's wart
rifle sling palsy
Scandinavian blubber finger
sealers' finger
shearer's knuckle
silk weavers' nails
spaek finger
speck finger
spekk finger
spring finger
staple finger syndrome
tanners' ulcers
tenpin finger
trigger finger
tulip finger
violinist's calluses

TRADE DISEASES

washerwoman's finger
wet winders' acroasphyxia
whale finger
white finger
window cleaner's finger
vibration syndrome

Foot
aesthete's foot
athlete's foot
aviators' astragalus
basketball heel
black heel
electric feet
fatigue fracture
flip flop dermatitis
footballers' foot
foot slogger's nodule
golfer's foot
guitarist's foot drop
hollow foot
Hong Kong foot
immersion foot
jogger's heel
march foot
march fracture
march tumor
motorist's heel
paddy field foot
pantie girdle syndrome
policeman's heel
pump bumps
runner's cramp
salt water sores
satellite feet
shelter foot
ski boot neuropathy
soldiers' feet
surfers' foot
surfers' knot
swell foot
tailor's bunion
tango foot

tennis blisters
toilet seat neuropathy
trench bite
trench foot
trench frostbite
tropical immersion foot
war frostbite
yoga foot drop

Gastrointestinal
air controllers' syndrome
aviator's stomach
back packer's diarrhea
banking clerk's dyspepsia
blast injury
camp diarrhea
camp jaundice
change of shift syndrome
copper colic
executives' disease
founders' colic
green tobacco sickness
harvest fever
holiday typhoid
jet tummy
painters' colic
pig breeders' disease
player's liver
plumbers' colic
potter's colic
sailor's stomach
seat belt syndrome
ship sickness
shoemaker's ulcer
stress dyspepsia
tight girdle syndrome
TNT jaundice
tobacco croppers' sickness
tourista
tourist hepatitis
tourist's disease
toxigenic tourista
tractor sickness

traveler's diarrhea
trench diarrhea
trench enteritis
wartime pot belly

Genitourinary
cello scrotum
chimney sweep's cancer
cyclists' neurosis
Derbyshire droop
electroplaters' eczema
mule spinners' cancer
mule spinners' disease
scrotal soot cancer
spinners' cancer
working wife syndrome
zip injury
zipper trauma

Hand
barbers' nodules
beat hand
blackjack disease
boxer's fracture
bull men's hand
cabinet makers' callosities
carpenter's hand
celery itch
chauffeur's fracture
chauffeur's palm
cheese worker's itch
chicken pickers' dermatitis
cornpicker hand
crocodile hand
cyanogen sores
dishpan hands
eczema rimosum
electroplaters' eczema
fish tank granuloma
frozen meat impetigo
gas workers' epithelioma
gold spinners' hand
grease gun injury

grocers' itch
grocery bag neuropathy
hammer hand
hammer syndrome
handball palm
handlebar neuropathy
helium tremors
hooked hands
hopper's gout
housewive's hands
immersion hand
ironing machine injury
joiner's hand
karate hand
KP dermatitis
leather workers' ulcers
lover's palsy
masons' eczema
milker's granuloma
milkers' hands
milkers' panaritium
milkers' vaccinia
nickel platers' rash
planker's hand
planker's segs
plasterer's bunions
pneumatic drill disease
pneumatic hammer disease
potters' eczema
psychoanalyst's disease
pumpkin carvers' palm
rifle sling palsy
roentgenologist's cancer
rose pickers' dermatoses
salt water sores
silk winders' dermatosis
spinners' eczema
stud gun injury
tailor's callosities
tennis blisters
trench hand
vibration disease
vibration syndrome

VWF
washermen's itch
washerwoman's dermatitis
washerwoman's hand

Head
academy headache
assembly headache
Covent Garden hummy
dynamite head
dynamite headache
effort migraine
footballers' migraine
gunshot headache
miner's headache
Monday head
Monday headache
nitrate head
nitroglycerine head
nitroglycerine headache
powder headache
punch drunk syndrome
red out
sightseers' headache
slug happiness
sweat band dermatitis
wind screen headache

Heart
angina electrica
athlete's heart
athletic heart syndrome
aviator's heart
bicycle heart
choristers' heart
doctors' disease
doctors' heart syndrome
dynamite heart
effort syndrome
holiday heart syndrome
liftman's heart
soldiers' heart
soldier's spot

television angina
vasodilator disease
war heart
writer's angina

Hip
coachman's bursitis
dashboard dislocation
hot pants syndrome
hyperbaric arthralgia
lightermen's bursitis
motor driver's spine

Kidney
army nephritis
athlete's albuminuria
athlete's kidney
athletic pseudonephritis
conga drummer's pigmenturia
exercise myoglobinuria
exertional hemoglobinuria
karate myoglobinuria
march hemoglobinuria
stock car kidney
trench nephritis
war nephritis

Knee
bakers' knee
beat knee
carpet layer's knee
chauffeur's knee
clergyman's bursitis
football knee
housemaid's knee
hunter's knee
hyperbaric arthralgia
knobbies
lawn tennis knee
motorist's knee
nun's bursitis
nun's knee
parson's knee

splitter's knee
  twist injuries

Leg

  bathing cramp
  beet sugar worker's neuritis
  bumper fracture
  charley horse
  deck legs
  dentists' leg
  desert sores
  divers' paralysis
  dustman's bursa
  economy class syndrome
  fender fracture
  fertilizer sores
  gun fighter's wound
  Halifax legs
  jake paralysis
  knobbies
  lawn tennis leg
  maladie de plongeurs
  Malibu disease
  march fracture
  mother of pearl worker's
    osteomyelitis
  motorist's fracture
  pantie girdle syndrome
  paratrooper's fracture
  pearl worker's disease
  pearl worker's osteomyelitis
  ping pong tenosynovitis
  quick draw leg
  shin splints
  spinners' folliculitis
  strawberry picker's peroneal
    palsy
  sugar worker's neuritis
  surfer's knobs
  surfers' knots
  surfers' nodules
  tango foot
  television legs

  tennis leg
  trap drummer's neurosis
  trench leg
  trench shin

Lip

  bird stuffers' disease
  fishermen's sore
  lipstick dermatitis

Lung

  air conditioner pneumonitis
  allergic alveolitis
  aluminosis
  aluminum dust lung
  aluminum lung
  apple pickers' disease
  arc welder's disease
  arc welder's lung
  arc welder's siderosis
  ax grinder's disease
  bagassosis
  bakers' asthma
  baryta grinders' disease
  baryta miners' disease
  bauxite workers' disease
  bauxite workers' lung
  bird breeders' lung
  bird fanciers' lung
  bird feather pickers' disease
  bird rearers' lung
  black lung
  black phthisis
  black spit
  blast chest
  blast lung
  brown lung
  budgerigar fanciers' lung
  builders' phthisis
  carders' asthma
  cardroom workers' asthma
  carpenter's disease
  cave sickness

chaff cutter's lung
cheese washer's asthma
cheese washer's disease
cheese washer's lung
chili grinders' disease
chokes
coal miner's lung
coal worker's pneumoconiosis
coal workers' melanosis
coal workers' pneumoconiosis
coffee worker's disease
coffee worker's lung
colliers' anthracosis
colliers' asthma
colliers' black spit
colliers' lung
colliers' phthisis
colliers' tuberculosis
comber's fever
coppermen's chest
corundum smelters' lung
corundum workers'
    pneumoconiosis
cotton carders' asthma
cotton grinders' asthma
cotton mill asthma
cotton mill fever
cotton spinners' phthisis
cotton strippers' asthma
detergent worker's lung
doghouse disease
elevator disease
elevator laugh
factory fever
farmer's lung
feather picker's disease
ferroalloy workers' disease
file cutter's phthisis
fire-eater's asbestosis
firemen's lung
flax dressers' disease
flax dressers' phthisis
flax dust byssinosis

flax fever
flax workers' phthisis
flock fever
foundry worker's
    pneumoconiosis
french millstone maker's lung
french millstone maker's
    phthisis
furrier's lung
ganister miner's disease
gerbil keeper's lung
glass blower's emphysema
gold dust complaint
gold miner's disease
gold miner's phthisis
grain handler's asthma
grain handler's
    pneumoconiosis
grain porter's fever
grain threshing catarrh
granite mason's phthisis
granite worker's lung
grinders' asthma
grinders' complaint
grinders' consumption
grinder's disease
grinder's lung
grinders' phthisis
grinders' rot
grinders' silicosis
grinders' tuberculosis
hacklers' disease
hacklers' lung
hacklers' Monday
hackling fever
hard metal disease
hard metal lung
harvester's lung
hay maker's lung
hematite miner's lung
hemp worker's disease
hemp disease
horn blower's disease

humidifier lung
iron dust lung
iron lung
iron miner's lung
iron oxide lung
Kieselguhr lung
knife grinders' phthisis
knife grinders' rot
lead miners' lung
lung rot
malt worker's disease
malt worker's lung
maple bark stripper's disease
marble cutter's phthisis
mason's disease
mason's lung
mason's trouble
mattress maker's disease
mattress makers' fever
meat worker's asthma
meat wrapper's asthma
metal polisher's disease
miller's asthma
miller's bronchitis
mill fever
millstone maker's asthma
millstone maker's lung
millstone maker's phthisis
millstone maker's tuberculosis
millworker's asthma
millworker's lung
miners' asthma
miners' consumption
miners' disease
miners' dyspnea
miner's lung
miners' lung disease
miners' melanosis
miners' phthisis
miners' rot
miners' tuberculosis
mold machine pneumonia
Monday diseases
Monday fever
Monday syndrome
Monday tightness
moulder's bronchitis
moulder's tuberculosis
mummy unwrapper's lung
mushroom grower's lung
mushroom picker's lung
mushroom worker's lung
mushroom worker's pneumonitis
nailers' consumption
needle grinder's siderosis
oyster shuckers' asthma
paprika splitter's lung
pearl grinders' phthisis
pigeon breeder's lung
pigeon fancier's lung
potters' asthma
potters' consumption
potters' disease
potters' lung
potters' phthisis
potters' rot
potters' tuberculosis
pottery worker's silicosis
poucey chest
poultry keeper's lung
printer's asthma
printers' phthisis
rag picker's disease
rag sorter's disease
Rand miners' phthisis
rouge polisher's lung
Salem sarcoid
sandblaster's asthma
sandblaster's lung
sandblaster's phthisis
sandblaster's silicosis
sandblaster's tuberculosis
sauna taker's disease
Schneeberg tumor
scissor grinder's disease

sewer disease
Sheffield grinders' disease
shoddy fever
silo filler's disease
silo filler's lung
silo worker's asthma
silver polishers' lung
slag cough
slate dresser's lung
slate miner's lung
slate miner's phthisis
slate worker's lung
smallpox handler's lung
smelter pneumoconiosis
soot lung
spinners' phthisis
steam fitter's asthma
steel grinder's disease
steel grinder's phthisis
stone cutter's asthma
stone cutter's consumption
stone cutter's lung
stone cutter's phthisis
stone hewer's phthisis
stone mason's asthma
stone mason's disease
stone mason's lung
stone mason's phthisis
stone mason's tuberculosis
sugar cane lung
tailors' phthisis
tea factory cough
tea maker's asthma
tea tasters' cough
tea taster's disease
thresher's disease
thresher's lung
threshing disease
threshing fever
tin miner's lung
tin smelters' pneumoconiosis
tobacosis
tonoko lung

town-dweller's lung
trench lung
vanadium lung
vineyard sprayers' lung
weavers' asthma
weavers' cough
welder's bronchitis
welder's disease
welders' lung
welders' siderosis
wheat millers' asthma
wood pulp worker's disease
woodworker's lung
wool sorter's disease
wool sorter's pneumonia
wool staplers' disease

Mouth
blue gum
glass blower's mouth
glass blower's tumor
hatters' sore mouth
Lucifer match makers' disease
musician's mouth
phossy jaw
salivation disease
trench mouth
trumpeter's parotitis

Neck
clay shoveler's disease
clay shoveler's fracture
dentist's neck
desk neck
fish porter's bursitis
hula hoop syndrome
humpers' lump
long scarf syndrome
maltster's itch
navvies' disease
porter's neck
root puller's fracture

shoveler's disease
shoveler's fracture
shovel sickness

Nervous System
apple thinners' disease
aviators' bends
aviator's blackout
barometer maker's disease
battery refiner's disease
bends
blackout
boxer's brain damage
boxer's encephalopathy
boxers' hemorrhage
boxing brains
caisson disease
Danbury shakes
dementia pugilistica
divers' palsy
divers' paralysis
file cutters' disease
hatters' shakes
hatters' tremor
helium tremors
niggles
punch drunk syndrome
sewer fume poisoning
slug happiness
sponge divers' disease
Taravana diving syndrome
television epilepsy
tractor sickness
tunnel disease
weight lifter's blackout
wood cutters' encephalitis

Neurasthenia
academy headache
aerasthenia
aerodromophobia
aeroneurosis
aerophobia

airmens' breakdown
arctic temper
assembly headache
aviation sickness
aviator's asthenia
aviator's disease
aviator's neurosis
aviator's sickness
back-to-school syndrome
barbed wire disease
battle exhaustion
battle fatigue
battle neurosis
boo-hoo fever
bureaupathy
change-of-shift syndrome
checkitis
cinematic neurosis
circadian dysrhythmia
combat fatigue
combat neurosis
compensation neurosis
concentration camp syndrome
index readers' syndrome
informational indigestion
jet engine sickness
jet lag
jet phobia
job stress
litigation neurosis
loser's psychosis
me-too syndrome
microwave neurosis
military carditis
military frenzy
night nurse's paralysis
pension disease
prison neurosis
radiowave sickness
railroad neurosis
railway brain
railway brain strain
railway strain

reflex horn syndrome
school phobia
shell shock
skating mania
soap wrapper jig
sonic boom stress
soldiers' heart
speakers' fright
stage fright
tank exhaustion
testitis
time zone syndrome
title mad
travel dysrhythmia
ultrasonic sickness
vocational phobia
war hysteria
war neurosis
war psychosis
war sailor syndrome
war shock
white-out syndrome
working wife syndrome
writers' syndrome

NEUROPATHY
backpack neuralgia
backpack palsy
back pocket sciatica
beet sugar worker's neuritis
cigar roller's neuritis
credit carditis
crutch palsy
driver's thigh
exhaustion paralysis
file cutters' paralysis
grocery bag neuropathy
guitarist's foot drop
guitarist's occupational palsy
gunbelt neuropathy
hammerman's paralysis
hammer palsy
handlebar palsy

knapsack paralysis
lover's palsy
minute man disease
pack palsy
pall bearer's palsy
poker player's palsy
printer's palsy
psychoanalyst's disease
rifle sling palsy
ruck sack paralysis
shoemakers' polyneuropathy
shoeworkers' neuropathy
shooting gallery lead
   poisoning
ski boot neuropathy
sling palsy
stone carrier's paralysis
strawberry picker's foot drop
strawberry picker's peroneal
   palsy
sugar worker's neuritis
tennis elbow
toilet seat neuropathy
tourniquet paralysis
war tremors
yoga foot drop

NOSE
apple packers' epistaxis
apple packers' nosebleeds
aviators' cancer
street car colds
sugar beet pollinosis
swimmer's nose

PROSTATE
banana seat hematuria
proof reader's prostatitis

SHOULDER
baseball shoulder
beat shoulder
bricklayer's shoulder

conveyer belt shoulder
deal runner's shoulder
dustman's shoulder
golf shoulder
hod carriers' shoulder
hodmens' shoulder
timber porter's shoulder
waiter's shoulder

Sinuses
aerosinusitis

Skin
acid bites
acne artificialis
alkali itch
apple sorters' disease
arc burn
army itch
bakers' acne
bakers' dermatitis
bakers' eczema
bakers' itch
bakers' psoriasis
bathers' itch
bikini dermatitis
bird's eyes
bluemen
bread bakers' itch
bricklayers' itch
brickmason's eczema
brine boils
broom maker's disease
bunches
burnishers' eczema
butchers' dermatitis
butchers' pemphigus
butchers' tubercle
butcher's wart
cable rash
camel itch
carpenter's dermatitis
caterpillar dermatitis

celery itch
cementers' itch
cement workers' dermatitis
cement workers' itch
cheese worker's itch
chicken pickers' dermatitis
chlorine acne
chrome cripples
chrome holes
clam digger itch
clam diggers' dermatitis
coal miners' dermatitis
conditioning dermatitis
coolie itch
corn itch
cotton spinners' cancer
cowpox
dairymen's itch
degreaser's flush
desert sores
dhobi itch
doffers' acne
Dogger Bank itch
drysalters' itch
electroplaters' eczema
farmers' skin
fertilizer sores
flash burn
flax soakers' eczema
flax workers' eczema
flower pickers' dermatitis
flutter board dermatitis
football impetigo
furniture polisher's eczema
galvanizers' eczema
gardeners' mycosis
gas workers' epithelioma
golf course dermatitis
grinder's dermatitis
grocers' itch
hair worker's disease
harvester's disease
harvest itch

herpes gladiatorum
hop dermatitis
hot pants syndrome
housewife's dermatitis
housewife's eczema
housewife's lime dermatitis
housewive's eczema
hula hoop dermatitis
KP dermatitis
laundrymen's itch
lime holes
lithographers' dermatitis
lumberman's itch
machinist's furunculosis
maladie de plongeurs
maltster's itch
masons' eczema
metal plater's dermatitis
miners' bunches
miners' dermatitis
miner's itch
money counters' disease
mosquitos
nickel platers' rash
nickel refiner's itch
paraffin plukes
paraffin workers' cancer
parsnip ill
peasant's skin
phosphoritis
photographer's dermatitis
photographer's eczema
photographer's skin disease
pitch worker's cancer
pitch worker's papilloma
polishers' nodules
potters' eczema
poultryman's itch
printer's ink dermatitis
radiologist's cancer
rice paddy dermatitis
rose pickers' dermatosis
sailor's skin

salt water boils
school dust dermatitis
scrum pox
sea bather eruption
shoemaker's breast
silk handler's disease
silk winders' dermatosis
smarts (the)
smelters' itch
soda ulcer
solders' dermatitis
spinners' cancer
spinners' folliculitis
sponge divers' disease
sponge fisher's disease
stucco boils
sugar boils
sugar maker's lymphadenitis
sugar worker's itch
sweat band dermatitis
swimmer's dermatitis
swimmers' itch
swimming pool granuloma
swimming pool rash
tar smarts
tar workers' cancer
tar workers' dermatitis
telephoner's impetigo
tennis blisters
threshers' itch
toilet seat dermatitis
trade cancers
trade dermatitis
trade holes
vagabonds' disease
vagabonds' pigmentation
vagrants' disease
veldt sore
Volkswagon dermatitis
warehouseman's itch
washerman's mark
washermen's itch
washerwoman's dermatitis

washerwoman's itch
washerwoman's scall
washerwomen's eczema
wood cutters' disease
wood cutters' eczema
wood worker's dermatitis
wrestler's herpes
zinc pox

Teeth
aerodontalgia

Thigh
backpack neuralgia
backpocket sciatica
butcher's thigh
cavalry bone
cavalryman's leg
cavalryman's osteoma
cricket thigh
credit carditis
driver's thigh
exercise bone
fencer's pubialgia
guitarist's groin
gunbelt neuropathy
gunfighter's wound
march fracture
motor scooter handlebar
   syndrome
pillion rider's pelvic split
pope
pulled jockey muscle
rider's bone
rider's bursa
rider's hygroma
rider's leg
rider's sprain
rider's tendon
rider's thigh
sports pubic osteoarthropathy
sprinter's fracture

Throat
blackboard sore throat
boilermaker's laryngitis
clergyman's sore throat
clergyman's throat
cyclist's sore throat
depot sore throat
dysphonia clericorum
hospital throat
ministers' ail
minister's sore throat
preachers' voice
schoolboard laryngitis
schoolboard sore throat
singer's knots
singer's nodes
singer's nodule
speaker's throat
teacher's node
teacher's nodule
telephone paralysis
weavers' tonsils

Thumb
ampoule snapper's thumb
bowler's thumb
boxers' thumb
drummer's palsy
drummer's thumb
flax soakers' eczema
football keeper's thumb
gamekeeper's thumb
leather buffers' nodes
pig's feet
tennis thumb
vaccinator's thumb

Toe
ballet dancer's toe
down hill toe jam
pheasant hunter's toe

TRADE DISEASES

    tennis toe
    turf toe

Tongue
    label lickers' tongue
    stamp lickers' tongue

Wrist
    crutch palsy
    espresso wrist
    file cutters' paralysis
    golfer's wrist
    hammer palsy
    hopper's gout
    hyperbaric arthralgia
    jack hammer arthropathy
    lawn tennis wrist
    midwife's disease
    parsnip ill
    salt water boils
    strikers' arthritis
    tennis wrist
    washermen's itch
    washerwoman's dermatitis

Ref
RB
115
P58

OCT 3 0 1980